Total Ankle Replacement

Editor

NORMAN ESPINOSA

FOOT AND ANKLE CLINICS

www.foot.theclinics.com

Consulting Editor
MARK S. MYERSON

December 2012 • Volume 17 • Number 4

ELSEVIER

1600 John F. Kennedy Blvd. • Suite 1800 • Philadelphia, PA 19103-2899

http://www.theclinics.com

FOOT AND ANKLE CLINICS Volume 17, Number 4
December 2012 ISSN 1083-7515, ISBN-13: 978-1-4557-4953-9

Editor: David Parsons

Foot and Ankle Clinics (ISSN 1083-7515) is published quarterly by Elsevier, Inc., 360 Park Avenue South, New York, NY 10010-1710. Months of issue are March, June, September, and December. Periodicals postage paid at New York, NY, and additional mailing offices. Subscription price per year is $295.00 (US individuals), $386.00 (US institutions), $146.00 (US students), $336.00 (Canadian individuals), $456.00 (Canadian institutions), $201.00 (Canadian students), $433.00 (foreign individuals), $456.00 (foreign institutions), and $201.00 (foreign students). To receive student/resident rate, orders must be accompanied by name of affiliated institution, date of term, and the *signature* of program/residency coordinator on institution letterhead. Orders will be billed at individual rate until proof of status is received. Foreign air speed delivery is included in all *Clinics* subscription prices. All prices are subject to change without notice. **POSTMASTER:** Send address changes to *Foot and Ankle Clinics*, Elsevier Health Sciences Division, Subscription Customer Service, 3251 Riverport Lane, Maryland Heights, MO 63043. **Customer Service: 1-800-654-2452 (US and Canada). From outside of the United States and Canada, call 314-447-8871. Fax: 314-447-8029. E-mail: JournalsCustomerService-usa@elsevier.com (for print support); JournalsOnlineSupport-usa@elsevier.com (for online support).**

Reprints. For copies of 100 or more, of articles in this publication, please contact the Commercial Reprints Department, Elsevier Inc., 360 Park Avenue South, New York, NY 10010-1710. Tel.: 212-633-3812; Fax: 212-462-1935; E-mail: reprints@elsevier.com.

Printed and bound by CPI Group (UK) Ltd, Croydon, CR0 4YY

Transferred to digital print 2012

Contributors

CONSULTING EDITOR

MARK S. MYERSON, MD
Director, Institute for Foot and Ankle Reconstruction at Mercy, Mercy Medical Center, Baltimore, Maryland

GUEST EDITOR

NORMAN ESPINOSA, MD
Head of Foot and Ankle Surgery, Department of Orthopaedics, University of Zurich, Balgrist Hospital, Zurich, Switzerland

AUTHORS

MATHIEU ASSAL, MD, PD
Associate Professor, Service de Chirurgie Orthopédique et Traumatologie, Hôpital La Tour, Geneva, Switzerland

ALEXEJ BARG, MD
Senior Resident, Clinic of Orthopaedic Surgery, Kantonsspital Liestal, Liestal, Switzerland; Attending Surgeon, Orthopaedic Department, University Hospital of Basel, University of Basel, Basel, Switzerland; Research Fellow, Harold K. Dunn Orthopaedic Research Laboratory, University Orthopaedic Center, University of Utah, Salt Lake City, Utah

M. BONNIN, MD
Centre Orthopédique Santy, Lyon, France

J.A. COLOMBIER, MD
Clinique de l'Union, Saint Jean, France

MARK E. EASLEY, MD
Department of Orthopaedic Surgery, Duke University Medical Center, Durham, North Carolina

NORMAN ESPINOSA, MD
Head of Foot and Ankle Surgery, Department of Orthopaedics, University of Zurich, Balgrist Hospital, Zurich, Switzerland

F. GAUDOT, MD
Centre Hospitalier Raymond Poincaré, Garches, France

MATTHEW HARRISON, MD
Foot and Ankle Fellow, Counties Manukau District Health Board, Auckland, New Zealand

HEATH B. HENNINGER, PhD
Assistant Professor, Harold K. Dunn Orthopaedic Research Laboratory, University Orthopaedic Center, University of Utah, Salt Lake City, Utah

BEAT HINTERMANN, MD
Associate Professor and Chief, Clinic of Orthopaedic Surgery, Kantonsspital Liestal, Liestal, Switzerland

MARTIN HUBER, MD
Department of Foot and Ankle Surgery, Schulthess Klinik, Zurich, Switzerland

HYUK JEGAL, MD
Foot and Ankle Service, KT Lee's Orthopedic Hospital, Seoul, Korea

JACQUES HEINRICH JONCK, MB, ChB, FC Orht SA
Consultant, Department of Orthopaedics, Windhoek Central Hospital, Namibia, Windhoek, Namibia

TH. JUDET, MD, PhD
Centre Hospitalier Raymond Poincaré, Garches, France

MARKUS KNUPP, MD
Attending Surgeon, Clinic of Orthopaedic Surgery, Kantonsspital Liestal, Liestal, Switzerland

FABIAN G. KRAUSE, MD
Department of Orthopaedic Surgery, Inselspital, University of Berne, Freiburgstrasse, Berne, Switzerland

KYUNG TAI LEE, MD, PhD
Foot and Ankle Service, KT Lee's Orthopedic Hospital, Seoul, Korea

ANDRÉ G. LEUMANN, MD
Attending Surgeon, Orthopaedic Department, University Hospital of Basel, University of Basel, Basel, Switzerland

ANDREAS M. MÜLLER, MD
Attending Surgeon, Orthopaedic Department, University Hospital of Basel, University of Basel, Basel, Switzerland

MARK S. MYERSON, MD
Medical Director, Institute for Foot and Ankle Reconstruction at Mercy, Baltimore, Maryland

FLORIAN D. NAAL, MD
Department of Foot and Ankle Surgery, Schulthess Klinik, Zurich, Switzerland

GEERT I. PAGENSTERT, MD
Senior Attending Surgeon, Orthopaedic Department, University Hospital of Basel, University of Basel, Basel, Switzerland

YOUNG UK PARK, MD, PhD
Foot and Ankle Service, KT Lee's Orthopedic Hospital, Seoul, Korea

JOCHEN PAUL, MD
Resident, Orthopaedic Department, University Hospital of Basel, University of Basel, Basel, Switzerland

PASCAL F. RIPPSTEIN, MD
Department of Foot and Ankle Surgery, Schulthess Klinik, Zurich, Switzerland

TIMO SCHMID, MD
Department of Orthopaedic Surgery, Inselspital, University of Berne, Freiburgstrasse, Berne, Switzerland

NG Y.C. SEAN, MD
Clinical Fellow, Service de Chirurgie Orthopédique et Traumatologie, Hôpital La Tour, Geneva, Switzerland

JESS G. SNEDEKER, PhD
Department of Orthopedics, University Hospital Balgrist, Zurich; Institute for Biomechanics, ETH Zurich, Switzerland

YASUHITO TANAKA, MD, PhD
Professor & Chairman, Department of Orthopaedic Surgery, Nara Medical University, Kashihara, Nara, Japan

MATTHEW TOMLINSON, MBChB, FRACS
Consultant Orthopaedic Surgeon, Counties Manukau District Health Board, Auckland, New Zealand

VICTOR VALDERRABANO, MD, PhD
Professor and Chairman, Orthopaedic Department, University Hospital of Basel, University of Basel, Basel, Switzerland

STEPHAN H. WIRTH, MD
Department of Orthopedics, University Hospital Balgrist, Zurich, Switzerland

CREVOISIER XAVIER, MD, PD
Associate Professor, Unité d'orthopédie, Centre Hospitalier Universitaire Vaudois, Lausanne, Switzerland

LUKAS ZWICKY, MSc
Research Fellow, Clinic of Orthopaedic Surgery, Kantonsspital Liestal, Liestal, Switzerland

Contents

the design rationale and explains the surgical technique with the Mobility implant, as well as offering technical tips and pitfalls gained through personal experiences and literature review. The tibial component has a flat articular surface and a conical intramedullary stem on the tibial side.

Treatment of the Arthritic Valgus Ankle **647**

Alexej Barg, Geert I. Pagenstert, André G. Leumann, Andreas M. Müller, Heath B. Henninger, and Victor Valderrabano

The ankle joint is part of a biomechanical hindfoot complex. Approximately 1% of the world's adult population is affected by ankle osteoarthritis (AO). Trauma is the primary cause of ankle OA, often resulting in varus or valgus deformities. Only 50% of patients with end-stage ankle OA have a normal hindfoot alignment. The biomechanics and morphology of the arthritic valgus ankle is reviewed in this article and therapeutic strategies, including joint preserving and nonpreserving modalities are presented. Pitfalls are discussed and the literature is reviewed regarding outcomes in patients with valgus deformity who underwent total ankle replacement.

Surgical Treatment of the Arthritic Varus Ankle **665**

Mark E. Easley

Within the past several years, the arthritic varus ankle has been addressed extensively in *Foot and Ankle* Clinics, with numerous excellent reviews by particularly knowledgeable authors. To support these outstanding contributions, this article provides a practical approach to this challenging constellation of foot and ankle abnormalities. Varus ankle arthritis exists on a continuum that prompts the treating surgeon to be familiar with a spectrum of surgical solutions, including joint-sparing realignment, arthroplasty, and arthrodesis. Each of these treatment options is addressed with several expanded case examples and supports the management approaches with the available pertinent literature.

Revision Total Ankle Replacement **687**

Jacques Heinrich Jonck and Mark S. Myerson

This review of the current literature regarding total ankle replacement (TAR) revision surgery focuses on the causes for implant failure, how to deal with the clinical dilemmas of pain and stiffness following TAR, the management of asymptomatic peri-implant cyst formation, and the management of the distal tibia and talus during revision surgery.

Management of Specific Complications Related to Total Ankle Arthroplasty **707**

Pascal F. Rippstein, Martin Huber, and Florian D. Naal

Total ankle arthroplasty (TAA) has evolved over time and modern 3-component implants offer good and reliable clinical results. Despite recent improvements, TAA is still associated with a relatively high incidence of complications. Surgeon experience seems to play the most important role. This review highlights the most common intraoperative and postoperative complications, such as malleolar fracture, impingement, cyst formation, malalignment, and loosening, and offers a differentiated concept for their management.

The New Zealand Joint Registry: Report of 11-Year Data for Ankle Arthroplasty **719**

Matthew Tomlinson and Matthew Harrison

This article describes the results of the first 11 years of ankle arthroplasty data for the New Zealand Joint Registry. The main purpose is to collect accurate outcome information regarding these procedures and to guide orthopedic surgeons in the care of their patients. Trends can often be identified early, and implants with higher revision rates can be identified. In addition, individual surgeons can be given data that compare their performance with the collective data, providing invaluable feedback. Patient-based questionnaires are highly important for gauging the results of surgery. Patient response rates have been less than optimal, particularly after revision surgery.

Index **725**

FOOT AND ANKLE CLINICS

FORTHCOMING ISSUES

March 2013
Treatment of Osteochondral Defects
Mark S. Myerson, MD, *Guest Editor*

June 2013
Sporting Injuries of the Foot & Ankle
James Calder, MD, *Guest Editor*

RECENT ISSUES

September 2012
Foot and Ankle Innovations in Latin America
Cristian Ortiz, MD, and
Emilio Wagner, MD, *Guest Editors*

June 2012
Adult Flatfoot
Steven M. Raikin, MD, *Guest Editor*

March 2012
Management of the Varus Foot
Alastair S. Younger, MD, ChB, FRCSC, *Guest Editor*

December 2011
Current Management of Lesser Toe Disorders
John T. Campbell, MD, *Guest Editor*

Preface

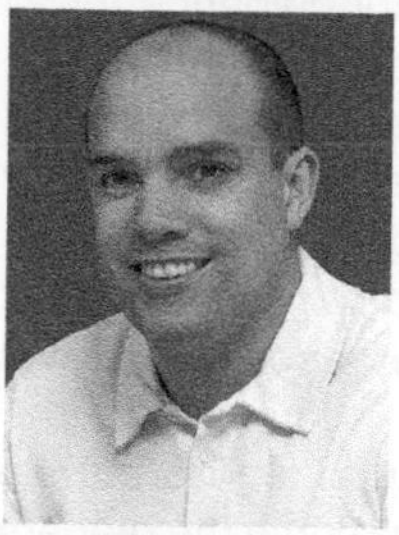

Norman Espinosa, MD
Guest Editor

Surgical treatment of end-stage arthritis has considerably changed over the last two decades. For more than a century, ankle arthrodesis has remained the gold standard in the treatment of symptomatic ankle arthritis with good-to-excellent clinical and subjective outcomes in the short and mid term. However, as a consequence to altered hindfoot biomechanics, long-term sequels as progressive deterioration of the adjacent joints and functional limitation must be expected. Alternative treatments that preserve ankle function and prevent or halt adjacent joint arthritis would be preferable to postpone or avoid ankle fusion.

With the development of new total ankle replacement designs and the recognition of asymmetric ankle arthritis and its treatment, ankle arthrodesis has started to face new treatment strategies that attempt to preserve hindfoot joints and function: total ankle replacement and corrective osteotomies.

During the last decade total ankle replacement has seen significant improvements, including more anatomical design, better biomechanical behavior, and accurate instrumentation. Thanks to the growing scientific interest in analyzing the performance of total ankle replacement and their modes of failure, the longevity of current total ankle replacements has improved. It seems no longer to be questioned that total ankle replacement has become one of the most dynamic areas of change in orthopedic surgery.

The influence of deformity on the development of ankle arthritis and its potentially detrimental effect on mechanics of the native and replaced ankle joint represent a current hot spot of scientific attention. The goal is to achieve a well-balanced hindfoot to allow for proper force transmission and function. Osteotomies have become important players in the treatment of deformity. Based on several studies in the past, different algorithms and treatment strategies have been formulated to understand adequate indications and techniques of corrective ostoetomies and to balance the hindfoot properly.

It's all about indications. The main question to answer is: who is the ideal candidate for fusion, joint preserving surgery, or total ankle replacement? Selecting the correct indication of treatment represents a fundamental key of success.

Foot Ankle Clin N Am 17 (2012) xiii–xiv
http://dx.doi.org/10.1016/j.fcl.2012.09.001

The current issue is an excellent compilation of scientific up-to-date review articles that deal with the surgical management of symptomatic end-stage arthritis. Experts with a vast experience and knowledge in this field provide a useful guidance for all of us who have to deal with those difficult and complex conditions.

I have to thank and congratulate all authors who have contributed to this issue and who have invested so much time and effort in preparing their articles. It is not an easy job and I think this should always be appreciated. A special thanks goes to my teacher, mentor, and friend, Mark Myerson, who kindly invited me to work as a guest editor. It has been an honor. I would also like to thank everybody at Elsevier, especially David Parsons, for helping me put this issue together.

Finally, I hope that this condensed form of expertise will help us to ameliorate the treatment of patients and to improve their quality of life and that it will serve the readers as a base for future research.

Norman Espinosa, MD
Head of Foot and Ankle Surgery
Department of Orthopaedics
University of Zurich
Balgrist Hospital
Forchstrasse 340
8008 Zurich

E-mail address:
norman.espinosa@balgrist.ch

Biomechanics of the Normal and Arthritic Ankle Joint

Jess G. Snedeker, PhD[a,b,*], Stephan H. Wirth, MD[a], Norman Espinosa, MD[a]

KEYWORDS

• Osteoarthritis • Ankle joint • Biomechanics • Arthroplasty

KEY POINTS

- OA of the ankle can be debilitating and has a significant impact on quality of life.
- When compared with the hip and knee joint where primary OA is more common, the ankle seems less susceptible to onset of primary OA. Onset of OA can be related to altered mechanical loading patterns of the cartilage, and downstream changes in tissue metabolism and joint structure.
- Understanding biomechanics of the normal and arthritic ankle joint can aid in the analysis of an underlying clinical problem and provide a strategic basis for a more optimal management.

INTRODUCTION

Osteoarthritis (OA) of the ankle can be debilitating and has a significant impact on quality of life. When it comes to the decision that treatment should be considered, physicians can choose among conservative and surgical measures. The palette of treatment is manifold and should always be tailored to the needs of patient and the degree of disease. To select the most appropriate treatment for a given patient, it is often helpful to understand the biomechanics (functional anatomy) of the normal ankle joint, how pathology can alter normal function, and the biomechanical consequences that a given surgical intervention will provoke.

When compared with the hip and knee joint where primary OA is more common, the ankle seems less susceptible to onset of primary OA. Onset of OA can be related to altered mechanical loading patterns of the cartilage, and downstream changes in tissue metabolism and joint structure. Altered joint loading patterns have been associated with aging and trauma. In contrast to the knee and hip, a high degree of joint surface congruency and correspondingly constrained kinematics, combined with

[a] Department of Orthopedics, University Hospital Balgrist, Zurich, Switzerland; [b] Institute for Biomechanics, ETH Zurich, Switzerland
* Corresponding author.
E-mail address: snedeker@ethz.ch

Foot Ankle Clin N Am 17 (2012) 517–528
http://dx.doi.org/10.1016/j.fcl.2012.08.001
1083-7515/12/$ – see front matter

a generally more limited range of motion may make the cartilage of the intact ankle joint less sensitive to age-related changes that can play a role in primary OA. This is supported by the fact that nearly 70% of cases of ankle (OA) are secondary to a traumatic event, most frequently involving ankle fractures and subsequently unaddressed chronic ankle instability. Here disruption or injury to cartilage tissue itself, or injury-related changes in loading of the cartilage surfaces can thus initiate a progressive degeneration of the joint that eventually requires operative intervention.

Understanding biomechanics of the normal and arthritic ankle joint can undoubtedly aid in the analysis of an underlying clinical problem and provide a strategic basis for a more optimal management. The challenge to the clinician and the biomechanist is that the mechanical (and for that matter, physiologic) complexity of the ankle joint still clouds current understanding. This article provides the reader with an overview of current understanding of functional ankle anatomy, how this function can be altered in the degenerated ankle, and how surgical intervention further affects foot and ankle biomechanics. The intention is to provide the reader with insight to the mechanopathophysiology of degenerative cartilage tissue remodeling, how it can affect the kinetics and kinematics of the ankle joint, and the postoperative implications of a tibiotalar surgical intervention. Here the focus is on how altered (often increased) loading of neighboring joints in the midfoot and hindfoot may induce postoperative joint remodeling and can manifest in secondary clinical problems.

FUNCTIONAL ANATOMY OF THE HINDFOOT

To understand the biomechanics of the hindfoot a thorough knowledge of its anatomy is essential. During gait the hindfoot distributes forces from a vertical position into a horizontal one and vice versa This is a complex kinematic process and requires the tibiotalar, subtalar, and distal tibiofibular joints to act as a combined osseous and soft tissue (ligaments, capsule, retinacula) support complex, which provides proprioception, stabilization, and control over the movement of the talus and calcaneus around their axes of motion. A stable ankle results from a perfect interplay of static (bones, ligaments, retinaculum) and dynamic anatomic structures (muscles, tendons).

The ankle joint is a highly constrained articulation, composed of the tibia, talus, and fibula, which provide stability together with the tendons, ligaments, and syndesmoses. Tendons and ligaments attribute to dynamic stabilization of the joint. Motion at the ankle is multiplanar and linked to the tibia. The course of movement within the ankle joint is predominantly from plantarflexion to dorsiflexion, but contains mild degrees of internal and external rotation.

The talus articulates with the tibial plafond superiorly, the tibia medially, and the fibula laterally. The talus has a convex dome and is wider anteriorly than posteriorly, thus the greatest contact between tibiotalar and tibiofibular surfaces is achieved during midstance phase. As such, the ankle in dorsiflexion is in its most stable condition.[1] Despite this the talus exhibits a cone-shape nature with a greater radius of its medial part than the lateral. The strongest part of the tibial plafond is found posteromedially. Resection of the subchondral layer reduces the compressive resistance of the bone by 30% to 50%. When resecting 1 cm of the distal tibia compressive resistance is reduced 70%–90%).[2]

Passive stability of the ankle depends on congruity of its articular surfaces and the integrity of the ligamentous and retinacular complexes.[3–6] Under weightbearing conditions the congruency of bones provides 100% of stability for eversion and inversion but only 30% of rotational stability. The ligamentous complexes predominantly control rotatory stability and anterioposterior tibiotalar shifting. Under nonweightbearing conditions, stability in the frontal plane is supported by the malleoli and in the sagittal, frontal, and transversal plane by the collateral ligaments together with the musculature.[3] The anterior talofibular ligament (ATFL) originates at the distal anterior fibula and inserts on the body of the talus and blends into the anterior joint capsule, approximately 18 mm above the subtalar joint line.[7–9] It is approximately 20 mm long, 8 mm wide, 2 mm thick, and spans the anterior ankle joint. The angle in relation to the floor averages approximately 75 degrees. The ATFL primarily restricts internal rotation of the talus in the mortise. The ATFL has the highest degree of deformation (ie, greatest strain) but the lowest load to failure when compared with the calcaneofibular ligament (CFL). The CFL originates from the anterior border of the distal lateral malleolus, close to the origin of the ATFL and attaches to a small tubercle posterior and superior to the peroneal tubercle of the calcaneus approximately 13 mm distal and posterior to the subtalar joint line. It is confluent with the peroneal tendon sheath. The CFL is 20 to 30 mm long, almost 5 mm wide, and 3 to 5 mm thick. Together, the ATFL and CFL form an angle of about 105 degrees in the sagittal plane and an angle averaging 90 to 100 degrees in the frontal plane The CFL stabilizes the subtalar joint and inhibits adduction and exerts its greatest effect in the neutral and dorsiflexed position. In dorsiflexion, the CFL approaches a vertical position with respect to the subtalar joint and acts as a true collateral ligament, preventing talar tilting. The PTFL is a strong ligament with broad insertion on the talus and the fibula.[10] It originates at the posteromedial aspect of the fibula and runs in a horizontal direction to insert at the posterolateral aspect of the talus.[9] The PTFL becomes taught during dorsiflexion of the ankle and rarely ruptures.[11–14]

The inferior extensor retinaculum adds mechanical support to the ATFL and CFL. It is divided into three bands (lateral, intermediate, and medial roots) that retain the extensor digitorum longus, extensor digitorum brevis, and peroneus tertius. The inferior extensor retinaculum is attached to the lateral talus and calcaneus. Together with the CFL, the lateral root of the inferior extensor retinaculum constitutes the superficial ligamentous support of the subtalar joint.

On the medial side the deltoid ligament or medial collateral ligament (MCL) provides a strong ligamentous support to the ankle joint. It is divided into two portions: the superficial and deep layers.[10,15,16] According to Milner and Soames's classification the MCL complex consists of six ligaments.[17,18] The superficial layer of the deltoid is made up of the tibiospring; the tibionavicular; the superficial posterior tibiotalar, and tibiocalcaneal ligaments. The differentiation between these structures is difficult. The superficial layer is a broad, fanshaped, and continuous structure arising from the anterior colliculus of the medial malleolus. The tibionavicular component attaches to the navicular bone medially and blends with its fibers into the superomedial component of the spring ligament.[19,20] The tibiospring ligament extends to the superior border of the plantar calcaneonavicular ligament (spring ligament).[21] The tibiocalcaneal ligament runs in a vertical direction and inferiorly to insert onto the sustentaculum tali.[8] The deep layer of the MCL includes the deep posterior tibiotalar and deep anterior tibiotalar ligaments. Both are intra-articular but extrasynovial. Therefore, deep portion and superficial portion of the MCL complex are anatomically separated. The anterior tibiotalar ligament arises from the lateral anterior colliculus and inserts on the medial aspect of the talus just distal to the articular surface. The posterior tibiotalar ligament originates from the intercollicular groove to extend posterolateraly to its attachment on the medial tubercle of the talus.[8] The MCL complex acts equally to resist valgus tilting of the talus and as a secondary restraint against anterior translation. The deep layer of the MCL provides the greatest restraint against lateral translation.[22,23]

Considering the ligamentous support for the subtalar joint there is no consensus found in the literature regarding precise terminology of the ligaments or function. However, some agreement has been reached in classifying the subtalar ligaments into three layers: (1) a superficial layer containing the lateral root of the inferior retinaculum, the lateral talocalcaneal ligament, and the CFL; (2) an intermediate layer containing the intermediate root of the inferior retinaculum and the cervical ligament; and (3) a deep layer containing the medial root of the inferior retinaculum and the interosseous talocalcaneal ligament.[7,21,24] The interosseous talocalcaneal ligament ensures adequate function of the hindfoot and is a strong bond between the calcaneus and talus. It originates at the most medial part of the sinus tarsi (some fibers attach to the deep portion of the deltoid ligament), courses downward and lateral to the sulcus calcanei, where it blends with the most medial fibers of the cervical ligament.[8] The cervical ligament is located within the sinus tarsi and runs in an oblique fashion from the neck of the talus to the superior surface of the calcaneus and separates the anterior from the posterior joint capsule The cervical ligament is a resistive bundle connecting talus and calcaneus. It is thought that the cervical ligament together with the interosseous talocalcaneal ligament might play an important role in subtalar instability.

There are three axes of motion: one in the transversal, one in the frontal, and one in the sagittal plane (**Fig. 1**). Each of these axes generates a rotatory plane perpendicular to that axis. According to Huson,[25] rearfoot motion is often described as motion according to these cardinal planes (**Fig. 2**). However, it is important to understand that rearfoot motion does not happen in these isolated planes only. The ankle and subtalar joint both have oblique axes of motion. With regard to the ankle joint Kelikian[26] stated that "the axis of motion is the imaginary line through which motion occurs. It can be static, dynamic, single or multiplanar." Sarrafian[9] described two concepts: the single axis of motion and multiple axis of motion. According to the work of Inman,[27,28] the empiric axis of the ankle joint runs slightly distal to the tip of the medial malleolus (5 mm ± 3 mm) and distal (3 mm ± 2 mm)-anterior (8 mm ± 5 mm) through the tip of the lateral malleolus. Related to the frontal plane the axis is inclined downward and laterally and in relation to the horizontal plane it is rotated posterolaterally. The angle between axis of the tibial plafond and the midline bisecting the tibial shaft projected to the frontal plane is 82.7 degrees (± 3.7 degrees). Projected to the transverse plane the angle of the empiric axis of the ankle joint with the transverse axis of the knee is 20 to 30 degrees.[27,28] Barnett and Napier[29] and Hicks[30] were first to introduce the concept of multiple axes at the hindfoot and recognized that the axis of

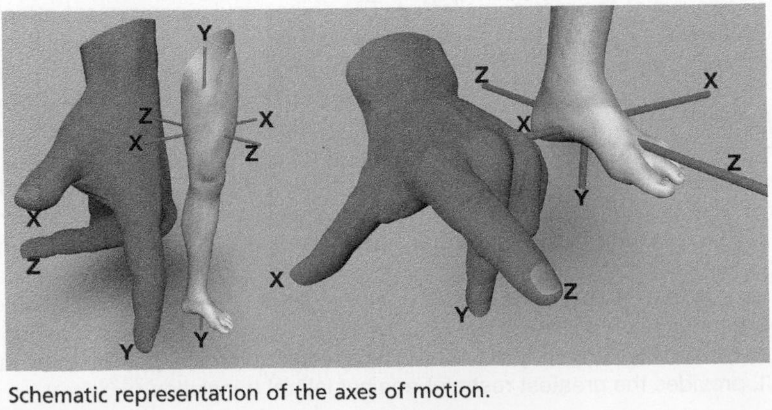

Fig. 1. Schematic representation of the axes of motion.

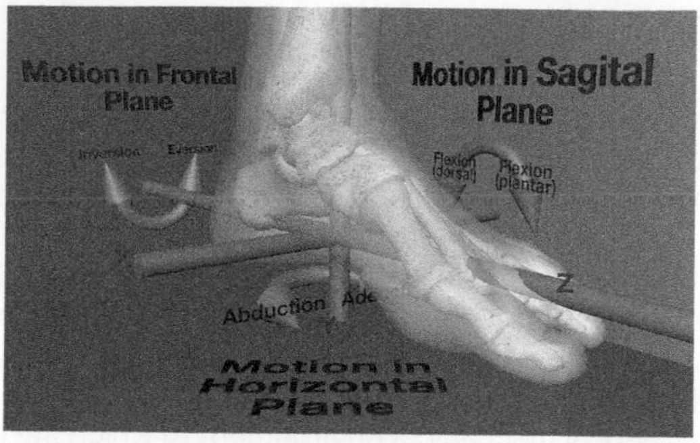

Fig. 2. Rearfoot motion is often described as according the cardinal anatomical planes.

motion at the ankle is inclined downward and laterally at dorsiflexion and downward and medially in plantarflexion. The different curvatures of the talar trochlea have been found to be responsible for this phenomenon. The medial curvature radius of the marginal profile of the trochlea tali is higher posteriorly than ventral. The opposite is found on the lateral marginal profile of the trochlea tali.[31] The lateral profile is almost a true circle, whereupon the medial profile is formed by an arc of two circles with different radii.[29] A virtual line connecting the center of these arcs specified by the curvature radius of the medial and lateral marginal profile of the talar trochlea represents the axis of motion.

The subtalar joint consists of an anterior, medial, and posterior joint, each of them having its own capsule and separated by the sinus tarsi and the tarsal canal. As mentioned, the axis of the subtalar joint is also oblique.[32–35] According to Perry and Schoneberger[36] and Viladot and colleagues,[37] the posterior subtalar joint and the anterior subtalar joint have a different center of rotation. The resulting axis of the subtalar joint is oriented upward, anteriorly and medially. Close[32] and coworkers reported a 42-degree (± 9 degrees) upward tilt and 23-degree (± 11 degree) medial deviation in the horizontal plane to the perpendicular axis of the foot (**Fig. 3**). Van Langelaan[38] was able to show that subtalar joint motion followed a helical character. The calcaneus rotates around the interosseus ligament, resulting in a screw-like motion associated with translation and rotation. According to Inman,[39] motion at the subtalar joint is triplanar, comprised of inversion (calcaneus turns inward) and eversion (calcaneus turns outward).

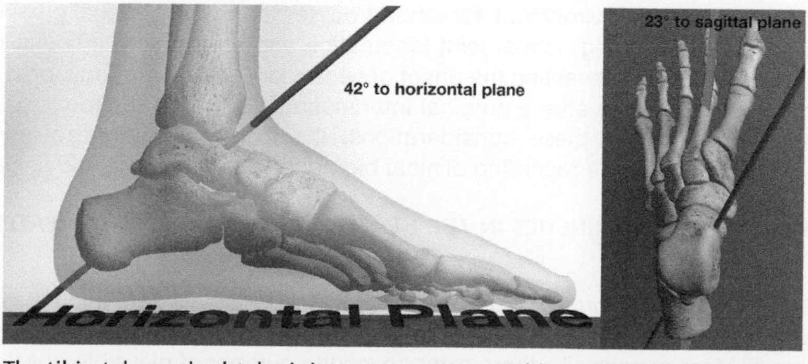

Fig. 3. The tibio-talar and subtalar joints cooperate to yield complex joint kinematics. These are visualized here in the neutral position by an instantaneous axis of rotation.

A BRIEF REVIEW OF THE POTENTIALLY CRUCIAL ROLE OF JOINT BIOMECHANICS IN ONSET OF OA

Details regarding the initiation and mid-stage progression of OA remain largely unclear, at least partly because human studies have focused on late and end stages of the disease. However, it is thought that the initiation and progression of OA is centrally related to the composition and structural organization of articular cartilage, and depends heavily on the molecular mechanisms that regulate metabolic activity (and extracellular matrix synthesis) of chondrocytes. In addition to strong dependence of chondrocyte behavior on their local biochemical environment (eg, oxygen tension), it is clearly established that the anabolic and catabolic activity of chondrocytes depends heavily on the local mechanical environment to which the cells are exposed. Both of these facts have implications to the orthopedic surgeon, who should concern himself or herself with ensuring adequate tissue blood supply and normal mechanical tissue loads.

The onset of OA represents a progression of cartilage calcification (from the subchondral bone toward the articular surface) that is often characterized as a so-called tidemark advance. The tidemark is identifiable in histologic analysis under a microscope as a rough delineation between normal hyaline articular cartilage and calcified cartilage in the deeper layers. The process of advancing calcification could possibly depend on abnormally high proangiogenic cell signaling in the joint tissues. It has also been related to aberrant cell-mediated repair of microdamage. Here, very small cracks form in the extracellular matrix as a result of normal joint loads during daily activity. This damage should initiate a targeted remodeling response to repair the matrix. For largely unknown reasons, cells seem to lose their ability to adequately respond to this microdamage as the body ages. This insufficient response is widely thought to rely on a breakdown on appropriate cell-matrix interplay.

This interplay is largely mechanics driven, with cells synthesizing matrix toward the goal of restoring a normative local mechanical environment. As the advancement of OA corresponds to the thinning of the hyaline cartilage layer, the mechanical stresses in the cartilage matrix typically increase (less tissue is available to support joint loads). Thus begins a spiraling cycle of degeneration, whereby aberrant mechanical feedback drives a chronic and pathologic remodeling process accelerating the progression of OA.

In this sense, normal articular cartilage tissue loads are essential to maintaining a healthy joint. Trauma to the periarticular bone or the constraining ligaments can be sufficient to alter the mechanical loading profile of the cartilage, and this can lead to a similarly mechanics-driven degenerative modeling process. Trauma often also directly involves the articular cartilage itself, creating a much more challenging mechanical/molecular environment for chondrocytes attempting (usually vainly) to repair the tissue. Restoring normal joint kinematics and consequent articular tissue loads may be critical to preventing the onset of secondary OA after trauma, or in slowing the progression of OA after a surgical intervention. To enable the foot and ankle surgeon to better weigh these considerations, the following section reviews the current state of knowledge regarding clinical biomechanics of the arthritic ankle.

JOINT KINEMATICS AND KINETICS IN THE HEALTHY, PATHOLOGIC, AND TREATED ANKLE

The chief obstacle to a thorough biomechanical understanding of foot and ankle function is the huge number of potential kinematic degrees of freedom presented by these structures.[40] More specifically, there exist an infinite number of plausible possibilities for stabilization of these motions by ligaments and active musculature.[41] Thus, despite enormous technologic improvements in osteokinematic assessment (in vivo biplanar fluoroscopy being the current gold standard[42]), understanding of how soft and hard, active and passive skeletal structures interact to provide foot and ankle function remains limited.

Nonetheless, biomechanical descriptions of foot and ankle function have drastically evolved over the last 30 years. Descriptive models have advanced from extremely rudimentary (and functionally incorrect) modeling of the joint as two rigid bodies revolving around a skewed axis hinge, to more accurate and complex models that include numerous interacting joint articulations.[43–46] Such models have been developed and tested against a large body of experimental studies. The most salient findings of these studies are briefly summarized next. In particular, the focus is on joint function (walking velocity, cadence, stride length), and the underlying biomechanics of these measures (kinematics and kinetics).

Humans adopt a wide range of self-selected walking styles, with similarly ranging velocities.[47,48] In this sense self-selected (preferred) walking speed is a product of the stride length and cadence, and can be viewed as being characteristic of a given style. The painful ankle is generally associated with reduced velocity and an altered style (shorter strides, slower cadence, adoption of an asymmetric stance phase, with less time spent on the painful limb).[49–52] When the painful, degenerated ankle is treated using arthrodesis, walking velocity may be partially restored, although visible alterations in cadence and stride length generally persist.[53–57] Although early efforts using total ankle replacement (TAR) to treat the degenerated ankle generally failed to restore normal gait cadence or stride length,[50,58] results using second-generation TARs have proved more effective, but these metrics still seem to be generally reduced compared with normal controls.[51,59,60]

Similarly, ankle joint kinetics (the forces that result in a joint movement) are altered in patients with an osteoarthritic ankle.[49–51] In asymptomatic patients, kinetic analysis indicates that foot-ground reaction forces perpendicular to the ground reach a characteristic peak of approximately 120% body weight on heel strike, dropping to about 80% during mid-stance (while the opposite leg swings forward), finalized by a second peak of 120% body weight during push-off.[61] In patients with a degenerated ankle, the magnitudes of these peak forces are diminished (corresponding to an off-loading of the joint), but the spatiotemporal shape characteristics of the force-time curve remain generally unchanged.[50,51] Ground reaction forces in the transverse plane (shear forces) have been reported to be unaltered in patients with ankle degeneration.[62]

Although comparisons of ground reaction forces and corresponding joint loads is complicated by a need to control for individual walking style (cadence and stride length),[63] analysis of ground reaction forces in the arthodesed ankle has indicated generally lower forces than normal, with an anteriorly shifted center of pressure.[53,56,57] These altered kinetics have been suggested to potentially contribute to postoperative onset of mid-foot OA.[55] Ankle arthroplasty achieved using various implant designs has been shown to retain normal peak force associated with heel strike, but with diminished ground reaction forces afterward in the gait cycle.[51,59,64] This has been attributed to diminished muscle tone and an altered muscle recruitment strategy designed to protect the painful joint.[52,60,63] Whatever the cause, kinetic analysis indicates that along with diminished ground reaction forces, joint reaction moments (plantar flexion, adduction, and inversion) are similarly reduced.

Such altered gait and loading patterns are also generally reflected in joint kinematics that differ from the normal state. Exactly what constitutes normal is a problematic benchmark; the kinematic movements between bones of the foot and ankle are not only difficult to accurately quantify, but are also highly variable within the population.[65–67] Nonetheless, some ankle pathologies have been associated with altered kinematic patterns compared with those in the asymptomatic ankle. For instance, several studies have characterized ankle kinematics in patients presenting with joint degeneration, reporting altered sagittal motion with a predisposition for maintaining the foot in a plantar-flexed posture during the swing and stance phases of gait.[50,51] Kinematic analysis of the hindfoot in patients with ankle arthrosis have shown reduced ranges of motion in all functional planes, but with sagittal plane motion reduction being the most dominant characteristic.[49]

More sophisticated kinematic analyses of the foot and ankle have indicated that the degenerated ankle joint is associated with substantially altered subtalar joint motions. Here the normally coordinated kinematic coupling of tibiotalar and subtalar joints is altered, with both joints possibly undergoing an external rotation during the stance phase of gait.[68] Thus, not only the magnitude, but even the directionality of normal subtalar motion seems to be affected by degeneration at the tibiotalar joint. This secondary alteration in subtalar joint loading seems to have implications for a "knock-on" effect that may predispose the eventual onset of degeneration in the subtalar joint. This knock-on effect may similarly follow ankle arthrodesis, by which even larger changes are required at the subtalar joint to compensate for reduced sagittal motions at the tibiotalar joint.

The downstream kinematic implications of tibiotalar fusion are not only limited to the subtalar joint. Compensatory hyperextension of the knee has been observed,[54,55] presumably to extend the duration of the midstance phase of gait. The duration of this phase of gait critically limits walking cadence and stride length. Although evidence of kinematic alterations in the neighboring midfoot joints is inconsistent,[53,54,69,70] rates of degeneration secondary to arthrodesis in these joints are relatively high,[71] and may be attributed to an adopted strategy of kinematically compensatory midfoot hyperextension.

Ankle joint motion preservation by TAR presents a more complex picture, with a wide range of reported postoperative joint kinematics that seem to be heavily dependent on implant design, and that do not always positively correlate to long-term implant survival. More specifically, first-generation TARs were reported to better preserve ankle kinematics compared with arthrodesis, but were simultaneously characterized by unacceptably short implant survival rates.[50,58] Conversely, modern design TARs are only inconsistently linked to improved ranges of sagittal ankle motion, yet are increasingly reported to yield favorable clinical outcomes with encouragingly high rates of implant survival.[51,52,59,60,72] Reduced mid- to long-term complications in modern TAR implants may be caused by many operative and nonoperative factors.[73,74] Whether these factors include a better preservation of hindfoot and midfoot joint biomechanics lacks supporting quantitative kinematic evidence, primarily because of the technical challenge of quantifying small kinematic differences at these joints in vivo.[51,59,60] However, some limited evidence exists to suggest that onset of hindfoot and midfoot OA secondary to TAR can increase after joint arthroplasty.[75]

SUMMARY

The preservation (or restoration) of normal joint kinematics and kinetics is paramount to the long-term success of a therapeutic course of action. Altered joint loads can induce and accelerate the progression of OA, and this must be considered with respect to the most appropriate course of treatment. More specifically, the unstable ankle must be considered with care, because chronic instability can create pathomechanical joint loads leading to the onset of OA.[76] Surgical modification of the tibiotalar joint leads to altered joint loads in the midfoot and hindfoot that can be similarly problematic. In tailoring a therapy according to individual patient anatomy and presentation, the clinician and patient profit when the clinician incorporates these concerns into his or her decision-making process.

A solid grasp of foot and ankle structure and function is thus imperative to improving clinical treatment at the level of the individual patient and in setting standards of care. Historically, understanding has been hindered by the sheer complexity of this anatomic system, and limits on the ability to quantitatively measure in vivo joint motions. However, recent advances in experimental and analytical techniques have yielded drastic increases in the quality of data one can obtain, and corresponding advances in understanding have followed.

The tried-and-true clinical approach of tibiotalar fusion remains an attractive option for many patients. However, along with an ever increasing understanding of ankle biomechanics, it is not coincidental that viable last-line operative treatment of the painful arthritic ankle has expanded to include TAR. Promising reports of mid- to long-term success of next-generation TAR continue to emerge, as indications and techniques for the use of these devices become better defined and the designs of the implants themselves continue to evolve and improve. Regardless of the chosen treatment strategy, the surgeon must weigh the options that are available and the benefits that a patient is likely to derive from each. To properly weigh this balance the surgeon must consider the biomechanics at play, including downstream changes in neighboring joints that inevitably accompany any surgical intervention.

REFERENCES

1. Espinosa N, Brodsky JW, Maceira E. Metatarsalgia. J Am Acad Orthop Surg 2010;18(8):474–85.
2. Hintermann B, Valderrabano V. Total ankle joint replacement. Zeitschrift für ärztliche Fortbildung und Qualitätssicherung 2001;95(3):187–94 [in German].
3. Espinosa N, Smerek J, Kadakia AR, et al. Operative management of ankle instability: reconstruction with open and percutaneous methods. Foot Ankle Clin 2006; 11(3):547–65.
4. McKinley TO, Tochigi Y, Rudert MJ, et al. Instability-associated changes in contact stress and contact stress rates near a step-off incongruity. J Bone Joint Surg Am 2008;90(2):375–83.
5. Tochigi Y, Rudert MJ, McKinley TO, et al. Correlation of dynamic cartilage contact stress aberrations with severity of instability in ankle incongruity. J Orthop Res 2008;26(9):1186–93.
6. Stormont DM, Morrey BF, An KN, et al. Stability of the loaded ankle. Relation between articular restraint and primary and secondary static restraints. Am J Sports Med 1985;13(5):295–300.
7. Harper M. The lateral ligamentous support of the subtalar joint. Foot Ankle 1991; 11:354–8.
8. Kelikian AS, Sarrafian S. Sarrafian's anatomy of the foot and ankle. Philadelphia: Lippincott Williams & Wilkins; 2011.
9. Sarrafian SK. Anatomy of the foot and ankle: descriptive, topographic, functional. Philadelphia: JB Lippincott; 1983.
10. Tochigi Y, Rudert MJ, Amendola A, et al. Tensile engagement of the peri-ankle ligaments in stance phase. Foot Ankle Int 2005;26(12):1067–73.
11. Rasmussen O. Stability of the ankle joint. Analysis of the function and traumatology of the ankle ligaments. Acta Orthop Scand Suppl 1985;211:1–75.

12. Attarian DE, McCrackin HJ, DeVito DP, et al. Biomechanical characteristics of human ankle ligaments. Foot Ankle 1985;6(2):54–8.
13. Siegler S, Block J, Schneck CD. The mechanical characteristics of the collateral ligaments of the human ankle joint. Foot Ankle 1988;8(5):234–42.
14. Attarian DE, McCrackin HJ, DeVito DP, et al. A biomechanical study of human lateral ankle ligaments and autogenous reconstructive grafts. Am J Sports Med 1985;13(6):377–81.
15. Hintermann B, Knupp M, Pagenstert GI. Deltoid ligament injuries: diagnosis and management. Foot Ankle Clin 2006;11(3):625–37.
16. Tornetta P III. Competence of the deltoid ligament in bimalleolar ankle fractures after medial malleolar fixation. J Bone Joint Surg Am 2000;82(6):843–8.
17. Milner CE, Soames RW. Anatomy of the collateral ligaments of the human ankle joint. Foot Ankle Int 1998;19(11):757–60.
18. Milner CE, Soames RW. The medial collateral ligaments of the human ankle joint: anatomical variations. Foot Ankle Int 1998;19(5):289–92.
19. Mengiardi B, Pfirrmann CW, Vienne P, et al. Medial collateral ligament complex of the ankle: MR appearance in asymptomatic subjects. Radiology 2007;242(3):817–24.
20. Mengiardi B, Zanetti M, Schottle PB, et al. Spring ligament complex: MR imaging-anatomic correlation and findings in asymptomatic subjects. Radiology 2005; 237(1):242–9.
21. Golanó P, Vega J, Leeuw PA, et al. Anatomy of the ankle ligaments: a pictorial essay. Knee surgery, sports traumatology. Arthroscopy 2010;18(5):557–69.
22. Ferran NA, Oliva F, Maffulli N. Ankle instability. Sports Med Arthrosc 2009;17(2): 139–45.
23. Boss AP, Hintermann B. Anatomical study of the medial ankle ligament complex. Foot Ankle Int 2002;23(6):547–53.
24. van den Bekerom MP, Oostra RJ, Alvarez PG, et al. The anatomy in relation to injury of the lateral collateral ligaments of the ankle: a current concepts review. Clin Anat 2008;21(7):619–26.
25. Huson A. Joints and movements of the foot: terminology and concepts. Acta Morphol Neerl Scand 1987;25(3):117–30.
26. Kelikian AS. Operative treatment of the foot and ankle. Appleton and Lange, Stamford Connecticut; 1999.
27. Inman. The joints of the ankle. In: Inman VT, editor. The joints of the ankle. Williams & Wilkins, Baltimore; 1976.
28. Inman VT. The human foot. Manit Med Rev 1966;46(8):513–5.
29. Barnett CH, Napier JR. The axis of rotation at the ankle joint in man; its influence upon the form of the talus and the mobility of the fibula. J Anat 1952;86(1):1–9.
30. Hicks JH. The mechanics of the foot. I. The joints. J Anat 1953;87(4):345–57.
31. Riede UN, Heitz P, Ruedi T. Studies of the joint mechanics elucidating the pathogenesis of posttraumatic arthrosis of the ankle joint in man. II. Influence of the talar shape on the biomechanics of the ankle joint. Langenbecks Arch Chir 1971;330(2):174–84 [in German].
32. Close JR, Inman VT, Poor PM, et al. The function of the subtalar joint. Clin Orthop Relat Res 1967;50:159–79.
33. Wyller T. The axis of the ankle joint and its importance in subtalar arthrodesis. Acta Orthop Scand 1963;33:320–8.
34. Lapidus PW. Subtalar joint, its anatomy and mechanics. Bull Hosp Joint Dis 1955; 16(2):179–95.
35. Weindel S, Schmidt R, Rammelt S, et al. Subtalar instability: a biomechanical cadaver study. Arch Orthop Trauma Surg 2010;130(3):313–9.

36. Perry J, Schoneberger B. Gait analysis: normal and pathological function. Thorofare (NJ): Slack Inc; 1992.
37. Viladot A, Lorenzo JC, Salazar J, et al. The subtalar joint: embryology and morphology. Foot Ankle 1984;5(2):54–66.
38. van Langelaan EJ. A kinematical analysis of the tarsal joints. An X-ray photogrammetric study. Acta Orthop Scand Suppl 1983;204:1–269.
39. Inman VT. The influence of the foot-ankle complex on the proximal skeletal structures. Artif Limbs 1969;13(1):59–65.
40. Halloran JP, Ackermann M, Erdemir A, et al. Concurrent musculoskeletal dynamics and finite element analysis predicts altered gait patterns to reduce foot tissue loading. J Biomech 2010;43(14):2810–5.
41. Favre P, Snedeker JG, Gerber C. Numerical modelling of the shoulder for clinical applications. Philos Transact A Math Phys Eng Sci 2009;367(1895):2095–118.
42. de Asla RJ, Wan L, Rubash HE, et al. Six DOF in vivo kinematics of the ankle joint complex: application of a combined dual-orthogonal fluoroscopic and magnetic resonance imaging technique. J Orthop Res 2006;24(5):1019–27.
43. van den Bogert AJ, Smith GD, Nigg BM. In vivo determination of the anatomical axes of the ankle joint complex: an optimization approach. J Biomech 1994; 27(12):1477–88.
44. Leardini A, O'Connor JJ, Catani F, et al. A geometric model of the human ankle joint. J Biomech 1999;32(6):585–91.
45. Kitaoka HB, Crevoisier XM, Hansen D, et al. Foot and ankle kinematics and ground reaction forces during ambulation. Foot Ankle Int 2006;27(10):808–13.
46. Bruening DA, Cooney KM, Buczek FL. Analysis of a kinetic multi-segment foot model. Part I: model repeatability and kinematic validity. Gait Posture 2012; 35(4):529–34 [Epub 2012 Mar 14].
47. Egerton T, Danoudis M, Huxham F, et al. Central gait control mechanisms and the stride length-cadence relationship. Gait Posture 2011;34(2):178–82.
48. Hartmann A, Murer K, de Bie RA, et al. Reproducibility of spatio-temporal gait parameters under different conditions in older adults using a trunk tri-axial accelerometer system. Gait Posture 2009;30(3):351–5.
49. Khazzam M, Long JT, Marks RM, et al. Preoperative gait characterization of patients with ankle arthrosis. Gait Posture 2006;24(1):85–93.
50. Stauffer RN, Chao EY, Brewster RC. Force and motion analysis of the normal, diseased, and prosthetic ankle joint. Clin Orthop Relat Res 1977;(127):189–96.
51. Valderrabano V, Nigg BM, von Tscharner V, et al. Gait analysis in ankle osteoarthritis and total ankle replacement. Clin Biomech 2007;22(8):894–904.
52. Dyrby C, Chou LB, Andriacchi TP, et al. Functional evaluation of the Scandinavian total ankle replacement. Foot Ankle Int 2004;25(6):377–81.
53. Mazur JM, Schwartz E, Simon SR. Ankle arthrodesis. Long-term follow-up with gait analysis. J Bone Joint Surg Am Vol 1979;61(7):964–75.
54. Wu WL, Su FC, Cheng YM, et al. Gait analysis after ankle arthrodesis. Gait Posture 2000;11(1):54–61.
55. Beyaert C, Sirveaux F, Paysant J, et al. The effect of tibio-talar arthrodesis on foot kinematics and ground reaction force progression during walking. Gait Posture 2004;20(1):84–91.
56. Thomas R, Daniels TR, Parker K. Gait analysis and functional outcomes following ankle arthrodesis for isolated ankle arthritis. J Bone Joint Surg Am Vol 2006;88(3): 526–35.
57. Piriou P, Culpan P, Mullins M, et al. Ankle replacement versus arthrodesis: a comparative gait analysis study. Foot Ankle Int 2008;29(1):3–9.

58. Demottaz JD, Mazur JM, Thomas WH, et al. Clinical study of total ankle replacement with gait analysis. A preliminary report. J Bone Joint Surg Am Vol 1979; 61(7):976–88.
59. Doets HC, van Middelkoop M, Houdijk H, et al. Gait analysis after successful mobile bearing total ankle replacement. Foot Ankle Int 2007;28(3):313–22.
60. Ingrosso S, Benedetti MG, Leardini A, et al. GAIT analysis in patients operated with a novel total ankle prosthesis. Gait Posture 2009;30(2):132–7.
61. Chao EY, Laughman RK, Schneider E, et al. Normative data of knee joint motion and ground reaction forces in adult level walking. J Biomech 1983;16(3):219–33.
62. Shih LY, Wu JJ, Lo WH. Changes in gait and maximum ankle torque in patients with ankle arthritis. Foot Ankle 1993;14(2):97–103.
63. Detrembleur C, Leemrijse T. The effects of total ankle replacement on gait disability: analysis of energetic and mechanical variables. Gait Posture 2009; 29(2):270–4.
64. Zerahn B, Kofoed H. Bone mineral density, gait analysis, and patient satisfaction, before and after ankle arthroplasty. Foot Ankle Int 2004;25(4):208–14.
65. Lundberg A, Svensson OK, Bylund C, et al. Kinematics of the ankle/foot complex. Part 2: Pronation and supination. Foot Ankle 1989;9(5):248–53.
66. Carson MC, Harrington ME, Thompson N, et al. Kinematic analysis of a multi-segment foot model for research and clinical applications: a repeatability analysis. J Biomech 2001;34(10):1299–307.
67. Conti S, Lalonde KA, Martin R. Kinematic analysis of the agility total ankle during gait. Foot Ankle Int 2006;27(11):980–4.
68. Kozanek M, Rubash HE, Li G, et al. Effect of post-traumatic tibiotalar osteoarthritis on kinematics of the ankle joint complex. Foot Ankle Int 2009;30(8):734–40.
69. Coester LM, Saltzman CL, Leupold J, et al. Long-term results following ankle arthrodesis for post-traumatic arthritis. J Bone Joint Surg Am 2001;83(2):219–28.
70. Morgan CD, Henke JA, Bailey RW, et al. Long-term results of tibiotalar arthrodesis. J Bone Joint Surg Am 1985;67(4):546–50.
71. Sheridan BD, Robinson DE, Hubble MJ, et al. Ankle arthrodesis and its relationship to ipsilateral arthritis of the hind- and mid-foot. J Bone Joint Surg Br 2006; 88(2):206–7.
72. Valderrabano V, Hintermann B, Nigg BM, et al. Kinematic changes after fusion and total replacement of the ankle. Part 1: range of motion. Foot Ankle Int 2003;24(12):881–7.
73. Cracchiolo A III, Deorio JK. Design features of current total ankle replacements: implants and instrumentation. J Am Acad Orthop Surg 2008;16(9):530–40.
74. Espinosa N, Walti M, Favre P, et al. Misalignment of total ankle components can induce high joint contact pressures. J Bone Joint Surg Am 2010;92(5):1179–87.
75. Knecht SI, Estin M, Callaghan JJ, et al. The Agility total ankle arthroplasty. Seven to sixteen-year follow-up. J Bone Joint Surg Am 2004;86(6):1161–71.
76. Anderson DD, Chubinskaya S, Guilak F, et al. Post-traumatic osteoarthritis: improved understanding and opportunities for early intervention. J Orthop Res 2011;29(6):802–9.

Ankle Arthrodesis versus Total Ankle Replacement: How Do I Decide?

Fabian G. Krause, MD*, Timo Schmid, MD

KEYWORDS

• Ankle • Arthrodesis • Replacement • Decision-making

KEY POINTS

- End-stage ankle arthritis is a debilitating condition that results in functional limitation and poor quality of life.
- Balancing the criteria that are discussed in consideration of the recent relevant literature and evidence available, the surgeon is directed to the correct individual decision.
- Because end-stage ankle arthritis rarely occurs in isolation, any intra- and extra-articular pathologic condictions that may require additional surgery (ie, subtalar arthrodesis) and affect the outcome must be determined before surgery.

INTRODUCTION

End-stage ankle arthritis is a debilitating condition that results in functional limitation and poor quality of life.[1–3] Ankle arthrodesis (AA) and total ankle replacement (TAR) are standard treatments when nonoperative management has failed and the success of a joint-preserving operation is very unlikely.

AA results are predictable with a consistent pain relief once fusion is achieved.[4,5] In most cases, good and excellent intermediate-term results are reported for modern arthrodesis techniques.[5,6] Long-term reliability, however, is questioned because AA has been associated with premature arthritis, pain, and dysfunction of the adjacent hindfoot joints.[1] Radiographic changes of arthritis after AA, though, do not necessarily correlate with symptoms, and only a few patients will undergo adjacent joint arthrodeses.[7,8] Recent modifications in TAR designs have challenged the perception that AA is the treatment of choice for end-stage ankle arthritis.[9,10] The preservation of ankle motion in TAR is a theoretical advantage over AA.[9,11] Because gait is less affected, adverse effects on the adjacent joints are not expected to occur.[9]

The authors have nothing to disclose.

Department of Orthopaedic Surgery, Inselspital, University of Berne, Freiburgstrasse, 3010 Berne, Switzerland

* Corresponding author.

E-mail address: fabian.krause@insel.ch

Foot Ankle Clin N Am 17 (2012) 529–543

http://dx.doi.org/10.1016/j.fcl.2012.08.002

foot.theclinics.com

1083-7515/12/$ – see front matter

For both procedures, high complication rates of up to 50% at intermediate- and long-term follow-up and mean revision rates of 11% for AA and 21% for TAR at intermediate follow-up have been reported.[8,9,12–15] At present, appropriate evidence of objective, prospective, and controlled data for both procedures on intermediate- and long-term outcomes is still lacking.[11]

Taking into account numerous individual criteria, the correct indication, however, substantially influences the outcome of patients with end-stage ankle arthritis treated with AA or TAR. The purpose of this report is to assist the foot and ankle surgeon or orthopedic surgeon in decision making regarding AA versus TAR. Balancing the criteria that are discussed in consideration of the recent relevant literature and evidence available, the surgeon is directed to the correct individual decision.

DECISION MAKING

General Considerations

Patients with end-stage ankle arthritis will benefit most from AA and TAR after a long-standing course of ankle pain and functional disability refractory to nonoperative treatment including nonsteroidal anti-inflammatory drugs, bracing, and shoe wear modifications.[16] Therefore, patients should be encouraged to postpone surgery, if quality of life, soft tissues and bone stock, and general health allow waiting. In addition, joint-preserving surgery (ie, supramalleolar osteotomy) should always be considered for moderate or even severe ankle arthritis as either a temporizing or final solution.

Because end-stage ankle arthritis rarely occurs in isolation, any intra- and extra-articular pathologic conditions that may require additional surgery (ie, subtalar arthrodesis) and affect the outcome must be determined before surgery.[17] The preoperative Candian Orthopaedic Foot and Ankle Society end-stage ankle arthritis classification distinguishes isolated ankle arthritis (type 1), ankle arthritis with intra-articular varus or valgus deformity, hindfoot instability and/or a tight heel cord (type 2), ankle arthritis with hindfoot deformity, tibial malunion, midfoot abductus or adductus, supinated midfoot, plantarflexed first ray, etc (type 3), and types 1 to 3 plus subtalar, calcaneocuboid, or talonavicular arthritis (type 4).[17] When applied to patient's clinical and radiographic picture, the classification helps to correctly assess intra- and extra-articular ankle and hindfoot deformities and facilitates the decision of whether AA or TAR is to be recommended.

The ideal indication for TAR is a lightweight individual with a body mass index (BMI) ranging from 20 to 25 kg/m^2, little or no hindfoot deformity (ie, varus or valgus), low demand, severe pain secondary to ankle arthritis, and preservation of more than two thirds of normal ankle range of motion. Patients with arthritis or previous arthrodesis of the adjacent joints (ie, subtalar and talonavicular joint) are also considered good candidates for TAR because pantalar arthrodesis would be an undesirable alternative. However, only 10%–20% of patients meet these criteria and most TAR candidates have at least 1 or 2 relative contraindications.

Relative contraindications for TAR are a high activity level, BMI greater than 25 kg/m^2, coronal deformity greater than 15°, partial areas of avascular bone, traumatic bone loss, osteoporosis, poor motion, diabetics without angiopathy, or a history of previous infections. Absolute contraindications for TAR are Charcot arthropathy, advanced angiopathy with or without diabetes, ongoing infection or skin ulcers near the ankle, and drop- or clubfeet. Although there is only little evidence in the literature that the outcome of TAR is more impaired than of AA, most surgeons select an AA for these patients.

Information for the Patient

Patients with documented end-stage ankle arthritis, as noted on weight-bearing anteroposterior and lateral ankle radiographs, as well as on clinical presentation, should be counseled on advantages and disadvantages of the available treatment options. To avoid illusions and overdrawn expectations with regard to postoperative function, relief of pain, and return to sports after AA or TAR, the patient and the surgeon must be well informed on the expected outcomes.

The overall early- and intermediate-term outcomes after AA and TAR are comparable.[3,11,13,18,19] Because of the restricted ankle motion, the functional outcome is worse in AA, whereas TAR has a higher rate of complications with substantial need for repeat surgery.[3,11,13]

Patients designated for AA should be informed of the expected calf atrophy, decreased walking speed resulting from a shorter stride, and a restriction of up to two-thirds of their global sagittal midfoot and hindfoot motion.[5] Because most residual sagittal motion will then arise from the transversal tarsal and subtalar joints, degeneration of these joints in the long term is common but does not necessarily require sugery.[1,5] The patients should know about difficulties in jumping, running, and likely also jogging because of the mechanical restraints after an AA.[20]

According to the literature, complications after AA include nonunions, malunions, wound breakdown, and infections. With new open and percutanous fixation techniques allowing gentle soft tissue handling, the complication rate has substantially decreased within the past decade.[8] However, a higher risk of malunion and nonunion is seen with transmalleolar osteotomies, avascular necrosis of the talus, Charcot arthropathy, failed TAR, incomplete cartilage removal, and early weight-bearing.[21] The rehabilitation period after AA requires immobilization until there are clinical and radiographic signs of satisfactory fusion, generally averaging 12 to 20 weeks.[18]

Long-term results revealed that at an average of longer than 20 years after AA, 67% of patients were happy with their results and 92% would recommend it to someone else.[1] Furthermore, gait impairment following AA diminishes with shoe wear compared with walking barefoot.[22] In a recent study of 94 isolated AA for mainly posttraumatic ankle arthritis with a mean follow-up of 6 years, union occurred in 99%, the compensatory sagittal motion in the midtarsal joints averaged 24°, the rate of complications was 12% (only minor), and secondary arthritis of the subtalar and talonavicular joints developed in 17% and 11%, respectively.[8] Progression of preexisting arthritis occurred in 30% at the subtalar joint and in 19% at the talonavicular joint. None of these patients had an arthrodesis of the adjacent joints. There is consensus in the literature that a neutral position in the sagittal plane and neutral to slight valgus in the coronal plane is essential for a satisfactory functional outcome and puts less strain on the adjacent joints, including the knee.[8]

In the Swedish and Norwegian arthroplasty registers, the current published success rate for TAR including older designs ranges from 78% to 86% of 5-year survival and from 67% to 76% of 10-year survival.[23] The substantial rate of early and intermediate complications requiring repeat surgery does not necessarily imply a failure of TAR.[13] Some repeat surgery is for relieving impingement, improving alignment, bone-grafting cysts, and/or exchanging the polyethylene component to prolong implant survival.[24] The first 3 reasons associated with implant failure are aseptic loosening, malalignment, and deep infection.[25] After TAR persistent minor pain and discomfort is reported in 23% to 60%.[26]

A 10-year survival rate of 73% and 75% was reported for the mobile-bearing STAR (Skandinavian Total Ankle Replacement, Link Inc, Hamburg, Germany) prosthesis for patients with rheumatoid and primary end-stage ankle arthritis, respectively.[18,25] Average ankle range of motion after the STAR was 25° of plantarflexion and 5° of dorsiflexion, 54% of patients were pain free, and 46% had mild discomfort.[2]

The well-informed patient usually gives consent for the indicated procedure after decision making. Nevertheless, when the patient insists on the discarded procedure despite appropriate information, either a second opinion should be obtained to convince the patient or the operation may be refused. In cases when the surgeon performs an operation against his or her own conviction, the outcome is frequently poor.

Decision Making

The author's preferred approach to indicate AA versus TAR is to balance the patient's individual criteria and relative contraindications. Criteria for decision making should be evaluated with regard to their impact on the outcome after AA and TAR, according either to evidence in the literature or to personal experience of the surgeon. Major criteria in decision making regarding AA versus TAR in end-stage ankle arthritis are age, arthritis or arthrodesis of the adjacent joints, bilateral ankle affliction, underlying cause of ankle arthritis, and stability and deformity.

Age (Major Criterion)

Age is likely one of the most crucial criteria considering when AA versus TAR because there is appropriate evidence that age substantially affects the outcome of TAR. Many young patients are demanding in terms of postoperative function of their ankle joint, return to sports, and recreational activities. According to the literature, a minimum age of 50 years for TAR is recommended. Occasionally, strong arguments are required to convince these patients that an AA may be the better solution. However, also an AA for a younger patient should be considered a last option when joint-preserving surgery fails and for disabling pain, not for enhanced function.

In a Swedish study, younger age was associated with osteolysis, loosening, and subsequently an increased risk of later revision.[23] In a review of more than 300 TARs, the reported age was the only significant predictor of reoperation and failure after TAR, the 5-year implant survivorship was 74% and 89% for patients younger than and older than 54 years, respectively.[15] Patients with an age of 54 years or less had a 1.45-times greater risk for reoperation and a 2.65-times greater risk of implant failure than patients over the age of 54.

Nevertheless, TAR is occasionally also proposed for younger patients with bilateral ankle affliction, a low activity level caused by a medical condition other than ankle arthritis, and anticipated suffering from adjacent joint arthritis after AA (ie, rheumatoid patients).

Underlying Cause of Arthritis (Major Criterion)

The cause of end-stage ankle arthritis is an interesting criterion to indicate AA versus TAR and is closely related to age. Several studies revealed substantial differences of the outcome after TAR that correlated with the cause of arthritis.

As opposed to hip and knee osteoarthritis, a minority of end-stage ankle arthritis is primary and more often secondary to trauma and rheumatoid disease. Posttraumatic arthritis accounts for 65% to 80% and rheumatoid disease for 12 % to 15% of end-stage ankle arthritis.[2,27,28] Most posttraumatic end-stage ankle arthritis occurs in younger patients.

In cases of traumatic origin, the surgeon may have to deal with a varus or valgus deformity, loss of bone stock, and severe ankylosis. Higher complication rates and reoperation/revision rates after TAR for posttraumatic arthritis have been reported.[12,29] Studies have demonstrated less satisfaction of patients with posttraumatic ankle arthritis after TAR than of patients with primary and rheumatoid arthritis, likely because of significantly more pain during normal activities, previous operations, and younger age.[29,30]

Because rheumatoid arthritis affects not only the ankle bilaterally but also the adjacent hindfoot joints, and the activity level is usually low, patients with rheumatoid arthritis are thought to benefit from TAR. In patients with rheumatoid arthritis or other systemic collagen-type diseases, the factors to consider in determining AA versus TAR are the quality of the bone, the amount of bone remaining (ie, medial malleolus or lateral talar dome erosion), the soft tissue conditions (ie, will deformity correction lead to wound breakdown), and associated deformities of the midfoot and forefoot. Frequently, in these conditions, there is severe osteoporosis with weakening of the bone, thereby increasing the chance of intraoperative and postoperative fracture when corrective forces are applied.

A study that analyzed joint registry data and a separate meta-analysis reported a trend of less favorable implant survivorship in patients with inflammatory arthritis compared with those with osteoarthritis.[31,32] Other authors always consider TAR in patients with rheumatoid arthritis, when technically possible, and they reported identical or even better functional outcomes and less pain after TAR than in patients with primary and posttraumatic arthritis.[28,33] The difference in outcomes between patients with rheumatoid arthritis and particularly those with posttraumatic arthritis may be related to the differences in functional demands and expectations between these 2 groups.

Because of the generally younger age and the reported low postoperative satisfaction after TAR, patients with posttraumatic end-stage ankle arthritis are usually considered for AA, whereas older patients with primary and rheumatoid arthritis more likely profit with TAR.

A series of 21 TARs in 16 patients with hereditary hemochromatosis as the underlying cause of ankle arthritis was recently reported and was associated with a low risk of perioperative complications and good pain relief and function.[34] Hemophilic arthropathy of the ankle treated with 10 TARs in 8 patients has also led to good results in terms of pain relief and function without perioperative complications (**Fig. 1**A–C).[35]

End-stage ankle arthritis in association with neuromuscular dysfunction, particularly with spasticity (ie, cerebral palsy), is better treated with the more stable AA but has a high nonunion rate.

Deformity and Ligamentous Instability of the Hindfoot (Major Criterion)

The extents of clinical and radiographic deformities and ligamentous instabilities of the hindfoot are also used as criteria to decide whether TAR is technically feasible or may fail early because of persistent postoperative deformity, osteolysis, and subluxation or edge-loading of the polyethylene. In contrast, ligamentous instability is usually not a problem in AA, whereas bony hindfoot deformity may require compensating bone cuts during the procedure or additional realigning hindfoot or supramalleolar osteotomies.

The extent of hindfoot deformity and instability that can be adequately treated with TAR continues to increase.[10,36,37] However, despite recent advances, coronal plane deformity exceeding 10° to 15° remains a relative contraindication to TAR because implant failure correlates with increasing preoperative deformity.[9,38,39] A significantly increased failure rate at mean follow-up of 8 years was reported in TAR performed on ankles with a preoperative deformity of greater than 10° in the coronal plane.[9]

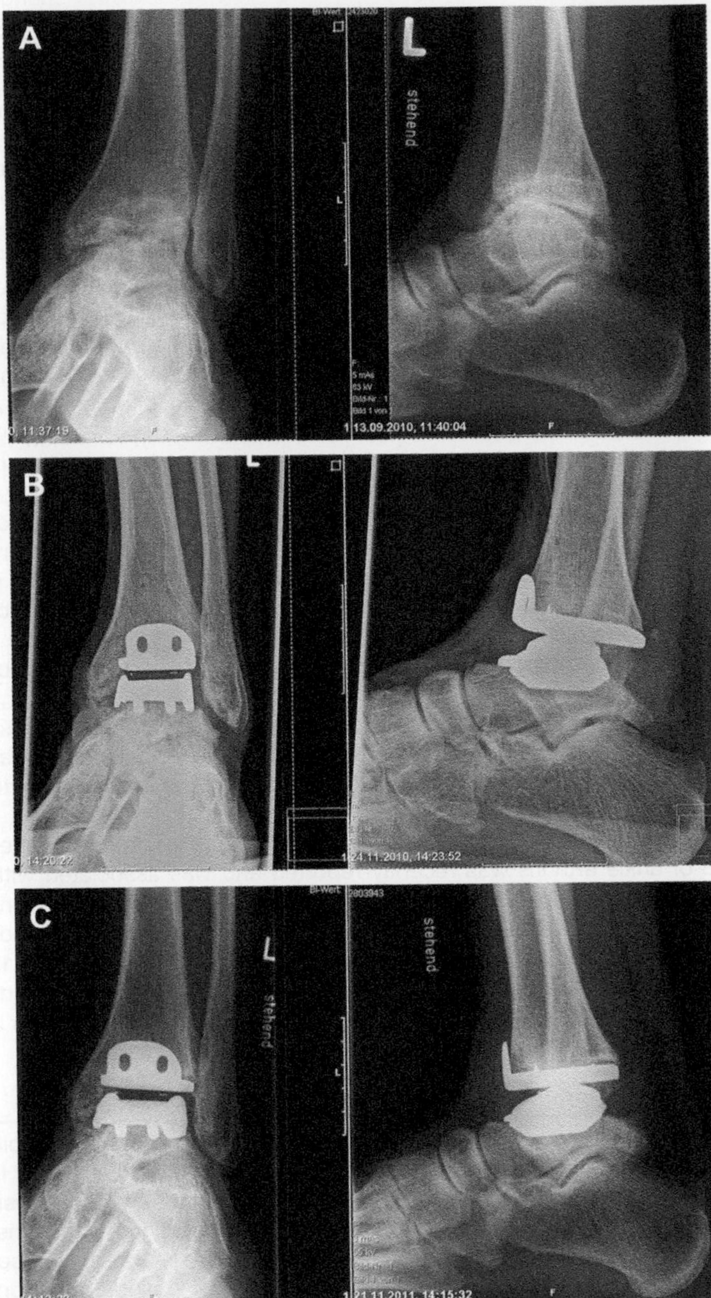

Fig. 1. (*A–C*) Preoperative anteroposterior and lateral weight-bearing radiographs of the ankle of a 60-year-old farmer who sustained an ankle fracture 30 years earlier (*A*). Criteria for the arthroscopic AA (*B*) were posttraumatic end-stage ankle arthritis with tenuous soft tissues, high activity level, no adjacent joint arthritis, unilateral affliction of the ankle joint, and medial ligamentous incompetence in combination with a moderate hindfoot valgus. At 1-year follow-up (*C*), he was entirely back to heavy work without pain. Global hindfoot motion amplitude was 20°.

The survival rate for ankles with preoperative varus or valgus deformity of more than 10° was 48% compared with a survival rate of 90% for ankles with neutral preoperative alignment. Sagittal plane deformity, typically with relative anterior translation of the talus on the tibia, or component malrotation may also result in potential early implant failure.

Between 30% and 40% of patients with end-stage ankle arthritis present with malalignment of greater than 10° in the coronal plane.[39] While the actual degree of angulation is important, the level of the angulation is also a consideration. The more proximal the angulation, the greater is the displacement of the foot and ankle from their functional position directly under the weight-bearing line of the leg. Varus angulation or medial displacement from the weight-bearing line and an extension angulation are more disabling and dysfunctional than valgus or flexion deformities. To prevent early TAR failure in these conditions, realigning hindfoot osteotomy or arthrodesis and supramalleolar osteotomy before or during TAR are recommended.[5,39] Minor deformities at the level of the ankle can be corrected with bone cuts during the operation.

Chronic lateral ankle instability with varus malalignment can result in ankle arthritis. In a recent study on the cause of ankle arthritis, end-stage ankle arthritis in 65 of 406 patients (13%) was determined to be the result of lateral ligamentous hindfoot instability.[40] Because the lateral ligaments are less powerful restraints, and by far more frequently injured, a straight or varus ankle is much more likely to become unstable and progress to arthritis. Ankle ligament imbalance should be corrected at the time of TAR, particularly in cases of longstanding varus or valgus deformities.[5] Without correct static (bony) alignment, ligament reconstruction will usually fail. Next to ligamentous incompetence, ankle instability may also be secondary to cartilage and bone wear on both sides of the joint.

Although lateral ligamentous hindfoot instability can normally be stabilized with lateral ligament repair and reconstruction, hindfoot realignment (ie, lateralizing calcaneal osteotomy), and release of the deltoid or a sliding osteotomy of the medial malleolus, medial ligamentous incompetence particularly in combination with a severe hindfoot valgus challenges even the experienced foot and ankle surgeon. Deltoid ligament incompetence, whether acquired or iatrogenic, is a relative contraindication for TAR. There is only scattered evidence of successful in vivo and in vitro deltoid ligament reconstructions in the literature.[41,42] Realignment of the hindfoot is also crucial to avoid failure of any deltoid reconstruction.

Ankle Range of Motion (Major Criterion)

Studies that investigated ankle range of motion before and after TAR revealed only little improvement, with the mean increase in the sagittal plane motion arc ranging from 3° to 14°.[11,26,29,32,33,37,39] Patients should be informed preoperatively that improvement in ankle motion is not one of the expected benefits from TAR. If the ankle is not capable of at least 5° of dorsiflexion, Achilles tendon lengthening is suggested. Failure to appropriately assess gastrocnemius-soleus tightness preoperatively was seen to lead to significant complications after TAR.[5,38] The downsides of TAR (ie, the number of complications and reoperations) may outweigh those of AA when there is preoperative ankle motion of less than 10°. However, even residual motion may be worth preserving by TAR in cases of severe adjacent joint arthritis.

Ipsilateral Arthritis of Adjacent Joints (Major Criterion)

AA is thought to place additional stress on the adjacent hindfoot joints. AA in combination with a talonavicular and/or subtalar arthrodesis or even pantalar arthrodesis substantially impairs physiologic gait and patient satisfaction. TAR is therefore indicated for patients with initial or advanced arthritis adjacent to the ankle joint that may eventually need additional arthrodeses of the hindfoot.

Although the association of AA and onset of or increase in adjacent joint arthritis is obvious, some studies suggest that even TAR does not fully protect the adjacent hindfoot from the development or progression of arthritis. One study showed worsening of subtalar arthritis in 25 of 167 TARs (15%) with a minimum follow-up of 5 years.[39] Reviewing 117 fixed-bearing TARs with a minimum follow-up of 2 years, progressive subtalar arthritis was noted in 22 (19%) in another study.[43]

However, radiographic assessment of subtalar arthritis is not always easy: if the x-ray beam is not perpendicular to the joint, overlap of osseous surfaces may obscure the joint space. When the clinical assessment and radiographs are not clear, computed tomography scan and/or diagnostic blocks are appropriate to investigate whether subtalar arthritis needs to be addressed at surgery.

Soft Tissues (Minor Criterion)

Obviously, the evaluation of soft tissues and vascularization is a major issue to obviate postoperative complications for AA and TAR. However, because the consequences will equally affect the outcome of either procedure, it is not considered as a major criterion for decision making regarding AA versus TAR.

Previous severe injury, unstable scar formations, or plastic reconstruction of the soft tissues surrounding the ankle joint may preclude both TAR and AA because of concerns for wound breakdown with subsequent deep infection or osteomyelitis. Appropriate vascularization of the ankle and hindfoot soft-tissues is also mandatory for both AA and TAR. To dispel any concerns, patients should be referred to angiology before surgery. In general, AA is preferred in cases of tenuous and unfavorable soft tissues and should be performed arthroscopically whenever feasible regarding the extent of bony defects and ankle or hindfoot deformity (**Fig. 2**A–C).

Activity Level (Minor Criterion)

Activity level is usually closely related to age; the younger the patient, the higher is the level of sports and labor. Patients with TAR are restricted in their activity level similar to other joint replacements and participation in impact-type sports is not recommended. To avoid unrealistic expectations, the young and active patient should be informed about this restriction. However, a recent study investigating the level of sports and recreational activities after AA and TAR showed a slight decrease in sports activities after AA, whereas patients of the TAR group were more likely to participate in high-demand activities of the ankle joint.[19] Neither procedure was found to be substantially superior in terms of improvement in overall activity profile.

Generally, the greater the frequency and intensity of weight-bearing activities, the greater is the likelihood that TAR will fail early. Those younger patients who want to return to full youthful activities and heavy laborers are therefore likely better served with an AA. However, at present there is no evidence in the literature that either impact or nonimpact sports correlate with early loosening and implant failure in TAR or early arthritis of adjacent joints in AA. Activity level is therefore considered as a minor criterion.

Infection/Osteomyelitis (Minor Criterion)

Like the aforementioned criterion "soft tissue," "infection/osteomyelitis" is a major concern when considering any operation but it is a minor criterion when it comes to the decision of AA versus TAR. Regardless of the operative procedure that was chosen,

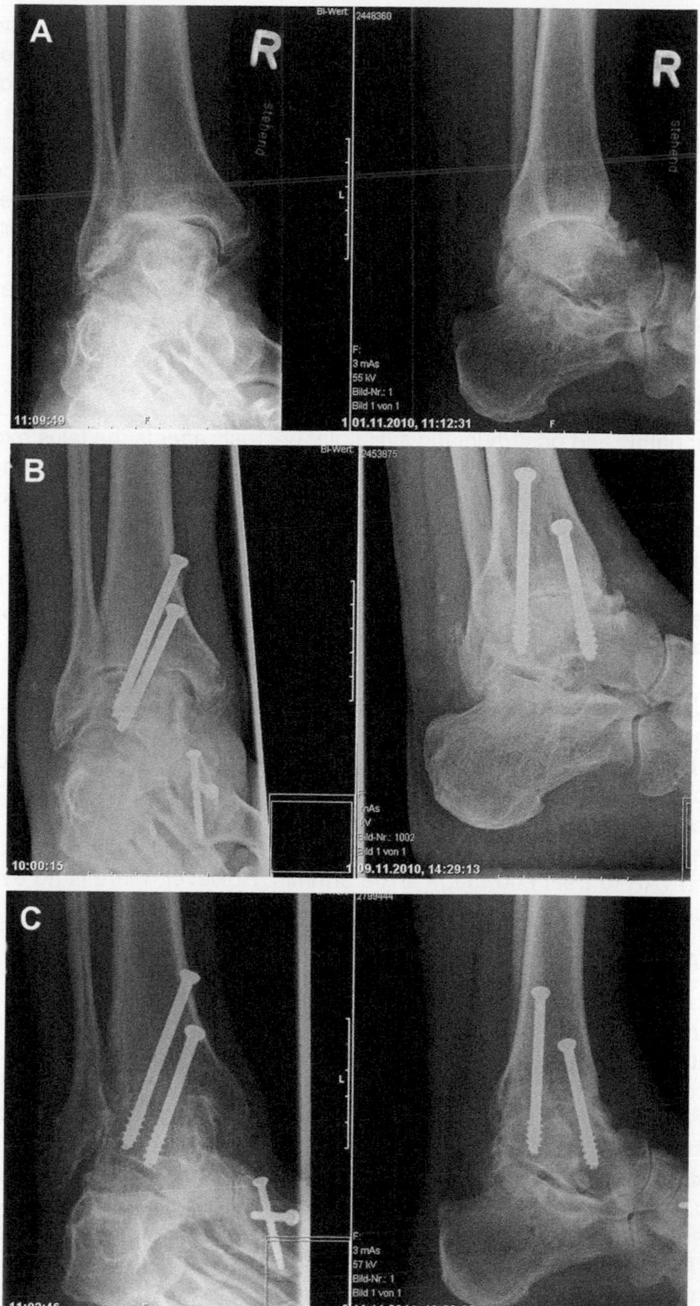

Fig. 2. (*A–C*) Preoperative anteroposterior and lateral weight-bearing radiographs of the ankle of a 44-year-old logistician (*A*). Criteria for TAR (*B*, Hintegra, Newdeal SA, Lyon, France) were hemochromatosis, possible bilateral ankle affliction, and adjacent joint arthritis that outmatched the relative contraindications of young age and a partial intraoperative avascular necrosis of the talus. The latter was removed and filled with cancellous bone graft. At 1-year follow-up (*C*), he was entirely back to heavy work without pain. Ankle motion was dorsiflexion/plantarflexion 10°/0°/20°.

earlier infection and osteomyelitis will likely impair the patient's average outcome as a result of previous operations, soft tissue scarring, need for bony defect reconstruction, and recurrence of osteomyelitis. Although an ongoing superficial and deep soft tissue infection or an ongoing osteomyelitis is an absolute contraindication for both AA and TAR, an earlier infection is not. After antibiotics have been paused for at least 2 weeks, persistent infection has to be ruled out with deep open or arthroscopic soft tissue samples and then laboratory blood work (ie, C-reactive protein) if necessary. Joint aspirations are less reliably and commonly lead to wrong negative results.

Although a previous infection or osteomyelitis is not a contraindication for TAR and there is no evidence in the literature that patients with previous infections are better served with an AA, again, most surgeons would elect an AA for these unfavorable cases.

Avascular Necrosis (Minor Criterion)

Usually, idiopathic and posttraumatic avascular necrosis affects the talus exclusively. Most tali with subtotal AVN will eventually develop subchondral collapse and secondary arthritis. This can occur at the ankle or subtalar joint or in both joints simultaneously. Typically, it involves the ankle joint first. Arthrodesis of the involved joint or joints is the treatment of choice. The risk of nonunion in AA can be increased up to 40% with avascular necrosis of the talus (>50% of the talar body).[21] The use of uncemented TAR is relatively contraindicated because the potential for appropriate implant osteointegration and component fixation is low.

Compliance (Minor Criterion)

We tend to associate drug addicts, alcoholics, homeless and unemployed individuals, and patients with a very low social status with malcompliance, but these prejudices do not always come true. Conversely, patients with a high social status (ie, physicians) may also present a surprisingly poor compliance.

Assuming malcompliance, most surgeons would prefer to recommend an AA instead of a TAR to treat end-stage ankle arthritis. However, there is no evidence in the literature that malcompliant patients do any better with an AA.

Diabetes (Minor Criterion)

Because of a high rate of infection and wound breakdown, TAR in patients with diabetic angiopathy and polyneuropathy is an absolute contraindication. However, postoperative complications in diabetic patients are also increased in AA.[44] Even if the incision for AA or TAR has healed uneventfully, unrecognized later ulcerations caused by a forefoot or midfoot deformity may cause infection that potentially spread into the hindfoot.

Because the osteointegration of uncemented TAR for end-stage ankle arthritis is thought to be poor and progression of the deformity is unpredictable, diabetic ankle Charcot arthropathy is a clear absolute contraindication for TAR. The primary indication for AA of a Charcot joint is salvage of the foot or leg, whereby the viability is threatened by the damage to the soft tissue envelope caused by the deformity. The clearest indication for realigning AA is to salvage the foot and to avoid an impending below-knee amputation. Also for AA, a high complication rate has to be anticipated in Charcot arthropathy of the ankle.

BMI (Minor Criterion)

There is no evidence in the literature that a high BMI is a criterion that impairs the outcome of either AA or TAR. Studies comparing AA and TAR that also reported the patient's BMI revealed no significant differences of the BMI in either group.[44] A high BMI obviously increases the lever arm at heel strike and push off that acts on the interface of TAR implants and the adjacent bone with the potential of early implant loosening. Furthermore, the elevated biomechanical stress may cause early failure of the polyethylene. In AA, the increased lever arm in patients with a high BMI may adversely affect union of the fusion site or cause tibial stress fracture later on, once the AA is healed. Conversely, that the activity level of these patients is usually low may compensate for the higher biomechanical stress. Despite the lack of evidence in the literature, most surgeons would recommend AA for patients with a BMI of greater than 25 or 30 kg/m^2 because the likelihood of failure seems to be higher for TAR.

Patient's Request (Minor Criterion)

The patient's request is to be considered in decision making if it does not grossly contradict the analysis of the individual criteria. When the patient insists on the inappropriate procedure despite comprehensive information, either a second opinion should be obtained to convince the patient or the operation may be refused. A wrong indication frequently leads to poor outcome.

Smoking (No Criterion)

Although smoking is reported to cause a nonunion rate in arthrodeses that is up to 16 times higher than that in nonsmokers,[44] its effect on TAR outcome has not been determined. However, in heavy smokers who cannot either stop or reduce smoking temporarily, the TAR implant osteointegration is likely impaired. Certainly, wound healing capacity is also diminished with nicotine abuse, and wound breakdown and infection are more common in these patients. Because the 3 procedures are equally affected, smoking is not considered as a criterion in decision making regarding AA versus TAR.

DISCUSSION

Decision making regarding AA versus TAR plays an important role for the successful treatment of end-stage ankle arthritis. Every patient's individual combination of criteria has to be assessed and balanced thoroughly before surgery. The author's personal major and minor criteria for decision making between AA versus TAR are listed in **Table 1**. Major criteria have shown evidence in the literature and are considered of equal value without a ranking among each other. When still in doubt after balancing the major criteria, minor criteria should be analyzed. Although they seem reasonable, solid evidence for the minor criteria from studies comparing the impact of these criteria on the outcome is lacking in the literature.

Balancing the criteria for decision making is not always easy and clear. For a patient with an age of 25 years, a high activity level, no adjacent joint arthritis, and posttraumatic end-stage ankle arthritis, an AA is clearly recommended by the authors. However, for a patient aged 50 years with a high activity level, some degree of subtalar arthritis, and posttraumatic end-stage ankle arthritis, a more thorough assessment and thoughtful balancing are required.

In a recent comparative study analyzing the impact of complications on AA and TAR outcome, patients with TAR were as satisfied and yielded scores as good as did the patients with AA despite having significantly more complications at a mean follow-up of 38 months.[13] This finding was thought to be associated with a better postoperative function and a selection bias. If any ankle range of motion is retained,

Table 1
Authors' major and minor criteria for decision making regarding AA versus TAR

	Criterion	AA	TAR
Major	Age, y	<50	>60
	Underlying cause of arthritis	Posttraumatic, neuromuscular disease (spasticity)	Primary, rheumatoid and collagen-type disease, hemophilia, hemochromatosis
	Bilateral ankle arthritis	No	Yes
	Ankle range of motion	Poor (<10°)	Appropriate (>15°)
	Ipsilateral arthritis or arthrodesis of adjacent joints	Absent	Present
	Deformity and ligamentous instability of the hindfoot	Varus/valgus >15°, severe instability	Varus/valgus <10°, mild instability
Minor	Soft tissues/vascularization	Moderate angiopathy, tenuous soft tissue	Intact
	Previous infection or osteomyelitis	Yes	No
	Compliance	Poor	Appropriate
	Diabetes	Unstable	Well controlled
	BMI, kg/m²	>25	<25
	Activity level	High	Low
	Avascular necrosis	Yes	No

If still in doubt after analyzing the major criteria, the minor criteria are also taken into consideration.

the patient's gait after TAR is less disturbed, and he or she will achieve better functional score results than those with AA.

There are by far more absolute and relative contraindication for TAR (ie, Charcot arthropathy or avascular necrosis of the talus) than for AA indicating a selection bias. Older and less demanding patients will have TAR, whereas younger and more active patients will have AA. Moreover, patients who are presumed to be less compliant and patients with complex hindfoot deformities or tenuous ankle soft tissue are more likely to undergo AA. This selection bias may account for a less desirable overall outcome after AA in comparative studies that do not consider the complexity of the cases.[2,13]

The authors also tend to involuntarily select AA for a patient, when negative criteria (ie, malcompliance, tenuous soft tissues) predominate, although evidence in the literature that TAR is more affected by these criteria than AA does not exist. TAR seems to be reserved for patients with an assumed uneventful healing and superior outcome.

This selection is likely because failure of TAR is more difficult and complex to reoperate or to salvage than is failure of AA. Once fusion is achieved, the risk of failure after AA is lower compared with TAR. If at all, adjacent joint arthritis after AA does usually not cause relevant symptoms within the first decade. Additionally, for implant-associated infections, the hardware can be easily removed in the stable AA. Conversely, TAR continues to be at risk for failure (ie, caused by polyethylene wear, aseptic loosening, or implant associated infections).

SUMMARY

Next to comprehensive patient information, the meticulous process of decision making regarding AA versus TAR is a prerequisite for superior outcomes. With the appropriate indication and a technically correct surgical procedure, patient satisfaction after AA and TAR is equally high. Incorrect indications lead to early failure and unsatisfied patients. If any doubt is left despite thorough decision making, the patient is usually better served with an AA.

REFERENCES

1. Coester LM, Saltzman CL, Leupold J, et al. Long-term results following ankle arthrodesis for post-traumatic arthritis. J Bone Joint Surg Am 2001;83:219–28.
2. Saltzman CL, Zimmerman MB, O'Rourke M, et al. Impact of comorbidities on the measurement of health in patients with ankle osteoarthritis. J Bone Joint Surg Am 2006;88:2366–72.
3. Soohoo NF, Zingmond DS, Ko CY. Comparison of reoperation rates following ankle arthrodesis and total ankle arthroplasty. J Bone Joint Surg Am 2007;89: 2143–9.
4. Stone JW. Arthroscopic ankle arthrodesis. Foot Ankle Clin N Am 2006;11:361–8.
5. Thomas R, Daniels TR, Parker K. Gait analysis and functional outcome following ankle arthrodesis for isolated ankle arthritis. J Bone Joint Surg Am 2006;88: 526–35.
6. Holt ES, Hansen ST, Mayo KA, et al. Ankle arthrodesis using internal screw fixation. Clin Orthop 1991;268:21–8.
7. Kitaoka HB. Arthrodesis of the ankle: technique, complications, and salvage treatment. Instr Course Lect 1999;48:255–61.
8. Zwipp H, Rammelt S, Endres T, et al. High union rates and function scores at midterm followup with ankle arthrodesis using a four screw technique. Clin Orthop Relat Res 2010;468:958–68.
9. Doets HC, Brand R, Nelissen RG. Total ankle arthroplasty in inflammatory joint disease with use of mobile-bearing designs. J Bone Joint Surg Am 2006;88: 1272–84.
10. Kofoed H. Scandinavian Total Ankle Replacement (STAR). Clin Orthop Relat Res 2004;24:73–9.
11. Haddad SL, Coetzee JC, Estok R, et al. Intermediate and long-term outcomes of total ankle arthroplasty and ankle arthrodesis. J Bone Joint Surg Am 2007;89: 1899–905.
12. Anderson T, Montgomery F, Carlsson A. Uncemented STAR total ankle prosthesis. Three- to eight-year follow-up of fifty-one consecutive ankles. J Bone Joint Surg Am 2003;85:1321–9.
13. Krause FG, Windolf M, Bora B, et al. Impact of complications in total ankle replacement and ankle arthrodesis analyzed with a validated outcome measurement. J Bone Joint Surg Am 2011;93:830–9.
14. Pyevich MT, Saltzman CL, Callaghan JJ, et al. Total ankle arthroplasty: a unique design. Two to twelve-year follow-up. J Bone Joint Surg Am 1998;80:1410–20.
15. Spirt AA, Assal M, Hansen ST. Complications and failure after total ankle arthroplasty. J Bone Joint Surg Am 2004;86:1172–8.
16. Demetriades L, Strauss E, Gallina J. Osteoarthritis of the ankle. Clin Orthop 1998; 349:28–42.
17. Krause FG, Di Silvestro M, Penner MJ, et al. Inter- and intraobserver reliability of the COFAS end-stage ankle arthritis classification system. Foot Ankle Int 2010;31:103–8.
18. Saltzmann CL, Mann RA, Ahrens JE, et al. Prospective controlled trial of STAR ankle replacement versus ankle fusion: initial results. Foot Ankle Int 2009;30: 579–96.

19. Schuh R, Hofstaetter J, Krismer M, et al. Total ankle arthroplasty versus ankle arthrodesis. Comparison of sports, recreational activities and functional outcome. Int Orthop 2011;36(6):1207–14 [Epub Nov 2011].
20. Vertullo CJ, Nunley JA. Participation in sports after arthrodesis of the foot and ankle. Foot Ankle Int 2002;23:625–8.
21. Frey C, Halikus NM, Vu-Rose T, et al. A review of ankle arthrodesis: Predisposing factors to non-union. Foot Ankle Int 1994;15:581–4.
22. Mazur JM, Schwartz E, Simon SR. Ankle arthrodesis. Long-term follow-up with gait analysis. J Bone Joint Surg Am 1979;61:964–75.
23. Henricsson A, Skoog A, Carlsson A. The Swedish ankle arthroplasty register: an analysis of 531 arthroplasties between 1993 and 2005. Acta Orthop 2007;78: 569–74.
24. Easley ME, Adams SB Jr, Hembree WC, et al. Results of total ankle arthroplasty. J Bone Joint Surg Am 2011;93:1455–68.
25. Zhao H, Yang Y, Yu G, et al. A systematic review of outcome and failure rate of uncemented Scandinavian total ankle replacement. Int Orthop 2011;35: 1751–8.
26. Gougoulias N, Khanna A, Maffulli N. How successful are current ankle replacements? A systematic review of the literature. Clin Orthop Relat Res 2010;468: 199–208.
27. Chou LB, Coughlin MT, Hansen S Jr, et al. Osteoarthritis of the ankle: the role of arthroplasty. J Am Acad Orthop Surg 2008;16:249–59.
28. Rippstein PF, Huber M, Coetzee JC, et al. Total ankle replacement with use of a new three-component implant. J Bone Joint Surg Am 2011;93:1426–35.
29. Wood PL, Deakin S. Total ankle replacement. The results in 200 ankles. J Bone Joint Surg Br 2003;85:334–41.
30. Hintermann B, Valderrabano V, Dereymaeker G, et al. The HINTEGRA ankle: rationale and short-term results of 122 consecutive ankles. Clin Orthop Relat Res 2004;424:57–68.
31. Fevang BT, Lie SA, Havelin LI, et al. 257 Ankle arthroplasties performed in Norway between 1994 and 2005. Acta Orthop 2007;78:575–83.
32. Stengel D, Bauwens K, Ekkernkamp A, et al. Efficacy of total ankle replacement with meniscal-bearing devices: a systematic review and meta-analysis. Arch Orthop Trauma Surg 2005;125:109–19.
33. Bonnin MP, Laurent JR, Casillas M. Ankle function and sports activity after total ankle arthroplasty. Foot Ankle Int 2009;30:933–44.
34. Barg A, Elsner A, Hefti D, et al. Total ankle arthroplasty in patients with hereditary hemochromatosis. Clin Orthop Relat Res 2011;469(5):1427–35 [Epub 2010 Jul 28].
35. Barg A, Elsner A, Hefti D, et al. Haemophilic arthropathy of the ankle treated by total ankle replacement: a case series. Haemophilia 2010;16(4):647–55 [Epub 2010 Mar 16].
36. Kim BS, Choi WJ, Kim YS, et al. Total ankle replacement in moderate to severe varus deformity of the ankle. J Bone Joint Surg Br 2009;91:1183–90.
37. Mann J, Mann R, Horton E. STAR ankle: long-term results. Foot Ankle Int 2011;32: 473–84.
38. Conti SF, Wong YS. Complications of total ankle replacement. Clin Orthop Relat Res 2001;391:105–14.
39. Wood PL, Sutton C, Mishra V, et al. A randomised, controlled trial of two mobile-bearing total ankle replacements. J Bone Joint Surg Br 2009;91:69–74.
40. Valderrabano V, Horisberger M, Russel I, et al. Etiology of ankle arthritis. Clin Orthop Relat Res 2009;457:1800–6.

41. Deland JT, Asla RJ, Segal A. Reconstruction of the chronically failed deltoid ligament: a new technique. Foot Ankle Int 2004;25:795–9.
42. Haddad SL, Dedhia S, Ren Y, et al. Deltoid ligament reconstruction: a novel technique with biomechanical analysis. Foot Ankle Int 2010;31:639–51.
43. Knecht SI, Estin M, Callaghan JJ, et al. The Agility total ankle arthroplasty. Seven to sixteen-year follow-up. J Bone Joint Surg Am 2004;86:1161–71.
44. Perlman MH, Thordarson DB. Ankle fusion in a high risk population: an assessment of nonunion risk factors. Foot Ankle Int 1999;20:491–6.

The Concept of Ankle Joint Preserving Surgery

Why Does Supramalleolar Osteotomy Work and How to Decide When to Do an Osteotomy or Joint Replacement

Yasuhito Tanaka, MD, PhD

KEYWORDS

- Joint-preserving surgery • Supramalleolar osteotomy • Varus-type osteoarthritis

KEY POINTS

- Joint-preserving surgical techniques include arthroscopic debridement, ligament reconstruction, distraction arthroplasty, and osteotomy.
- The mechanisms of action underlying supramalleolar osteotomy for varus-type osteoarthritis are believed to consist of correcting the medial displacement of the load line, laterally distributing the medial concentration of stress within the ankle.
- For the varus-type osteoarthritis, supramalleolar osteotomy is very effective for patients in stage 2 or stage 3a, but clinical results for patients with stage 3-b are unsatisfactory.
- Although indication of supramalleolar osteotomy is very limited, relieve of pain and retaining of joint function can be achieved simultaneously.

The structure of the ankle is stabilized by bone, and external force is distributed to the adjacent intertarsal joints, reducing the vulnerability of the joint to osteoarthritis. The load-bearing area of the ankle, however, is comparatively smaller than that of the knee, and the load per unit area is conversely high. Kimizuka and colleagues[1] reported that when a force of 500 N was applied, the area of contact in the ankle was 350 mm^2, compared with 1100 mm^2 in the hip and 1120 mm^2 in the knee. For this reason, osteoarthritis readily develops once a structural abnormality occurs. The ankle is frequently susceptible to trauma, and postfracture arthritis accounts for a high proportion of cases of osteoarthritis of the ankle.[2] This arthritis is most commonly caused by malleolar or plafond fracture.[3] Morphologic abnormality of the ankle due to varus deformity of the distal joint surface of the tibia or joint instability is another possible cause, as is morphologic abnormality of the foot such as flat or club foot.

Department of Orthopaedic Surgery, Nara Medical University, Kashihara, Nara 634-8522, Japan
E-mail address: yatanaka@naramed-u.ac.jp

Foot Ankle Clin N Am 17 (2012) 545–553
http://dx.doi.org/10.1016/j.fcl.2012.08.003

JOINT-PRESERVING SURGERY

Joint-preserving surgical techniques include arthroscopic debridement, ligament reconstruction, distraction arthroplasty, and osteotomy. Arthroscopic debridement yields good outcomes in terms of anterior impingement of the ankle by bone and soft tissue.[4] However, this approach is of limited therapeutic efficacy for advanced osteoarthritis of the ankle.[5] In patients with complete cartilage loss, symptoms cannot easily be improved using arthroscopic debridement alone.

Ligament reconstruction has been reported as effective for treating early-stage osteoarthritis with joint instability.[6] Noguchi[7] emphasized the contribution of lateral ligament instability as a cause of ankle osteoarthritis, given the presence of patients with mild varus deformity of the distal joint surface of the tibia. Löfvenberg and colleagues,[8] however, described the long-term natural course of 46 ankles with old lateral ligament injury over 18 to 23 years, reporting arthritic changes in only 6 (13%). This report indicates that ligament insufficiency does not necessarily lead to osteoarthritis and that morphologic causes such as varus deformity of the distal joint surface of the tibia also play an important role. Sugimoto and colleagues[9] stated that varus deformity of the distal joint surface of the tibia is frequently present in patients with a tendency to develop chronic lateral ligament injury of the ankle and that these may affect each other. The absence of bony misalignment is therefore a condition for the indication of ligament reconstruction.

Posttraumatic arthritis is common in the ankle joint, and distraction arthroplasty may also be considered as joint-preserving surgery for young patients with advanced arthritis caused by joint surface irregularity.[10] Normal leg alignment is a prerequisite for distraction arthroplasty, however, and as the authors' focus on realignment surgery in this article, they limit themselves to supramalleolar osteotomy.

HISTORY OF SUPRAMALLEOLAR OSTEOTOMY FOR OSTEOARTHRITIS OF THE ANKLE

Supramalleolar osteotomy to treat varus-type osteoarthritis of the ankle is also known as "low tibial osteotomy," as opposed to "high tibial osteotomy" to treat varus-type osteoarthritis of the knee.[11–14] Indications include residual deformities of poliomyelitis[11] and congenital equinovarus,[12] as well as valgus deformity of the ankle due to abnormality of the fibula.[13] This approach is also indicated for rheumatoid ankle arthritis[14] and hemophilic arthropathy.[15] As opinions are divided with respect to other conditions, however, this article focuses only on osteoarthritis of the ankle due to malalignment of the ankle joint. Supramalleolar osteotomy has been used to treat osteoarthritis of the ankle due to posttraumatic malunion. Graehl and colleagues[16] performed supramalleolar osteotomies on 8 patients who were symptomatic from a malunion of the distal two-thirds of the tibia. All of the patients had varus malunion with a mean angulation of 15°. Takakura and colleagues[17] used osteotomy to treat varus-type osteoarthritis of the ankle due to fracture, and Hintermann and colleagues[18] used osteotomy to treat valgus-type osteoarthritis of the ankle due to residual deformity following pronation-external rotation-type fracture, both with good results.

Idiopathic osteoarthritis shows both varus and valgus types. Takakura and colleagues[19] first reported the outcomes of supramalleolar osteotomy to treat varus-type osteoarthritis of the ankle in 5 patients, and this was followed by other reports from around Asia. Teramoto and colleagues[20] reported the use of distal tibial oblique osteotomy to treat the valgus type, but this technique is still at the case report level. Most cases involving valgus type in deformity comprise stage 4 posterior tibial tendon dysfunction, and the indications for supramalleolar osteotomy are limited.

Pagenstert and colleagues[21,22] took a comprehensive view of leg alignment and described methods including osteotomy at other sites, such as calcaneal osteotomy, in addition to supramalleolar osteotomy. Posttraumatic patients in particular may also have a range of degenerative elements, and an overall approach must of course be adopted. As the results of research in this area cannot yet be described as adequate, further studies are anticipated in the future.

WHY DOES SUPRAMALLEOLAR OSTEOTOMY WORK?

Unlike chondrocytes of the knee, those of the ankle are by nature resistant to degeneration and are easily repaired if damaged.[23,24] Hence, osteotomy is regarded as highly effective if a favorable biomechanical environment for cartilage repair is created within the joint.

As the level and pathology of degeneration differs between individual cases in posttraumatic arthritis, the authors here describe the mechanism whereby supramalleolar osteotomy produces effects in varus-type osteoarthritis of the ankle, which has been comparatively well studied in a large number of cases.

Varus-type osteoarthritis of the ankle is characterized morphologically by varus deformity of the distal joint surface of the tibia. With respect to the question of the extent to which varus deformity of the distal joint surface of the tibia is involved in the onset of ankle osteoarthritis, Oneda and colleagues[25] performed a biomechanical investigation using a rigid-body spring model. They stated that medial displacement of the load line was important, with varus deformity of the distal joint surface of the tibia by itself not resulting in medial stress concentration in the ankle. The subtalar joint plays a significant role in maintaining the talus in normal position relative to tibia.[26] Hayashi and colleagues[27] studied the subtalar joint in varus-type osteoarthritis, and failure of compensation function was observed in terminal stages.

This displacement of the load line is regarded as occurring because of the medial positioning of the foot below the talus in line with varus deformity of the distal joint surface of the tibia.

The mechanisms of action underlying supramalleolar osteotomy are believed to consist of correcting the medial displacement of the load line, laterally distributing the medial concentration of stress within the ankle. Simulations using the rigid-body spring model[28] and cadaveric studies[29,30] have shown the value of giving the distal joint surface of the tibia a valgus tilt. An investigation that tracked the position of the load line on whole-leg radiographic images also showed that correction in the neighborhood of the ankle was more useful than correction around the knee.[31]

As for sagittal plain, Tarr and colleagues[32] found that distal tibial deformities significantly alter total tibiotalar contact area, contact shape, and contact location. Greater changes were obtained with deformities as much as 42% for anterior bow of 15° and 40% for posterior bow of 15°.

INDICATION AND LIMITATION OF SUPRAMALLEOLAR OSTEOTOMY

For the varus-type osteoarthritis, classification is important for operative indication. The condition of varus-type osteoarthritis of the ankle is classified into 4 stages[33,34] (**Fig. 1**): no joint-space narrowing, but early sclerosis and osteophyte formation (stage 1), narrowing of the joint space medially (stage 2), obliteration of the joint space with subchondral bone contact medially (stage 3), and obliteration of the whole joint space with complete bone contact (stage 4). Stage 3 was further classified into stages 3a and 3b.[34] In the former, obliteration of the joint space was limited in the facet to medial malleolus, whereas in the latter, obliteration of the joint space was advanced

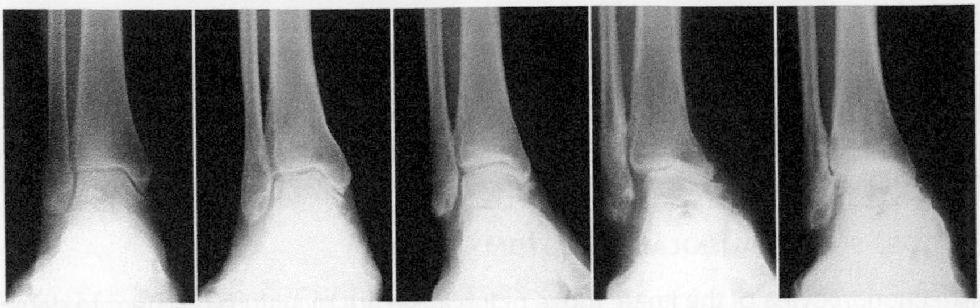

Fig. 1. Takakura-Tanaka classification for varus-type osteoarthritis.

to the roof of the talar dome. Low tibial osteotomy is effective for patients in stage 2 or stage 3a (**Fig. 2**), but clinical results for patients with stage 3b are unsatisfactory.[34] At least, retaining of the cartilage of the roof of the talar dome is necessary for the osteotomy.

Teramoto and colleagues[35] devised a distal tibial oblique osteotomy without fibular osteotomy and reported good results for the stage 3b osteoarthritic ankles. The ankle mortise in stage 3b osteoarthritis is sometimes enlarged and has large talar tilt. The purpose of this osteotomy is to shut enlarged ankle mortise. Stress distribution in the ankle is changed by making fibular osteotomy or not.[29] Research should be done about what kinds of osteotomies are most suitable for osteoarthritis.

Because supramalleolar osteotomy is realignment surgery, to obtain good result, accurate evaluation is necessary for structural malalignment of the osteoarthritic ankle. Radiographic evaluation was performed using anteroposterior (AP) and lateral images of the ankle under weight-bearing conditions. The angle between the tibial axis and the distal joint surface of the tibia on the AP view (tibial anterior surface [TAS] angle) and the same angle on the lateral view (tibial lateral surface [TLS] angle) were measured (**Fig. 3**).[36,37] These measurements indicated the varus angle and the amount of anterior opening of the joint, respectively. The tibial axis was defined as the line between the midpoints of the tibial shaft 8 cm and 13 cm above the tip of

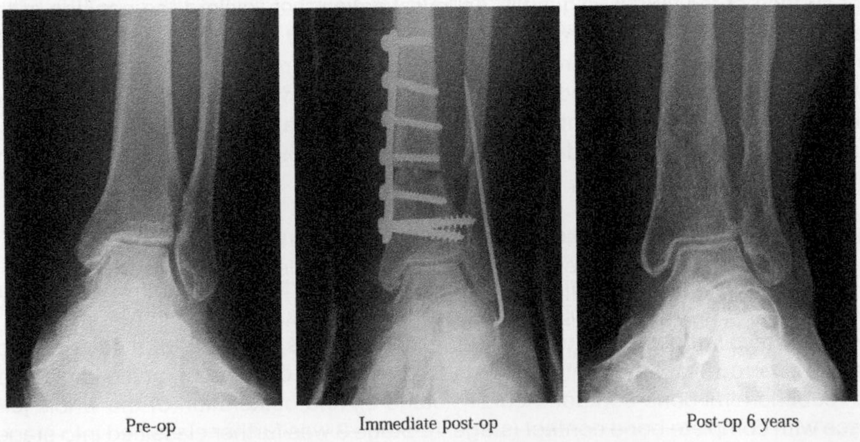

Fig. 2. Supramalleolar osteotomy for the ankle with stage 3a osteoarthritis. A 59-year-old woman completely satisfied with the result 6 years after the surgery.

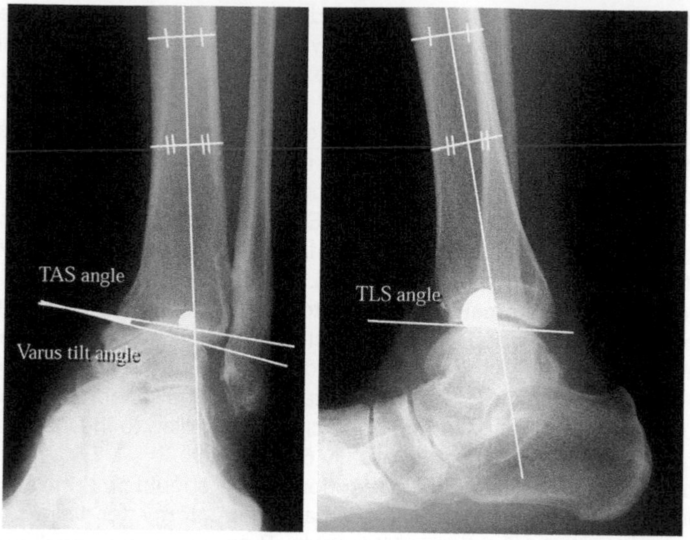

Fig. 3. Radiographic measurement. TAS, tibial anterior surface; TLS, tibial lateral surface.

the medial malleolus. In healthy Americans[38] and Japanese people,[9] the mean TAS angle is 93.3° and 88.1°, respectively. TLS angle is 81.0° in healthy Japanese people.[9]

Varus tilt of the talus is observed in some ankles with osteoarthritis. It is evaluated with the varus tilt angle in the weight-bearing AP radiograph, which is formed by the distal joint surface of the tibia and the upper surface of the talar dome (see **Fig. 3**).[34] If the varus tilt angle in the weight-bearing AP view was 5° or less, good results would be obtained by osteotomy alone. However, no joints with the varus tilt angle of more than 10° can attain a normal joint space. Lee and colleagues[39] said that the optimal threshold for predicting high postoperative talar tilt was 7.3° of preoperative talar tilt.

Improvement of range of motion of the ankle cannot be expected with supramalleolar osteotomy. Therefore, supramalleolar osteotomy should be indicated for the patients with retaining of the motion of the ankle. Although indication of this procedure is limited, relief of pain and retaining of joint function can be achieved simultaneously with this procedure.

KINDS OF OSTEOTOMY

An open wedge osteotomy,[33,34,39–42] a closed wedge osteotomy,[18,43] an oblique osteotomy,[44,45] and a dome osteotomy[16] were reported. As fixation device, plate[41] or external fixator[13,44] were used.

A lateral closed wedge osteotomy for varus-type osteoarthritis is technically difficult because of the presence of the fibula on the lateral side, and the method could weaken peroneal muscles because it will shorten the lateral side. They thought that an open wedge method would be better than a closed wedge method for varus-type osteoarthritis. An anteromedial open wedge osteotomy to correct the varus and anterior opening of the distal joint surface is planned for the varus-type osteoarthritis. Many surgeons[39–42] chose medial open wedge osteotomies for varus-type osteoarthritis.

Correction of the TAS angle should be limited within the normal value if there is no loss of cartilage in varus deformity caused by injury,[11] but if articular cartilage on the articular surface of the malleolus disappeared, overcorrection is considered appropriate because all load must be supported by the remaining cartilage on the lateral side of the joint. Overcorrection according to varus deformity brought much better results than undercorrection, especially for advanced osteoarthritis. There was discussion on how much overcorrection would be adequate. The authors aimed the TAS angle for 96° to 98°.[34] However, Lee and colleagues[39] reported that overcorrection did not correct large varus tilt of the talus and sometimes caused lateral foot pain. Therefore, they attempted to achieve a TAS angle of 95°, and if deformity was remained, they corrected it by calcaneal osteotomy. As for the TLS angle, overcorrection restricted dorsiflexion of the ankle. The TLS angle is aimed for 81° to 82°.[34]

The osteotomy site of this method is set up to 5 cm above from the tip of the medial malleolus (see **Fig. 2**). The degrees of correction were justified by the shape of the grafted bone. The lengths of the outer and side margins of the wedge-shaped graft bone were measured during preoperative drawing for the osteotomy. The grafted bone is usually harvested from the iliac bone crest. According to the varus-type osteoarthritis, medial height of the graft is usually 6 to 8 mm.

As for posttraumatic osteoarthritis, correction usually should be done at the injured site. Hintermann and colleagues[18] made varus osteotomy for valgus malunited pronation-external rotation fractures of the ankle. They aimed for correction to a varus position between 2° and 4°. When the ankle with malleolus fractures was operated, anatomic repair of the fibula was the key of the operation.[46] If the fibula was shortened at the fracture site, lateralization of the talus occurred. Therefore, lengthening of the fibula is necessary for adequate reduction.[29,47] Reidsma and colleagues[48] reported the long-term result of correction osteotomies for malunited fracture and showed that minor posttraumatic arthritis is not a contraindication but rather an indication for reconstructive surgery. They found that prolonged time to reconstruction is associated negatively with outcome.

HOW TO DECIDE WHEN TO DO AN OSTEOTOMY OR JOINT REPLACEMENT

Although there were many reports[49–51] of comparative studies between arthrodesis and total ankle arthroplasty, there was none between osteotomy and total ankle arthroplasty. It was thought that total ankle arthroplasty is difficult to be indicated for the ankle with severe malalignment. Therefore, a realignment surgery may be necessary before arthroplasty. On the contrary, there is no indication of supramalleolar osteotomy for normal aligned osteoarthritic ankles. Because long-term results of supramalleolar osteotomy were not clear, the author refer to results of high tibial osteotomies. It was said that the ideal candidate for a high tibial osteotomy is a young patient (<60 years of age), with isolated medial osteoarthritis, with good range of motion, and without ligamentous instability.[52] Same things may be true in supramalleolar osteotomy. Results of total knee arthroplasty are much better than those of total ankle arthroplasty. Therefore, indication of a supramalleolar osteotomy may be more widespread than a high tibial osteotomy. However, the literature review of high tibial osteotomy shows that the outcomes gradually deteriorate with time.[52] Further studies are needed concerning whether same things are happening in supramalleolar osteotomy or not.

REFERENCES

1. Kimizuka M, Kurosawa H, Fukubayashi T. Load-bearing pattern of the ankle joint. Contact area and pressure distribution. Arch Orthop Trauma Surg 1980;96:45–9.

2. Valderrabano V, Horisberger M, Russell I, et al. Etiology of ankle osteoarthritis. Clin Orthop 2009;467:1800–6.
3. Horisberger M, Valderrabano V, Hinterman B. Posttraumatic ankle osteoarthritis after ankle-related fractures. J Orthop Trauma 2009;23:60–7.
4. Hassouna H, Kumar S, Bendall S. Arthroscopic ankle debridement. 5-year survival analysis. Acta Orthop Belg 2007;73:737–40.
5. Glazebrook MA, Ganapathy V, Bridge MA, et al. Evidence-based indications for ankle arthroscopy. Arthroscopy 2009;25:1478–90.
6. Takao M, Komatsu F, Naito K, et al. Reconstruction of lateral ligament with arthroscopic drilling for treatment of early-stage osteoarthritis in unstable ankles. Arthroscopy 2006;22:1119–25.
7. Noguchi K. Biomechanical analysis for osteoarthritis of the ankle. J Jpn Orthop Assoc 1985;59:213–20.
8. Löfvenberg R, Kärrholm J, Lund B. The outcome of nonoperated patients with chronic lateral instability of the ankle: a 20-year follow-up study. Foot Ankle Int 1994;15:165–9.
9. Sugimoto K, Takakura Y, Aoki T, et al. A factor of chronic instability of the ankle. Seikeigeka 1990;41:1631–8.
10. Tellisi N, Fragomen AT, Kleinman D, et al. Joint preservation of the osteoarthritic ankle using distraction arthroplasty. Foot Ankle Int 2009;30:318–25.
11. McNicol D, Leong JC, Hsu LC. Supramalleolar derotation osteotomy for lateral tibial torsion and associated equinovarus deformity of the foot. J Bone Joint Surg Br 1983;65:166–70.
12. Napiontek M, Nazar J. Tibial osteotomy as a salvage procedure in the treatment of congenital talipes equinovarus. J Pediatr Orthop 1994;14:763–7.
13. Wiltse LL. Valgus deformity of the ankle: a sequel to acquired or congenital abnormalities of the fibula. J Bone Joint Surg Am 1972;54:595–606.
14. Heywood AW. Supramalleolar osteotomy in the management of the rheumatoid hindfoot. Clin Orthop 1983;177:76–81.
15. Pearce MS, Smith MA, Savidge GF. Supramalleolar tibial osteotomy for haemophilic arthropathy of the ankle. J Bone Joint Surg Br 1994;76:947–50.
16. Graehl PM, Hersh MR, Heckman JD. Supramalleolar osteotomy for the treatment of symptomatic tibial malunion. J Orthop Trauma 1987;1:281–92.
17. Takakura Y, Takaoka T, Tanaka Y, et al. Results of open-wedge osteotomy for the treatment of a post-traumatic varus deformity of the ankle. J Bone Joint Surg Am 1998;80:213–8.
18. Hintermann B, Barg A, Knupp M. Corrective supramalleolar osteotomy for malunited pronation-external rotation fractures of the ankle. J Bone Joint Surg Br 2011;93:1367–72.
19. Takakura Y, Aoki T, Sugimoto K, et al. The treatment for osteoarthritis of the ankle joint. Jpn J Joint Dis 1986;5:347–52.
20. Teramoto T, Makino Y, Takenaka N, et al. Two cases of valgus-type osteoarthritis of the ankle treated by distal tibial oblique osteotomy. J Jpn Soc Surg Foot 2010; 31:71–5.
21. Pagenstert GI, Hintermann B, Barg A, et al. Realignment surgery as alternative treatment of varus and valgus ankle osteoarthritis. Clin Orthop 2007;462:156–68.
22. Pagenstert G, Knupp M, Valderrabano V, et al. Realignment surgery for valgus ankle osteoarthritis. Oper Orthop Traumatol 2009;21:77–87.
23. Aurich M, Squires GR, Reiner A, et al. Differential matrix degradation and turnover in early cartilage lesions of human knee and ankle joints. Arthritis Rheum 2005;52: 112–9.

24. Kuettner KE, Cole AA. Cartilage degeneration in different human joints. Osteoarthritis Cartilage 2005;13:93–103.
25. Oneda Y, Sugimoto K, Takakura Y, et al. Three dimensional contact stress analysis of the ankle joint. J Jpn Soc Surg Foot 1989;11:91–3.
26. Ting AJ, Tarr RR, Sarmiento A, et al. The role of subtalar motion and ankle contact pressure changes from angular deformities of the tibia. Foot Ankle 1987;7:290–9.
27. Hayashi K, Tanaka Y, Kumai T, et al. Correlation of compensatory alignment of the subtalar joint to the progression of primary osteoarthritis of the ankle. Foot Ankle Int 2008;29:400–6.
28. Tanaka Y, Ohneda Y, Nakayama S, et al. Computer simulation of low tibial osteotomy using a three dimensional rigid body spring model. J Jpn Soc Surg Foot 1992;13:134–8.
29. Knupp M, Stufkens SA, van Bergen CJ, et al. Effect of supramalleolar varus and valgus deformities on the tibiotalar joint: a cadaveric study. Foot Ankle Int 2011; 32:609–15.
30. Stufkens SA, van Bergen CJ, Blankevoort L, et al. The role of the fibula in varus and valgus deformity of the tibia: a biomechanical study. J Bone Joint Surg Br 2011;93:1232–9.
31. Sugimoto K, Takaoka T, Kakiyama K, et al. Radiographical study of osteoarthritis of the ankle. J Jpn Soc Surg Foot 1992;13:139–42.
32. Tarr RR, Resnick CT, Wagner KS, et al. Changes in tibiotalar joint contact areas following experimentally induced tibial angular deformities. Clin Orthop 1985; 199:72–80.
33. Takakura Y, Tanaka Y, Kumai T, et al. Low tibial osteotomy for osteoarthritis of the ankle. Results of a new operation in 18 patients. J Bone Joint Surg Br 1995;77: 50–4.
34. Tanaka Y, Takakura Y, Hayashi K, et al. Low tibial osteotomy for varus-type osteoarthritis of the ankle. J Bone Joint Surg Br 2006;88:909–13.
35. Teramoto T, Otsuka K, Makino Y, et al. Dynamic assessments of the osteoarthritis of the ankle joint treated by distal tibial oblique osteotomy. J Jpn Soc Surg Foot 2006;27:48–53.
36. Katsui T, Takakura Y, Kitada C. Roentgenographic analysis for osteoarthritis of the ankle joint. J Jpn Soc Surg Foot 1980;1:52–7.
37. Monji J. Roentgenological measurement of the shape of the osteoarthritic ankle. Nippon Seikeigeka Gakkai Zasshi 1980;54:791–802.
38. Johnson J. Axis of rotation of the ankle. In: Stiehl J, editor. Inman's joints of the ankle. Baltimore (MD): Williams & Wilkins; 1991.
39. Lee WC, Moon JS, Lee K, et al. Indications for supramalleolar osteotomy in patients with ankle osteoarthritis and varus deformity. J Bone Joint Surg Am 2011;93:1243–8.
40. Cheng YM, Huang PJ, Hong SH, et al. Low tibial osteotomy for moderate ankle arthritis. Arch Orthop Trauma Surg 2001;121:355–8.
41. Lui TH. Opening wedge low tibial osteotomy: a minimally invasive approach. Foot Ankle Surg 2011;17:1–7.
42. Warnock KM, Johnson BD, Wright JB, et al. Calculation of the opening wedge for a low tibial osteotomy. Foot Ankle Int 2004;25:778–82.
43. Stamatis ED, Myerson MS. Supramalleolar osteotomy: indications and technique. Foot Ankle Clin 2003;8:317–33.
44. Horn DM, Fragomen AT, Rozbruch SR. Supramalleolar osteotomy using circular external fixation with six-axis deformity correction of the distal tibia. Foot Ankle Int 2011;32:986–93.

45. Elomrani NF, Kasis AG, Tis JE, et al. Outcome after foot and ankle deformity correction using circular external fixation. Foot Ankle Int 2005;26:1027–32.
46. Yablon IG, Heller FG, Shouse L. The key role of the lateral malleolus in displaced fractures of the ankle. J Bone Joint Surg Am 1977;59:169–73.
47. Weber BG, Simpson LA. Corrective lengthening osteotomy of the fibula. Clin Orthop 1985;199:81–7.
48. Reidsma II, Nolte PA, Marti RK, et al. Treatment of malunited fractures of the ankle: a long-term follow-up of reconstructive surgery. J Bone Joint Surg Br 2010;92:66–70.
49. Esparragoza L, Vidal C, Vaquero J. Comparative study of the quality of life between arthrodesis and total arthroplasty substitution of the ankle. J Foot Ankle Surg 2011;50(4):383–7.
50. Saltzman CL, Kadoko RG, Suh JS. Treatment of isolated ankle osteoarthritis with arthrodesis or the total ankle replacement: a comparison of early outcomes. Clin Orthop Surg 2010;2:1–7.
51. Haddad SL, Coetzee JC, Estok R, et al. Intermediate and long-term outcomes of total ankle arthroplasty and ankle arthrodesis. A systematic review of the literature. J Bone Joint Surg Am 2007;89:1899–905.
52. Amendola A, Bonasia DE. Results of high tibial osteotomy: review of the literature. Int Orthop 2010;34(2):155–60.

Total Ankle Replacement for Rheumatoid Arthritis of the Ankle

NG Y.C. Sean, MD[a], Crevoisier Xavier, MD, PD[b],
Mathieu Assal, MD, PD[a,*]

KEYWORDS

• Total ankle replacement • Rheumatoid arthritis • Tibiotalar arthritis

KEY POINTS

- Rheumatoid arthritis is an autoimmune disease that may affect multiple joints, both small and large, and leads to numerous complications.
- The standard surgical treatment for a rheumatoid arthritic ankle has been an arthrodesis.
- The ideal candidate for an ankle replacement in a rheumatoid patient is one who is moderately active, has a well-aligned ankle and heel, and a fair range of motion in the ankle joint.

Rheumatoid arthritis (RA) is an autoimmune disease that may affect multiple joints, both small and large, and leads to numerous complications. It is a debilitating disease, making it difficult for both patients and physicians to decide on the optimal course of treatment. Tibiotalar arthritis occurs in 15% to 52% of patients with adult-onset RA and 70% of patients with juvenile-onset RA over the course of the disease.[1–4] Patients usually have arthritic joints in the upper limbs and proximal lower limbs, which may have been treated with arthroplasty or arthrodesis, before changes are seen in the tibiotalar joint or other joints in the feet. In addition, patients also have other problems or comorbidities stemming from the medical treatment of RA, which involve drugs such as steroids and immunosuppressants. These patients also have osteopenic bones and a poor soft-tissue envelope around the joints, with fragile skin. Substantial deformity coupled with joint destruction will often lead to severe symptoms, and patients will present to the foot and ankle surgeon with pain, deformity, loss of function, and inability to walk. The tibiotalar joint is usually in neutral alignment in most rheumatoid patients, but often a valgus deformity may be observed. As observed by Kirkup,[2] valgus may be up to 3 times more frequent than a varus deformity.

The standard surgical treatment for a rheumatoid arthritic ankle has been an arthrodesis. Fusion allows for good pain relief, and acceptable long-term function and outcome.

[a] Service de Chirurgie Orthopédique et Traumatologie, Hôpital La Tour, Geneva, Switzerland;
[b] Unité d'orthopédie, Centre Hospitalier Universitaire Vaudois, Lausanne, Switzerland
* Corresponding author.
E-mail address: mathieu.assal@hcuge.ch

Foot Ankle Clin N Am 17 (2012) 555–564
http://dx.doi.org/10.1016/j.fcl.2012.08.004
1083-7515/12/$ – see front matter foot.theclinics.com

Some studies have shown that there are fewer complications following an arthrodesis compared with arthroplasty.[5] However, potential problems following arthrodesis include delayed or nonunion, decreased range of motion, and additional stresses on the adjacent midfoot and hindfoot joints, leading to midtarsal and subtalar arthritis.[4,6,7] The latter complication of adjacent arthritis often results from the multiple small joint involvement in patients with RA, and the fact that they have limited ability to compensate for a fused tibiotalar joint. A prolonged period of immobilization is also often needed following arthrodesis, with an average time to fusion of 17 to 19 weeks.[5] Although tibiotalar union rates in patients with RA might seem potentially high, ranging from 78% to 96%,[5,8,9] it is nonetheless a major concern because of pre-existing poor bone quality secondary to osteopenia and steroid usage. With these factors in mind, an arthroplasty might offer the better option, as this allows for preservation of motion (especially from new-generation uncemented, less constrained implants) and decreased stresses on adjacent joints. Gait becomes less compromised. In addition, it also allows for a quicker recovery compared with the potentially long fusion times in some cases of arthrodesis. In the authors' experience, a fair percentage of RA patients with an arthritic ankle also have simultaneous hindfoot and midfoot arthritis on presentation. An ankle arthroplasty might thus serve as a better option for this subset of patients.

PREOPERATIVE WORKUP AND CONSIDERATIONS

The rheumatoid patient has to be considered from a total-body point of view with the disease not only affecting the ankle joint, but frequently multiple other joints. The systemic effects of the disease, as well as that of the antiarthritic medication, must be thoroughly assessed.

The ideal candidate for an ankle replacement in a rheumatoid patient is one who is moderately active, has a well-aligned ankle and heel, and a fair range of motion in the ankle joint. The disease should be under control with medication, with no flare-ups. There often may be arthritic symptoms related to the foot, ankle, knee, or even hip in the ipsilateral or contralateral limb, but these should generally be under control with rest and medication. An arthrodesis of the ankle joint often leads to adjacent joint arthritis and aggravation of disease in other joints, and therefore should be avoided if at all possible.

The major contraindication to ankle arthroplasty is with regard to joint anatomy and severe deformity in the coronal plane. Severe preoperative valgus or varus deformity carries a high risk of postoperative failure because of recurrent deformity and instability.[7,10–13] Weight-bearing radiographs of the ankle joint are absolutely necessary to measure the amount of deformity in the coronal plane. If the joint line is visible on the anteroposterior (AP) radiograph, a deformity greater than 10° is often thought to be a contraindication to arthroplasty. Bony erosion is often seen in an RA patient, and the joint line becomes hard to estimate. Therefore, an alternative method is to use the side walls of the talus to estimate the axis of the talus, which can then be compared with the tibial axis to judge the amount of coronal plane deformity.[7] The radiographs are also valuable to assess other potential problems regarding an arthroplasty. Severe bone destruction, extensive cyst formation, and osteoporosis are all factors to consider, as they may not allow adequate bony support for the prosthesis. Clinical assessment may identify a disrupted deltoid ligament, considered to be a relative contraindication to ankle replacement. However, a well-aligned heel under the tibia with a relatively good mechanical axis would allow for a better functional result from an ankle replacement. If a planovalgus deformity is present, a viable option would be to carry out a 2-stage procedure.[14,15] First, a medical calcaneal osteotomy or distraction arthrodesis of the calcaneal-cuboid joint is performed to correct the planovalgus, followed by an ankle replacement after union of the fusion. A more aggressive approach would be a 1-stage procedure, incorporating both deformity correction and ankle replacement at the same surgery.[4,7,16] In the planning for surgery, the safer and most straightforward option would be to only fuse the hind foot, and a tibiotalocalcaneal nail would be an option for consideration.[17]

Arguments can be made for the alternative surgery, an ankle arthrodesis. A well-performed arthrodesis, getting the ankle joint as close as possible to a functioning, well-balanced joint, is highly desirable. Patients with severe systemic RA and polyarthritis may be better candidates for a fusion. Coexisting multiple problems and complications secondary to RA may make it difficult to restore normal activity for the patient, let alone normal function and range of motion of the ankle. Arthroplasty has its own problems, which often may be even more difficult to manage than those of an arthrodesis. Thus, it is practical to consider the option of an arthrodesis for certain types of patients, specifically whereby the ability to walk pain-free indoors would be sufficient to provide for an improved quality of life. An ankle that is already very painful and stiff might benefit more from an arthrodesis. While an arthroplasty restores some degree of ankle motion, this may be only slight and is dependent on the preoperative range of motion.[17–19] The procedure also requires a larger and more extensive surgical approach in contrast to an arthrodesis, and this increases the risk of wound breakdown and infection in an ankle already compromised by fragile soft tissue. The disadvantages of an arthrodesis have been previously discussed, including adjacent joint arthritis and a decreased range of motion and function.

The last point to consider in the preoperative evaluation is medication. The majority of these patients are on long-term suppressive therapy, including corticosteroids, disease-modifying antirheumatic drugs (DMARDs) and cytotoxic medications such as anti–tumor necrosis factor (TNF) agents. Analgesic medication such as nonsteroidal anti-inflammatory drugs (NSAIDs) or cyclooxygenase II (COX-II) inhibitors are often also prescribed. Potential complications with discontinuance of these medications include a flare-up of the disease, resulting in increased pain and therefore more difficult postoperative rehabilitation. An increased risk of infection is also a potential complication because these patients are often immunocompromised from the beginning and then made worse by these immunosuppressive drugs. Some studies have recommended maintaining patients on their usual preoperative dosages,[20,21] with generally good results thus far. The authors continue patients on their usual dosages intraoperatively and throughout the perioperative periods. Oral corticosteroids are converted to intravenous hydrocortisone when needed. Any patients who have had a recent change in their medication will also require a thorough assessment in consultation with the rheumatologist, and surgery is usually performed only when the requirements for medication have been stabilized.

Patients on cytotoxic therapy must often have their medication discontinued several weeks before surgery, to minimize the complications of wound breakdown and infection. If the surgical site is healing well at 2 to 3 weeks postoperatively, the medication may be resumed. Bibbo and Goldberg[22] demonstrated that there was no increased incidence of infection or wound breakdown in RA patients on TNF therapy undergoing foot and ankle surgery.

POSTOPERATIVE CONSIDERATIONS

Patients who undergo a total ankle arthroplasty are generally allowed immediate full weight bearing as tolerated while protected in a cast for 6 weeks. Patients are then begun on a physiotherapy program, which includes range-of-motion and strengthening exercises. An important consideration for these RA patients concerns the additional stresses placed on other joints, as this may sometimes cause considerable pain even in the presence of a well-functioning ankle arthroplasty.

Range-of-motion exercises are an important component of physiotherapy, and should be initiated as soon as tolerated. Prolonged inactivity will lead to stiffness, which defeats the whole purpose of an arthroplasty. Dorsiflexion is the more important motion, and the authors aim to achieve at least 10° of dorsiflexion in patients.

Dressing changes are done as necessary, more often in the early postoperative period. Sutures are removed at 3 weeks postoperatively, and patients are encouraged to wash their feet and keep the wound as clean as possible throughout this early period.

SURVIVORSHIP

Recent studies have reported on the survivorship of a total ankle arthroplasty. The primary end point is the failure of the prosthesis, necessitating a revision of one or more components, or conversion to an arthrodesis. Some studies have included only patients with RA, and some have compared RA patients with those with osteoarthritis. Most of these studies have a small series of patients, with 2 larger reports published by the Swedish Ankle Arthroplasty Register[12] and by Doets and colleagues.[7] The former included 261 RA patients with an 82% 5-year survivorship, and the latter reported on 93 patients with an 84% 8-year survivorship. In another study, Kofoed and Sorensen[23] reported a 75.5% survivorship of a cemented prosthesis at 14 years. In a separate subgroup of patients with well-aligned ankles, the survivorship has been shown to increase to 93%.[4,7,12,16,18] Other studies have reported on the results of a second-generation "mobile-bearing" ankle prosthesis. These prostheses are cementless and less constrained, allowing more natural motion and lowering the rates of aseptic loosening. Early results have been promising, with 94% survival of the Agility implant at 4.8 years,[24] and 95% survival of the Buechel-Pappas Low Contact Stress total ankle prosthesis at 10 years.[25] In addition, some studies have reported no difference in survival rates between patients with RA and those with osteoarthritis.[23]

COMPLICATIONS

Wound Dehiscence and Infection

Infection can be classified as early or late, as well as superficial or deep. The incidence of early or late deep infection is about 2%, similar to that following total knee arthroplasty.[2,10,18] Management includes arthrotomy and debridement, and intravenous antibiotics for at least 6 weeks. Implant removal, liner exchange, and possibly even conversion to an arthrodesis are all potential procedures that may be necessary, and must be discussed with the patient. Conversion to an arthrodesis has been reported in as many as 1 in 4 cases.[4,7]

Wound healing and delayed wound healing are also potential complications, but as surgical techniques and soft-tissue handling have improved, incidence rates have fallen concurrently. Soft-tissue coverage can be a major problem, and skin grafts and free flaps may be required in the management of soft-tissue problems.[26,27] Consultation with a plastic surgeon might be necessary in the more difficult cases.

Aseptic Loosening and Osteolysis

The durability and life span of modern second-generation total ankle implants have not been definitely determined. Data on long-term results have focused more on first-generation implants. These latter implants are cemented and highly constrained, and substantial rates of loosening, osteolysis, and subsidence have been noted, with tilt and subsidence as high as 80% in some reports.[7,11,23,28]

Second-generation prostheses were developed to address the problems and concerns with earlier implants. These prostheses are now cementless and less constrained, to reduce the bone stresses and hence the rate of aseptic loosening and osteolysis. Reports in the literature have been encouraging, with 94% survival of the Agility implant at 4.8 years, and 95% survival of the Buechel-Pappas Low-Contact Stress total ankle prosthesis at 10 years.[24,29]

The importance of good cortical support in both the tibial and talar components cannot be overemphasized. Any component that rests only on soft cancellous bone will inevitably subside, and therefore it is of utmost importance that any tibial or talar cut takes this into consideration. The authors aim to preserve as much of the cortical side walls as possible with minimal bony resection, so as to preserve the integrity and strength of the subchondral bone. This preservation has to be balanced with sufficient bone removal to create enough space for the implants, and also allow adequate ligamentotaxis to restore normal length and tension to the ankle ligaments. This approach implies a balance of soft tissues, thus making the procedure more complex, which is of greater importance in a rheumatoid ankle than in an osteoarthritic ankle. Even with good bony and soft-tissue balance and seating of the implants as optimally as possible, it has occasionally been noted that there is some tibial or talar subsidence in the first few months after surgery, after which the components become stable.[30] Some implants also have additional coatings to improve bony fixation, such as hydroxyapatite or calcium phosphate. These coatings allow for bony ingrowth and ongrowth, helping to further reinforce the implant-bone interface, and hence potentially reduce the rates of loosening. In some cases, stable radiolucent lines can also be seen around the tibial or talar components. These lines have been previously shown in uncemented implants to be either a result of imperfect apposition and stress shielding, or stable fibrous ingrowth similar to that seen in uncemented hip prostheses.[31]

Intraoperative Fractures

The inherent nature of RA results in osteopenia and weakened bones. A total ankle replacement thus places the medial and lateral malleoli at risk of fractures because of the nature of the procedure itself. An intraoperative malleolar fracture is the most frequent complication to occur at the time of surgery (**Fig. 1**), with the medial malleolus at greater risk.[7] Besides a fracture while preparing for the tibial component, they can occur from overdistraction with a laminar spreader while attempting to increase exposure of the posterior ankle joint, or by levering against the malleolus when using a rongeur to remove bony fragments from the distal tibial bone cuts. Extra attention has to be paid to the RA patient on corticosteroids, as this further weakens the bone and increases the risk of fractures.[32]

Keen awareness of the situation is absolutely vital while making the bone cuts. The incidence of fractures can be reduced by careful attention to the excursion of the saw blade to prevent from cutting too far medially or laterally, careful joint distraction and removal of debris, and avoiding the use of oversized trial implants and components. Some jigs allow the use of prophylactic pinning of the malleoli before making the

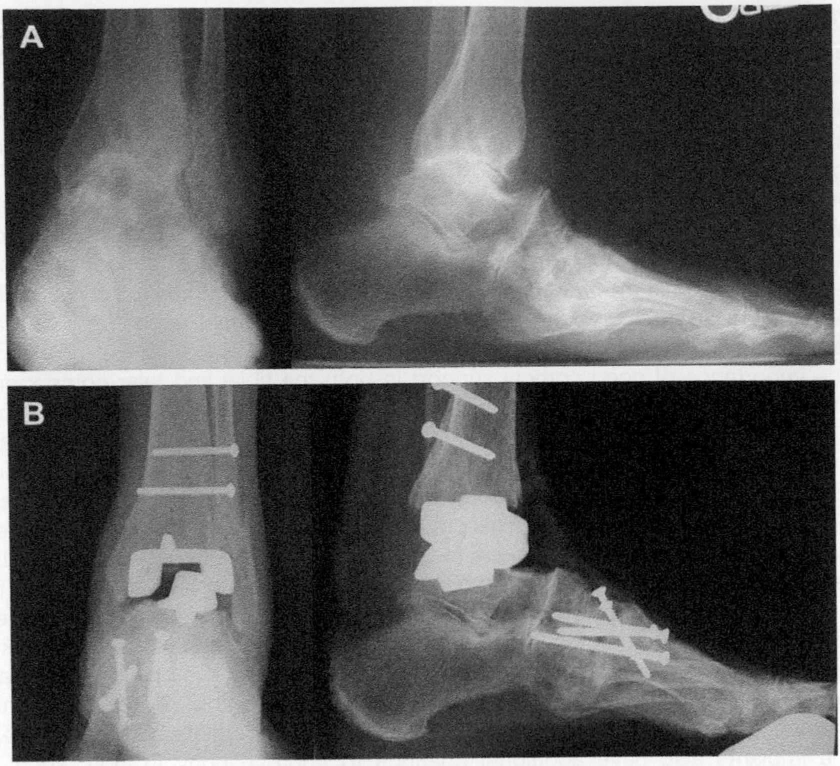

Fig. 1. (*A*) Rheumatoid arthritis of the ankle, AP and lateral views; (*B*) Following total ankle arthroplasty with intraoperative fracture of lateral maleolus.

bone cuts, and this is also useful. With experience, the incidence of iatrogenic intraoperative fractures should decrease.[26,27]

The management of intraoperative fractures depends on the nature and severity of the fracture. An undisplaced fracture with an intact soft-tissue sleeve can be treated nonoperatively with immobilization,[7] whereas a displaced fracture demands internal fixation. Accurate reduction to restore the joint line and interfragmentary compression to achieve absolute stability are necessary to reduce the rate of nonunion. Screw fixation or tension-band wiring are possible options. A fracture that occurs postoperatively may be an indication of a possible malalignment of the components, the latter leading to additional stresses and a failure of the arthroplasty. A revision arthroplasty or even a conversion to an arthrodesis may be required. In the event of a complication, it is always important to be aware that an arthrodesis must remain in the armamentarium of the orthopedic surgeon.

Subluxation and Dislocation

Correct implant sizing and accurate bony cuts are mandatory in performing an ankle arthroplasty. Ligamentotaxis plays an important role in ensuring adequate tension in the numerous ligaments that surround and support the tibiotalar joint. Subluxation or even frank dislocation of the ankle joint may occur if these factors are not taken into consideration during the operative procedure. Options for salvage would then

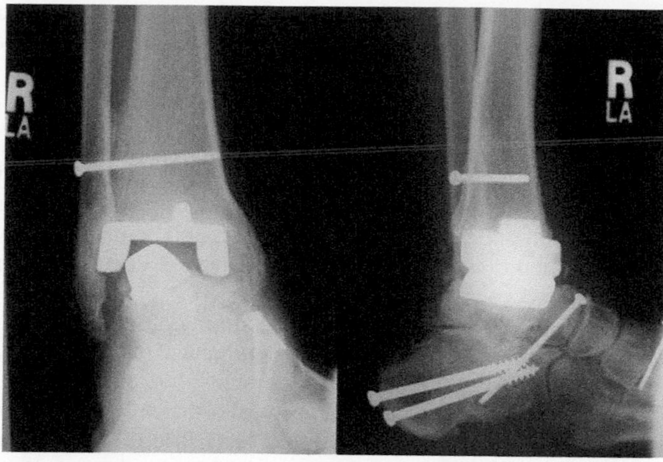

Fig. 2. Failed total ankle arthroplasty in varus.

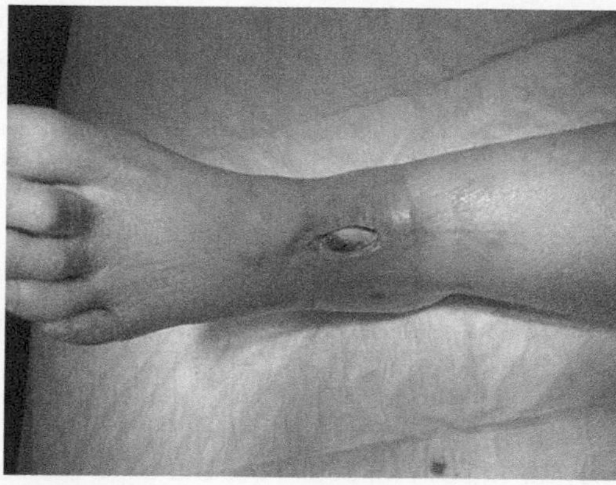

Fig. 3. Wound breakdown.

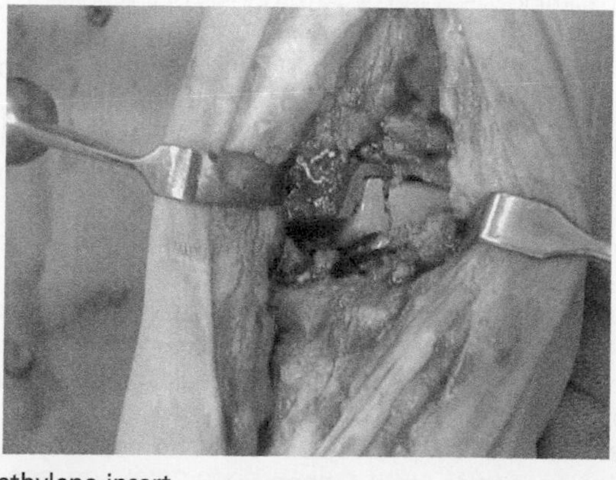

Fig. 4. Broken polyethylene insert.

include immobilization of the ankle joint, reconstruction of the ligaments, or even an arthrodesis, should the ankle joint remain unstable (**Figs. 2–4**).

SUMMARY

For patients with RA and symptomatic ankle arthritis, long-term studies still show that the gold standard is an arthrodesis. A well-performed ankle fusion is able to provide the RA patient with a substantially good quality of life and a high degree of satisfaction, with union rates that approach 96%. However, the risks and benefits of an arthrodesis must be considered when discussing the available choices with the patient, as ultimately the type of procedure is the patient's choice.

Good surgical technique and correction of any hindfoot deformity will result in satisfactory alignment of the ankle with regard to the mechanical axis, and this will lead to increased prosthetic longevity. The maximum amount of valgus or varus deformity with regard to the mechanical axis should be no greater than 10°, as greater malalignment leads to increased additional stresses and early failure of the implant.[33] The assessment of the soft tissues and bone stock are also very important to allow for uneventful healing of the wounds, as well as to ensure that there is adequate bone of sufficient strength to support the prostheses after implantation. Recent studies have shown a survival of total ankle prostheses of greater than 90% at 5 years and 80% at 10 years.[7,18] Patient satisfaction has also been high, even if objective measurements such as radiographs have not been ideal. One possible explanation could be the lower demands that RA patients place on their prostheses, owing to a generally lower level of activity and the lighter build of the patients as a result of the disease. These findings are encouraging overall, and provide the orthopedic surgeon with an additional option for patients with RA who present with a painful ankle.

REFERENCES

1. Lachiewicz PF. Total ankle arthroplasty: indications, techniques, and results. Orthop Rev 1994;23:315–20.
2. Kirkup J. Rheumatoid arthritis and ankle surgery. Ann Rheum Dis 1990;49(Suppl 2): 837–44.
3. Michelson J, Easley M, Wigley FM, et al. Foot and ankle problems in rheumatoid arthritis. Foot Ankle Int 1994;15(11):608–13.
4. Su EP, Kahn B, Figgie MP. Total ankle replacement in patients with rheumatoid arthritis. Clin Orthop Relat Res 2004;424:32–8.
5. Cracchiolo A III, Cimino WR, Lian G. Arthrodesis of the ankle in patients who have rheumatoid arthritis. J Bone Joint Surg Am 1992;74:903–9.
6. Dereymaeker GP, Van Eygen P, Driesen R, et al. Tibiotalar arthrodesis in the rheumatoid foot. Clin Orthop Relat Res 1998;349:43–7.
7. Doets HC, Brand R, Nelissen RG. Total ankle arthroplasty in inflammatory joint disease with use of two mobile-bearing designs. J Bone Joint Surg Am 2006; 88(6):1272–84.
8. Felix NA, Kitaoka HB. Ankle arthrodesis in patients with rheumatoid arthritis. Clin Orthop 1998;349:58–64.
9. Adam W, Ranawat C. Arthrodesis of the hind foot in rheumatoid arthritis. Orthop Clin North Am 1976;7:827–40.
10. Van der Heide HJ, Schutte B, Louwerens JW, et al. Total ankle prostheses in rheumatoid arthropathy. Acta Orthop 2009;80(4):440–4.
11. Neufeld SK, Lee TH. A review paper. Total ankle arthroplasty: indications, results, and biomechnical rationale. Am J Orthop 2000;29(8):593–602.

12. Henricson A, Skoog A, Carlsson A. The Swedish ankle arthroplasty register: an analysis of 531 cases performed 1993-2005. Acta Orthop 2007;78(5): 569–74.
13. Henricson A, Agren P. Secondary surgery after total ankle replacement. The influence of preoperative hind foot alignment. Foot Ankle Surg 2007;13:41–4.
14. Spirit AA, Assal M, Hansen ST Jr. Complications and failure after total ankle arthroplasty. J Bone Joint Surg Am 2004;86:1172–8.
15. Greisberg J, Assal M, Flueckiger G, et al. Takedown of ankle fusion and conversion to total ankle replacement. Clin Orthop Relat Res 2004;424:80–8.
16. Bonnin M, Bouysset M, Tebib J, et al. Total ankle replacement in rheumatoid arthritis: treatment strategy. In: Bouysset M, Tourne Y, Tillmann K, editors. Foot and ankle in rheumatoid arthritis. Paris: Springer-Verlag; 2006. p. 206–19.
17. Coetzee JC, Castro MD. Accurate measurement of ankle range of motion after total ankle arthroplasty. Clin Orthop Relat Res 2004;31:424–7.
18. Wood PLR, Crawford LA, Suneja R, et al. Total ankle replacement for rheumatoid ankle arthritis. Foot Ankle Clin 2007;12:497–508.
19. Anderson T, Montgomery P, Carlsson A. Uncemented STAR total ankle prostheses. Three- to eight-year follow-up of fifty-one consecutive ankles. J Bone Joint Surg Am 2003;85(7):1321–9.
20. Jam A, Witbreuk M, Ball C, et al. Influence of steroids and methotrexate on wound complications after elective rheumatoid hand and wrist surgery. J Hand Surg Am 2002;27(3):449–55.
21. Grennan DM, Gary J, Loudon J, et al. Methotrexate and early post-operative complications in patients with rheumatoid arthritis undergoing elective orthopaedic surgery. Ann Rheum Dis 2002;6(1):86–7.
22. Bibbo C, Goldberg JW. Infections and healing complications after elective orthopaedic foot and ankle surgery during tumor necrosis factor-alpha inhibition therapy. Foot Ankle Int 2004;25(5):331–5.
23. Kofoed H, Sorensen TS. Ankle arthroplasty for rheumatoid arthritis and osteoarthritis: prospective long-term study of cemented replacements. J Bone Joint Surg Br 1998;80:328–32.
24. Pyevich MT, Saltzman CL, Callaghan JJ, et al. Total ankle arthroplasty: a unique design: two to twelve-year follow-up. J Bone Joint Surg Am 1998; 80:1410–20.
25. Buechel FF, Pappas MJ. Survivorship and clinical evaluation of cementless, meniscal-bearing total ankle replacements. Semin Arthroplasty 1992;3: 43–50.
26. Myerson MS, Mroczek K. Perioperative complications of total ankle arthroplasty. Foot Ankle Int 2003;24(1):17–21.
27. Haskell A, Mann RA. Perioperative complication rate of total ankle replacement is reduced by surgical experience. Foot Ankle Int 2004;25(5):283–9.
28. Unger AS, Inglis AE, Mow CS, et al. Total ankle arthroplasty in rheumatoid arthritis: a long-term follow-up study. Foot Ankle 1988;8:173–9.
29. Buechel FF, Pappas MJ, Iorio LJ. New Jersey low contact stress total ankle replacement: biomechanical rationale and review of 23 cementless cases. Foot Ankle 1988;8:279–90.
30. Carlsson A, Markusson P, Sundberg M. Radiostereometric analysis of the double-coated STAR total ankle prosthesis. A 3-5 year follow-up of 5 cased with rheumatoid arthritis and 5 cases with osteoarthritis. Acta Orthop 2005; 76(4):573–9.

31. Wood PL, Clough TM, Jari S. Clinical comparison of two total ankle replacements. Foot Ankle Int 2000;21:546–50.
32. McGarvey WC, Clanton TO, Lunz D. Malleolar fracture after total ankle arthroplasty. Clin Orthop Relat Res 2004;424:104–10.
33. Assal M, Al-Shaikh R, Reiber BH, et al. Fracture of the polyethylene component in an ankle arthroplasty. Foot Ankle Int 2003;24(12):901–3.

Mobile- and Fixed-Bearing Total Ankle Prostheses

Is There Really a Difference?

Victor Valderrabano, MD, PhD[a,*], Geert I. Pagenstert, MD[a], Andreas M. Müller, MD[a], Jochen Paul, MD[a], Heath B. Henninger, PhD[b], Alexej Barg, MD[a,b]

KEYWORDS

- Total ankle replacement • Osteoarthritis • Biomechanics
- Survivorship of prosthesis components • 2-component total ankle replacement
- 3-component total ankle replacement

KEY POINTS

- Approximately 1% of the world's adult population is affected by ankle osteoarthritis.
- This article reviews the in vitro studies addressing the biomechanics and kinematics of the replaced ankle.
- A systematic literature review was conducted to assess possible differences in clinical outcomes, including prosthesis survivorship and postoperative range of motion, between mobile- and fixed-bearing total ankle prostheses.

SHORT HISTORY OF TOTAL ANKLE REPLACEMENT

Total ankle arthroplasty (TAR) is new compared with total replacement of the hip and knee.[1,2] Until the 1970s, ankle arthrodesis was the only "gold standard" therapy in patients with end-stage ankle osteoarthritis (OA).[3,4] In most articles addressing the history of TAR,[5–9] the report by Lord and Marotte[10] is described as the first clinical study of patients undergoing TAR. However, Muir and colleagues[11] described outcomes in a 71-year-old man who underwent talar dome resurfacing with a custom Vitallium implant for posttraumatic OA in 1962. The clinical examination at a 40-year follow-up showed mild hindfoot malalignment with slightly decreased range of motion (ROM) (25° plantar flexion), American Orthopaedic Foot and Ankle Society (AOFAS) score of 85, no pain, and no activity limitation.[11]

The authors have nothing to disclose.
[a] Orthopaedic Department, University Hospital of Basel, University of Basel, Spitalstrasse 21, Basel CH-4031, Switzerland; [b] Harold K. Dunn Orthopaedic Research Laboratory, University Orthopaedic Center, University of Utah, 590 Wakara Way, Salt Lake City, UT 84108, USA
* Corresponding author.
E-mail address: vvalderrabano@uhbs.ch

Foot Ankle Clin N Am 17 (2012) 565–585
http://dx.doi.org/10.1016/j.fcl.2012.08.005
foot.theclinics.com
1083-7515/12/$ – see front matter

Most first-generation TAR designs were 2-component prostheses.[7,12,13] Both types of prostheses, constrained and unconstrained, were available. Most TAR designs included a concave polyethylene tibial component and a convex metal component for the talus, usually made of cobalt chrome alloy. Cement fixation was used on both sides, talar and tibial. The reason for the cemented fixation was simple: in the 1970s, cementless fixation was not widely used in knee and hip prostheses, and cement fixation led to acceptable stability in patients who underwent total knee or hip replacement. In 1977, Evanski and Waugh[14] reviewed the early results in patients who underwent TAR using Howmedica (2-component unconstrained prosthesis; Howmedica, Rutherford, NJ) and Smith (2-component unconstrained prosthesis; Dow Corning, Arlington, TN) total ankle systems. The authors evaluated the TAR as an alternative to ankle arthrodesis in patients with end-stage ankle osteoarthritis and concluded that the results were "clinically comparable" to those of total hip replacement.[14] However, initial enthusiasm was dampened because of an extremely high complication rate, including loosening, wide osteolysis, subsidence, and mechanical failure of prosthesis components. Furthermore, the cement fixation required a larger bone resection, making the revision surgery a technically demanding procedure. The unsatisfactory results and extremely high failure rate substantially delayed the further development of total ankle designs and limited acceptance among foot and ankle surgeons. Hamblen[15] wrote in 1985 that "clearly the answer to the question of replacing the ankle joint using current techniques must be 'no.'"

TAR experienced a renaissance in the second half of the 1980s with 2 crucial aspects of the design: (1) the use of cementless fixation, resulting in more sparing bone cuts and a lower risk of prosthesis component loosening; and (2) the introduction of 3-component prostheses with a mobile bearing between the tibial and talar metal components, resulting in a lower mechanical failure rate of prosthesis. The Agility prosthesis (DePuy, Warsaw, IN) was the first of a new generation of ankle prostheses. It was designed by Dr Frank Alvine[16,17] and has been used since 1984, resulting in the longest follow-up of any fixed-bearing TAR. Second-generation TAR prostheses are the Buechel-Pappas ankle prosthesis (Endotec, Orange, NJ)[18] and the Scandinavian Total Ankle Replacement (STAR; Waldmar Link, Hamburg, Germany).[19]

Each second-generation TAR design—Agility, Buechel-Pappas, and STAR—has been implanted with encouraging mid- and long-term results.[20] Good clinical results, including preserved ROM of replaced ankle, high patient satisfaction, and acceptable initial and mid-term stability of prosthesis components, led to rethinking that ankle fusion many not be the only reasonable treatment option for patients with severe ankle OA.[13,21]

The continued critical review of second-generation implant failures and biomechanical studies provided important data that led to the development of modern TAR designs.

CLASSIFICATION SYSTEM OF TOTAL ANKLE ARTHROPLASTIES

Classification of TAR includes the following factors for consideration[22,23]:

- Fixation (cemented vs uncemented)
- Number of components (2- vs 3-components)
- Constraint type (constrained vs semiconstrained vs unconstrained)
- Congruency type (congruent vs incongruent)
- Component shape (anatomic vs nonanatomic)
- Bearing type (fixed vs mobile bearing)

Fig. 1 shows an overview of the most common total ankle designs classified by the number of components and constraint type. Currently, most TARs use a cementless

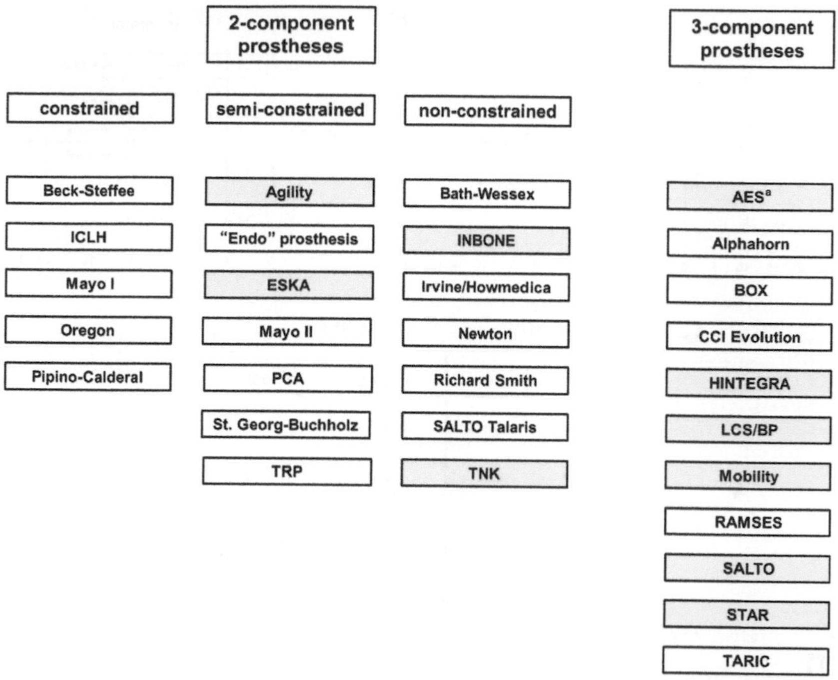

Fig. 1. Classification system of total ankle replacements regarding the number of components and constraint type. Yellow highlights the most commonly used prostheses. [a] Recent clinical studies[80,82,106,107] reported unacceptable high osteolysis rates, therefore the implant has been withdrawn by the manufacturer. (*Data from* Morgan SS, Brooke B, Harris NJ. Total ankle replacement by the Ankle Evolution System: medium-term outcome. J Bone Joint Surg Br 2010;92:61–5.)

implantation technique with biologic fixation (eg, hydroxyapatite coating). All 2-components ankle designs can be divided into 3 constraint groups: constrained, semiconstrained, and unconstrained prostheses. Most 3-components total ankles have a flat tibial component articulating with the flat superior surface of a mobile bearing.[24]

KINEMATICS OF A TOTAL ARTHROPLASTY OF THE ANKLE

Recent advances in understanding the anatomy and biomechanics of the complex hindfoot have been considered in the development of the new TAR designs and surgical techniques.[5,22] The kinematics and biomechanics of the replaced ankle remain important subjects of foot and ankle research.[25,26]

Valderrabano and colleagues[27] assessed kinematic changes in cadaveric ankles with fusion and TAR in regard to ROM, movement transfer,[28] and talar movement.[29] All measurements were performed in native ankles, then in ankles with 2-component (Agility) and 3-component prostheses (HINTEGRA [Newdeal, Lyon, France/Integra, Plainsboro, NJ] and STAR) and in fused ankles. Although the ROM in normal ankles was measured to be 14.7° ± 0.9° and 28.2° ± 0.8° for dorsiflexion and plantar flexion, respectively, the fused ankles showed significantly impaired ROM of 4.4° ± 0.4° and 8.1° ± 0.2° for dorsiflexion and plantar flexion, respectively (**Fig. 2**).[27] The ankle prosthesis almost achieved normal ROM, and similar findings were observed in other movement planes.[27] The authors stated that the prosthesis design that replicated the normal ankle joint ROM was the one with the most anatomic design.

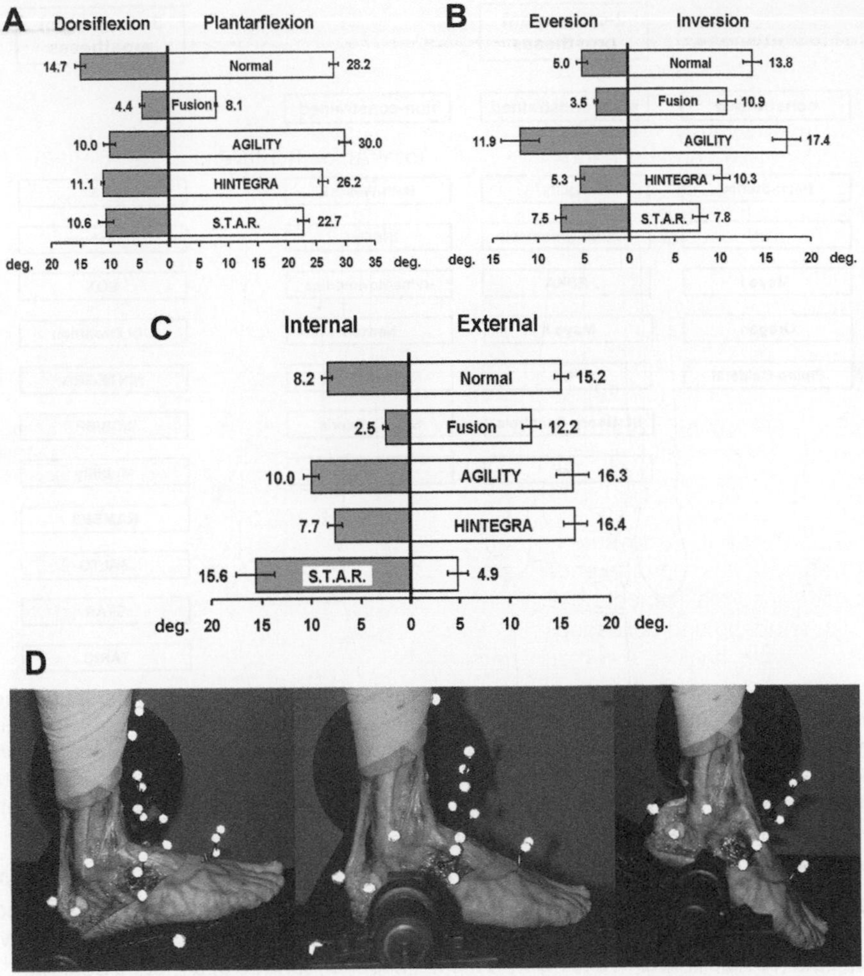

Fig. 2. ROM changes in ankle specimens with prostheses (Agility, HINTEGRA, and STAR). For comparison, the measurements were performed in native ankles and fused ankles. (*A*) Dorsiflexion, plantarflexion. (*B*) Eversion, inversion. (*C*) Internal rotation, external rotation. (*D*) All kinematics were measured using bone markers and a 4-camera high-speed video system. (*Data from* Valderrabano V, Hintermann B, Nigg BM, et al. Kinematic changes after fusion and total replacement of the ankle: part 1: range of motion. Foot Ankle Int 2003;24:881–7.)

Komistek and colleagues[30] used fluoroscopy to evaluate translational and rotational motions of the hindfoot in the sagittal and frontal planes in 10 subjects having a normal ankle and TAR on the opposite side (Buechel-Pappas prosthesis). The average ROM for normal and replaced ankles was 37.4° and 32.3°, respectively. In general, comparable kinematic patterns of motion were observed for normal and replaced ankles.[30]

Detrembleur and Leemrijse[31] addressed the effects of TAR on gait disability through analyzing energetic and mechanical variables. The study included patients who underwent TAR using 3-component implant designs: AES (Ankle Evolutive System, Biomet Merck, Valence, France) (n = 16), Mobility (DePuy International, Leeds, UK) (n = 3), and HINTEGRA prostheses (n = 1). All patients were analyzed before and approximately 7 months after surgery using instrumented motion analysis to assess spatiotemporal parameters, ankle kinematics, mechanical work, and electromyographic activity. In addition, energy expenditure was analyzed using an ergospirometer. The authors showed that TAR has a beneficial effect on locomotor function, resulting in improvement of AOFAS score, speed, spatiotemporal parameters, ankle amplitude instance, and vertical center of mass displacement.[31]

Valderrabano and colleagues[32] investigated patients' rehabilitation in the first year after TAR (**Fig. 3**). Fifteen patients with unilateral posttraumatic ankle OA were included in this study. All patients were matched to 15 persons without OA with the appropriate demographic factors as a control group. The study included assessment of clinical and functional status and 3-dimensional kinematic-kinetic analysis. All measurements were performed preoperatively, and at 3, 6, 9, and 12 months after TAR using HINTEGRA prosthesis. As expected, patients with ankle OA showed significant clinical and functional impairments preoperatively as assessed using the AOFAS and Short Form-36 (SF-36) scores. Gait analysis revealed a significant deficiency in 6 of 7 measured spatiotemporal variables: a decrease of the triplanar ankle movement, a decrease of the second active maximal vertical and the maximal medial ground reaction force, a reduction of the sagittal and transverse ankle joint moments, and a reduction of the ankle joint power. Patients with TAR experienced postoperative worsening of gait as measured 3 months after the surgery. However, at the last follow-up of 12 months, no differences in the spatiotemporal variables were detected with respect to normal subjects.[32]

Valderrabano and colleagues[33] also assessed changes in the lower leg muscles in patients with ankle OA. Fifteen patients with ankle osteoarthritis and 15 normal subjects were included in this prospective study. The investigators assessed clinical parameters (pain level, alignment, AOFAS score, ankle range of motion, calf circumference), radiologic parameters (ankle OA grading), and muscular-physiologic parameters (isometric maximal voluntary ankle torque, muscle surface electromyography) in all patients. The patients with ankle OA had increased pain level and reduced functional status. Furthermore, they showed significant atrophic changes of the lower leg muscles.[33] In another study Valderrabano and colleagues[34] addressed the muscle rehabilitation in patients who underwent TAR. TAR has been shown to normalize the muscle function (including torque and electromyography intensity) in OA ankles to a significant extent. However, after 1 year of rehabilitation, the level of function in the treated leg did not reach that of the contralateral unaffected leg.[34]

One of the demanding steps of the TAR procedure is achieving the correct positioning of the talar component. First, the original center of rotation of the tibiotalar joint may have changed because of joint degeneration or concomitant deformities. Second, even normal ankles have been shown to have different axes of rotation, which may change during the arc of motion.[35] Consequently, sagittal malposition of the talar component is a common intraoperative complication of TAR.[36,37] Lee and colleagues[36] reported that the number of malpositions may not decrease with increased surgeon experience.

Positioning of prosthesis components, especially the talus, has been shown to strongly affect the kinematics in the replaced ankle. Tochigi and colleagues[38] investigated the effect of talar component sagittal positioning on ROM using a specially modified STAR prosthesis. They found that anterior talar component displacement significantly decreased the plantar flexion, which was associated with bearing lift-off, whereas posterior displacement of the talar component significantly decreased the dorsiflexion.[38]

Saltzman and colleagues[39] addressed the effect of ankle prosthesis misalignment on the periankle ligament using an in vitro Agility prosthesis model. The anterior talofibular ligament was sensitive to transverse plane displacements, whereas the tibiocalcaneal ligament was sensitive to coronal plane displacements.[39] Sagittal

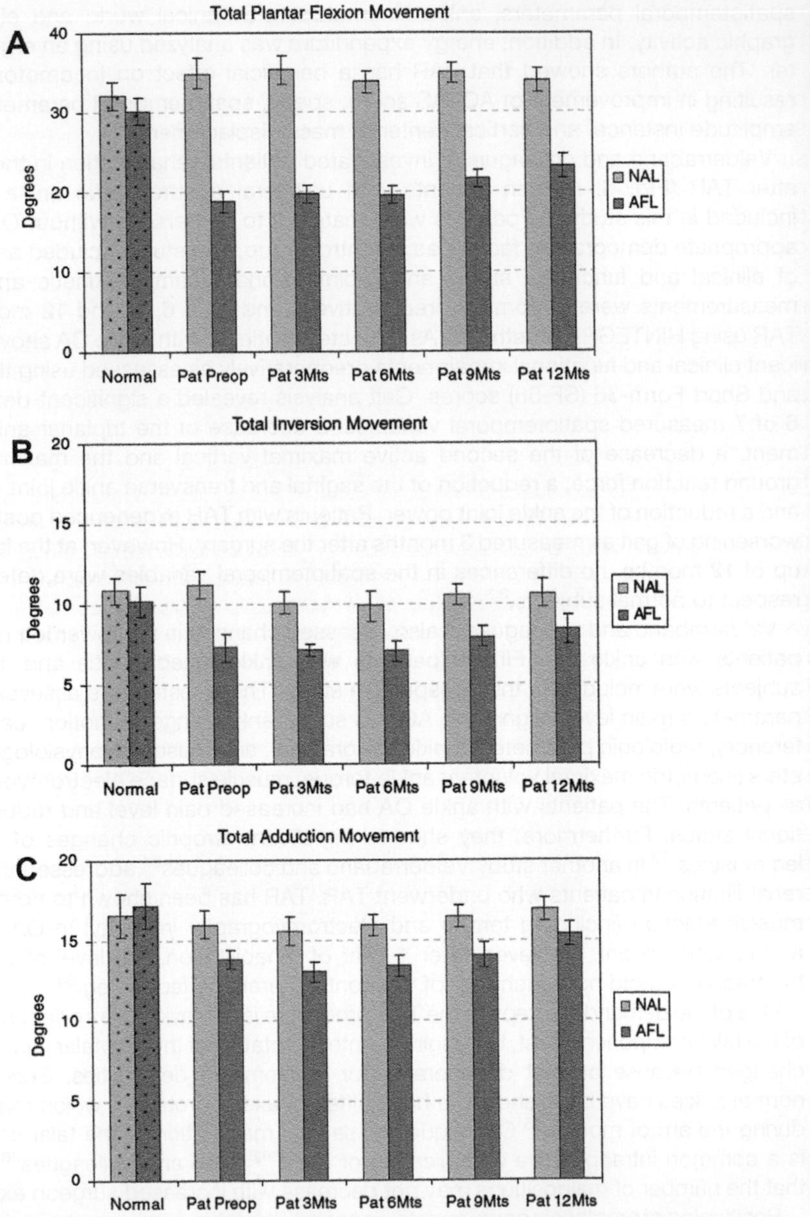

Fig. 3. Ankle joint complex gait kinematics during the 1st year rehabilitation. (*A*) Total plantar flexion movement. (*B*) Total inversion movement. (*C*) Total adduction movement. AFL, affected leg in patients, or nondominant leg in normal subjects; Mts, months; NAL, contralateral nonaffected leg in patients, or dominant leg in normal subjects; Pat, patients. (*From* Valderrabano V, Nigg BM, von Tscharner V, et al. Gait analysis in ankle osteoarthritis and total ankle replacement. Clin Biomech [Bristol, Avon] 2007;22:894–904; with permission.)

misalignment has been shown to have a negative influence on not only the biomechanics of the replaced ankle but also other factors, such as malrotation.

Nicholson and colleagues[40] used a cadaveric model to evaluate the joint contact characteristics in Agility prosthesis. The implanted 10 cadaveric specimens with the standard Agility prosthesis. Under an axial load of 700 N, the average contact pressure of 5.6 MPa with mean peak pressures of 21.2 MPa were measured. Contact pressures significantly decreased with larger components. The authors concluded that a heavy patient with a small ankle would not be expected to have a good outcome.[40]

Fukuda and colleagues[41] reported an in vitro study on the effect of talar component malrotation of the Agility prosthesis. They used 6 fresh-frozen cadaveric specimen with the following sequence of talar position (randomized): neutral position, 7.5° internal, and 7.5° external rotation. Contact pressure was measured using Tekscan ankle sensors. In all specimens, sequential static axial loadings (740 N) and 10 simulated dynamic strides under 650 N were applied. The talar component malrotation led to increased peak pressure, decreased contact area, and increased rotational torque, further supporting the need for accurate component placement.[41]

Recently, Espinosa and colleagues[42] reported on 2 finite-element models of Agility (2-component prosthesis) and Mobility (3-component prosthesis) ankles. Both models were validated through biomechanical testing of real prosthesis components using pressure-sensitive films. They modeled potential misalignments with respect to version of the tibial component, version of the talar component, and relative component rotation of the 2-component design. In the normally aligned prostheses, the simulation showed between 2- and 3-fold differences in average contact pressures between Agility (higher pressures) and Mobility ankles (**Fig. 4**). Pressures consistently increased with misalignment, suggesting that accurate positioning of prosthesis components is one of the most important requirements for procedure success. The highly congruent design of the 3-component Mobility prosthesis resulted in more evenly distributed and lower-magnitude joint contract pressures than the less-congruent 2-component Agility prosthesis. However, misalignments of more than 5° are critical in both prosthesis designs and may substantially influence the long-term results because of potential misalignment-induced wear.[42]

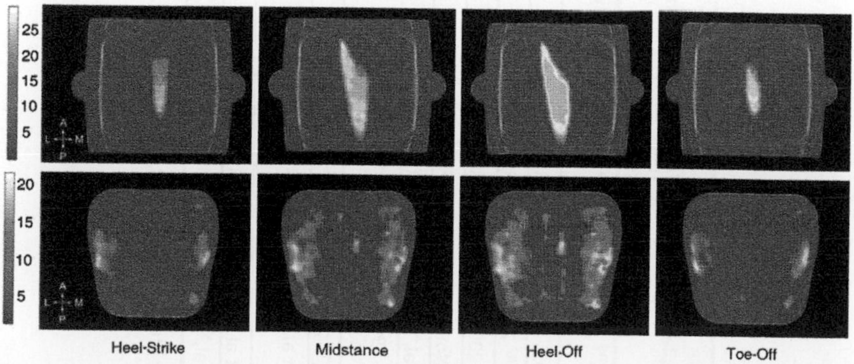

Fig. 4. Finite element simulation showing polyethylene contact pressure in normally aligned Agility (*top panel*) and Mobility prosthesis models (*bottom panel*) over the gait cycle, including heel-strike, midstance, heel-off, and toe-off (from left to the right). (*From* Espinosa N, Walti M, Favre P, et al. Misalignment of total ankle components can induce high joint contact pressures. J Bone Joint Surg Am 2010;92:1179–87; with permission.)

Table 1
Ankle arthroplasty results including survivorship and postoperative range of motion using 2-component prostheses

Study	Study Type	TAR	TAR Type	Ankles	Survivorship	Follow-up	Postoperative ROM
Pyevich et al,[46] 1998	RS, SC	Agility	2-components, semiconstrained	100	92% at 5 y	4.8 y	36° (10°–64°)
Alvine,[16] 2002	RS, SC			207	76% at 9 y	NR	NR
Knecht et al,[47] 2004	RS, SC			132	86% and 63% at 9 and 11 y	9.0 y	18° (2°–40°)
Spirt et al,[48] 2004	RS, SC			306	80% at 5 y	2.8 y	NR
Vienne and Nothdurft,[49] 2004	PS, SC			66	NR	2.4 y	40° (5°–60°)
Hurowitz et al,[50] 2007	RS, SC			65	95%, 70%, and 67% at 1, 3, and 6 y	NR	NR
Schill et al,[51] 1998	PS, SC	TPR	2-components, constrained	27	87% at 13 y	8.6 y	37°
Fevang et al,[52] 2007	PS, MC			32	90% at 5 y	4 y	NR
Shinomiya et al,[53] 2003	RS, SC	TNK	2-components, semiconstrained	20	NR	8 y	26°
Nishikawa et al,[54] 2004	RS, SC			32	77% at 14.1 y	6 y	16° (0°–40°)
Takakura et al,[55] 2004	RS, SC			70	NR	5.2 y	27.5°

Abbreviations: MC, multicenter; NR, not reported; PS, prospective; RS, retrospective; SC, single-center.

Table 2
Ankle arthroplasty results, including survivorship and postoperative ROM using 3-component prostheses

Study	Study Type	TAR	TAR Type	Ankles	Survivorship	Follow-up	Postoperative ROM
Buechel et al,[56] 1988	PS, SC	Buechel-Pappas	3-components, unconstrained	23	NR	2.9 y	29° (25°–34°)
Buechel et al,[57] 2003	PS, SC			50	93.5% at 10 y	5 y	28° (12°–46°)
Buechel et al,[58] 2004	PS, SC			40	92% and 74.2% at 12 and 20 y	12 y	25° (10°–47°)
Doets et al,[59] 2006	PS, SC			93	84% at 8 y	7.2 y	31.9°
San Giovanni et al,[108] 2006	RS, SC			31	93% at 8.3 y	8.3 y	23° (8°–40°)
Ali et al,[60] 2007	RS, SC			34	97% at 5 y	5 y	41° (5°–55°)
van der Heide et al,[61] 2009	PS, SC			21	83% at 5 y	2.7 y	NR
Wood et al,[62] 2009	PS, SC			100	79% at 6 y	4.5 y	NR
Kofoed,[63] 1995	PS, MC	STAR	3-components, unconstrained, cemented	28	70% at 12 y	NR	NR
Kofoed and Sorensen,[64] 1998	PS, SC			52	73.5% at 14 y	9 y	NR
Schill et al,[51] 1998	PS, SC			22	94.3% at 6 y	3.1 y	33.5°
Anderson et al,[65] 2003	RS, SC			51	70% at 5 y	5.2 y	28° (10°–55°)
Hagena et al,[66] 2003	PS, SC			78	NR	3.6 y	38.3°
Wood and Deakin,[67] 2003	PS, SC			200	92.7% and 87.9% at 5 and 8 y	3.8 y	27° (10°–60°)
Kofoed,[19] 2004	PS, SC			25	95.4% at 12 y	9.4 y	NR
Lodhi et al,[68] 2004	RS, SC			30	NR	2.2 y	35°
Valderrabano et al,[69] 2004	PS, SC			62.28	87% at 5 y	3.7 y	38.2° (10°–60°)
Murnaghan et al,[70] 2005	RS, SC			22	NR	2.2 y	28° (10°–51°)

(continued on next page)

Table 2
(*continued*)

Study	Study Type	TAR	TAR Type	Ankles	Survivorship	Follow-up	Postoperative ROM
Carlsson,[71] 2006	PS, SC		3-components, unconstrained, uncemented, single-coated	51	72.0% and 60.4% at 3 and 6 y	NR	NR
Carlsson,[71] 2006	PS, SC		3-components, unconstrained, uncemented, double-coated	57	93.7% at 5 y	NR	NR
Fevang et al,[52] 2007	PS, MC		3-components, unconstrained, uncemented	203	89% at 5 y	4 y	NR
Kumar and Dhar,[72] 2007	PS, SC			50	NR	3 y	27.2° (5°–45°)
Wood et al,[109] 2007	RS, MC			171	88% at 8 y	NR	NR
Schutte and Louwerens,[73] 2008	RS, SC			49	NR	2.3 y	27°
Wood et al,[74] 2008	PS, SC			200	93.3% and 80.3% at 5 and 10 y	7.3 y	NR
Hobson et al,[75] 2009	RS, SC			123	78% at 7 y	4 y	NR
van der Heide et al,[61] 2009	PS, SC			37	78% at 5 y	2.7 y	NR
Wood et al,[62] 2009	PS, SC			100	95% at 6 y	4.5 y	NR
Karantana et al, 2010	RS, SC			52	90% and 84% at 5 and 8 y	6.7 y	NR
Skyttä et al,[76] 2010	PS, MC			217	96%, 92%, 85%, and 80% at 1, 3, 5, and 7 y	3.2 y	NR
Mann et al,[77] 2011	PS, SC			84	96% and 90% at 5 and 10 y	9.1 y	39.5°
Nunley et al,[78] 2012	PS, SC			82	93.9% and 88.5% at 5 and 8.9 y	5.1 y	33°

Patsalis et al,[79] 2004	PS, SC	AES	3-components, unconstrained	15	NR	0.7 y	30° (20°–40°)
Besse et al,[80] 2009	PS, SC			50	96% at 3.3 y	3.3 y	38°
Anders et al,[81] 2010	RS, SC			93	90% at 5 y	3.5 y	NR
Morgan et al,[82] 2010	RS, SC			38	94.7% at 6 y	4.8 y	NR
Skyttä et al,[76] 2010	PS, MC			298	96% and 88% at 1 and 3 y	3.2 y	NR
Bonnin et al,[83] 2004	RS, SC	Salto	3-components, unconstrained	98	94.9% at 5.7 y	2.9 y	28.3°
Weber et al,[84] 2004	RS, MC			115	97.5% at 1.8 y	1.8 y	32.3°
Bonnin et al,[85] 2011	RS, SC			98	85% at 10 y	6.8 y	27°
Hintermann et al,[86] 2004	PS, SC	HINTEGRA	3-components, unconstrained	122	NR	1.6 y	39° (15°–55°)
Valderrabano et al,[87] 2006	PS, SC			152	NR	2.8 y	35° (10°–55°)
Kim et al,[88] 2009	PS, SC			45	NR	2.3 y	38.7°
Bai et al,[89] 2010	RS, SC			67	98.5% at 3.2 y	3.2 y	38°
Kim et al,[90] 2010	PS, SC			348	NR	3.3 y	34.3°
Barg et al,[91] 2011	PS, SC			52	78% and 91% at 5 and 8 y	5 y	38°
Wood et al,[92] 2010	PS, SC	Mobility	3-components, unconstrained	100	97% and 93.6% at 3 and 4 y	3.6 y	22° (2°–43°)
Rippstein et al,[93] 2011	PS, SC			240	97.7° at 4 y	2.7 y	21.9°
Giannini et al,[94] 2010	PS, MC	BOX	3-components, unconstrained	51	97.2% at 3 y	2.5 y	27.4° (16°–53°)

Abbreviations: MC, multicenter; NR, not reported; PS, prospective; RS, retrospective; SC, single-center.

CLINICAL OUTCOMES AFTER TAR

TAR is becoming more prevalent as a therapeutic joint sacrificing option in patients with end-stage ankle OA. Clinical outcomes, including stability of prosthesis components, are not yet comparable to those in hip or knee joint arthroplasty.[43,44]

Gougoulias and colleagues[45] recently performed a systematic review of the literature to analyze the outcome of TAR. Thirteen level IV studies reporting on at least 20 replaced ankles with a minimum follow-up of 2 years were included in this review. The total patient cohort included 1105 cases: 234 Agility, 344 STAR, 153 Buechel-Pappas, 152 HINTEGRA, 98 Salto (Tornier SA, Saint Ismier, France), 70 TNK (Kyocera, Kyoto, Japan), and 54 Mobility. The overall survivorship of prosthesis component was 90% at 5 years, with a wide range between 68% and 100% among different centers. Based on available data analysis, no superiority of an implant design could be deduced.[45]

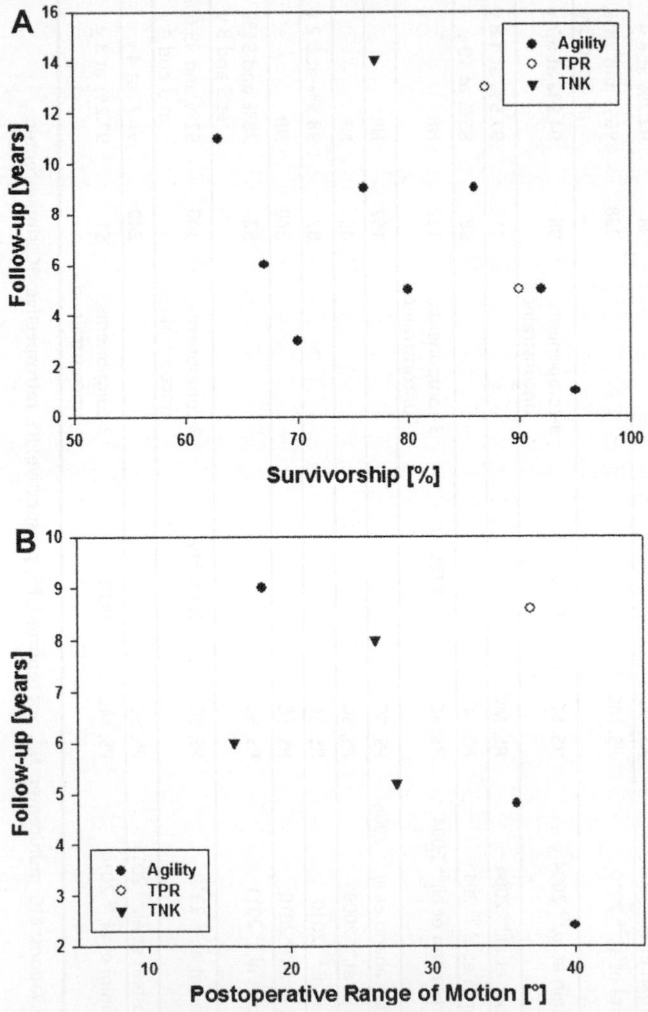

Fig. 5. (*A*) Prosthesis survivorship and (*B*) postoperative range of motion in patients who underwent TAR using 2-component total ankles: Agility, TPR, and TNK.

For this review, a literature search of MEDLINE, Cochrane, EMBASE, CINAHL, and ScienceDirect databases was conducted using following terms: "total ankle," "ankle replacement," and "ankle arthroplasty." In addition, electronic contents of the following journals were searched using these keywords: *Foot and Ankle International*, *Journal of Bone and Joint Surgery (American and British Volumes)*, *Clinical Orthopedics and Related Research*, *Foot Ankle Clinics of North America*, and *Journal of Foot and Ankle Surgery*.

Included were publications relevant to TAR using following ankle designs:

- Two-component prostheses: Agility, TPR, and TNK
- Three-component prostheses: Buechel-Pappas, STAR, AES, HINTEGRA, Mobility, and BOX (Finsbury Orthopaedics Limited, Leatherhead, UK)

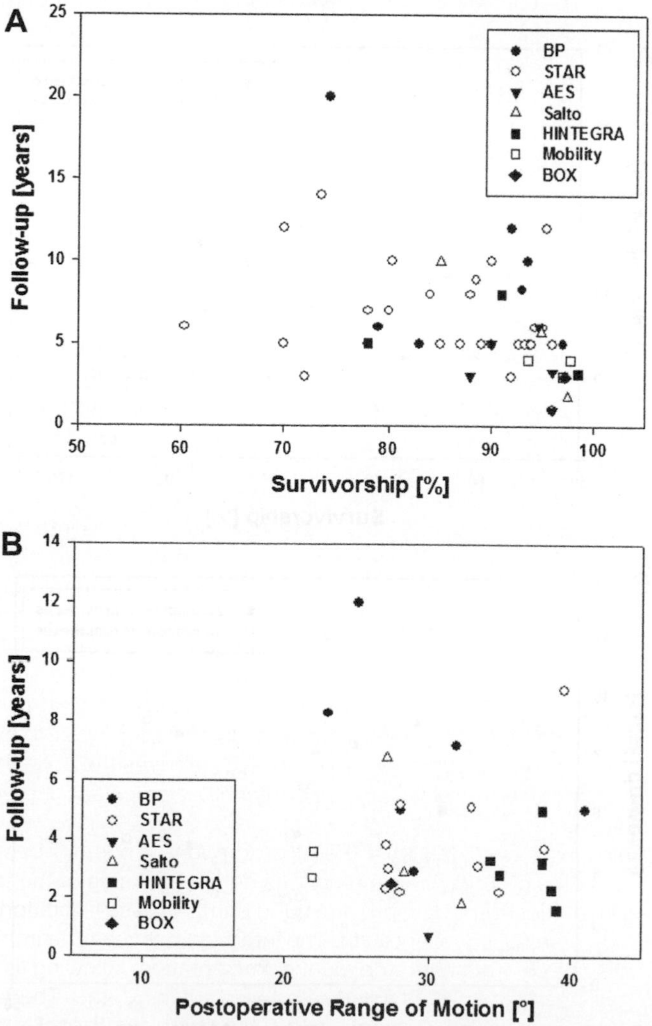

Fig. 6. (*A*) Prosthesis survivorship and (*B*) postoperative ROM in patients who underwent TAR using 3-component total ankles: Buechel-Pappas, STAR, AES, HINTEGRA, Mobility, and BOX.

No randomized trials were included. All included studies were graded as level IV evidence. The mean follow-up of included publications ranged between 0.7 and 12 years (**Tables 1** and **2**).

Kaplan-Maier survivorship analysis data in patients who underwent TAR using Agility, TPR, and TNK ankle systems were provided by 5, 2, and 1 study, respectively (see **Table 1**). The survivorship ranged from 63% at 11 years (Agility ankle) to 95% at 1 year postoperatively (Agility ankle) (**Fig. 5**A). The mean postoperative ROM ranged from 16° (TNK ankle) to 40° (Agility ankle) (see **Fig. 5**A). The survivorship of 3-component total ankles ranged from 60.4% at 6 years (uncemented, single-coated STAR ankle) to 98.5% at 3.2 years (HINTEGRA ankle) (**Fig. 6**A). The mean postoperative ROM ranged from 23° (Buechel-Pappas ankle) to 41° (Buechel-Pappas ankle) (see **Fig. 6**B). No substantial or significant differences were observed between 2- and

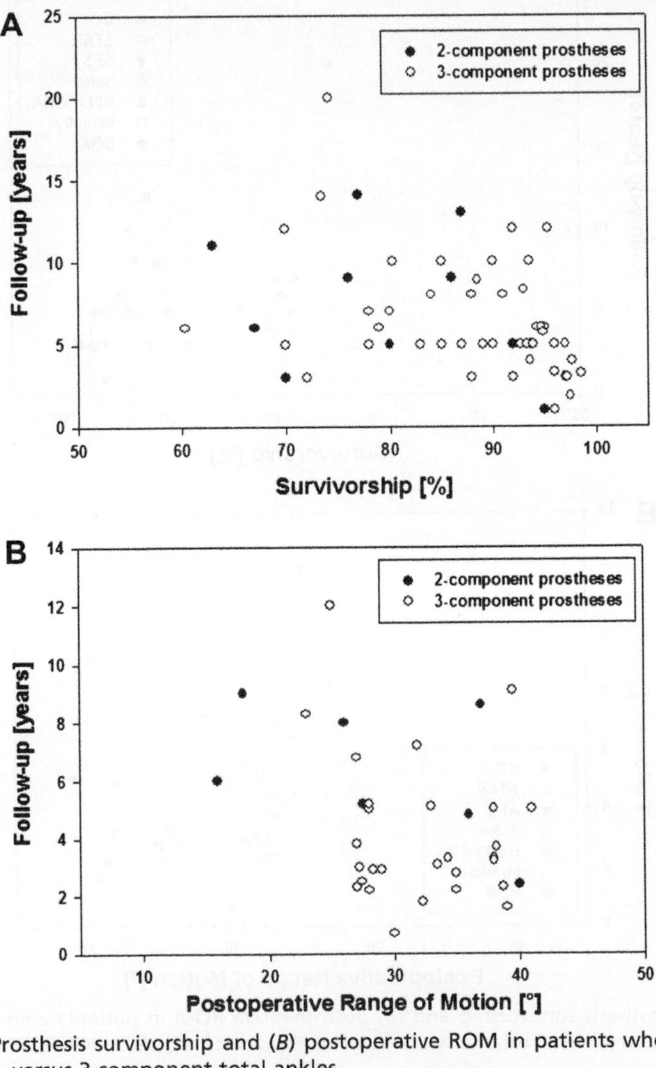

Fig. 7. (*A*) Prosthesis survivorship and (*B*) postoperative ROM in patients who underwent TAR using 2- versus 3-component total ankles.

3-component total ankle designs regarding prosthesis survivorship (**Fig. 7**A) and postoperative ROM (see **Fig. 7**B).

The analysis of the literature review should be interpreted carefully. First, the results presented in the current literature may be influenced by the surgeons' experience. A steep learning curve has been shown to be associated with performing TAR.[95,96] Experience, as a key factor for success in mid-term, has been also identified in Swedish Joint Arthroplasty Register data: the 5-year survival increased from 70% (95% CI, 57%–77%) for the first 90 cases to 86% (95% CI, 80%–93%) for the following 132 cases.[97] Second, variability in patient cohort with different underlying causes may be a confounding factor. Third, heterogeneity in outcome measures and nonuniform study designs complicate the direct comparison between the studies. Naal and colleagues[98] performed a systematic review of the literature and identified 15 outcome metrics. The most commonly used measures were the AOFAS hindfoot score, the Kofoed ankle score, a visual analog scale assessing pain, and the generic SF-36.[98] AOFAS hindfoot score is nonvalidated score, and the research committee of the AOFAS recently published a policy statement recommending not to use this instrument.[99] Fourth, many studies reporting the outcome in patients who underwent TAR are published by persons involved with the development of the prosthesis, which may raise some concern about possible conflict of interest. In fact, publications by some research groups, particularly those by TAR inventors, have shown significantly more superior outcomes than those published by other users or those shown in registry data.[44]

SUMMARY

TAR is undoubtedly gaining acceptance among foot and ankle surgeons as a valuable treatment option in patients with end-stage ankle OA. Current reports of this procedure show consistently good to excellent mid-term results with substantial pain relief, good functional outcome, and high patient satisfaction.[45] The unacceptable high failure rate of the first-generation ankle prostheses has been thoroughly analyzed, and the TAR designs have been significantly improved. Current fixation without cement has become the gold standard using biologic surfaces (eg, introduction of hydroxyapatite in the 1990s) for better and faster osseous integration of metallic prosthesis components.[100,101]

A variety of prosthesis designs are available. Although in the United States the STAR prosthesis is the only 3-component total ankle design with FDA approval,[2,77,102] in Europe the most common ankle prostheses are 3-component.[7,102–104] The mobile anatomic, nonconstrained, 3-component total ankle designs also predominate in available national arthroplasty registers.[52,76,97,105] The question remains regarding which prosthesis design philosophy is better, 2- or 3-component. Although biomechanical studies show advantages of 3-component prosthesis design regarding biomechanics and kinematics,[27–29,42] no obvious differences in clinical outcome between prosthesis types could be identified in the current literature.

REFERENCES

1. Glazebrook M, Daniels T, Younger A, et al. Comparison of health-related quality of life between patients with end-stage ankle and hip arthrosis. J Bone Joint Surg Am 2008;90:499–505.
2. Saltzman CL, Mann RA, Ahrens JE, et al. Prospective controlled trial of STAR total ankle replacement versus ankle fusion: initial results. Foot Ankle Int 2009; 30:579–96.

3. Muir DC, Amendola A, Saltzman CL. Long-term outcome of ankle arthrodesis. Foot Ankle Clin 2002;7:703–8.
4. Nihal A, Gellman RE, Embil JM, et al. Ankle arthrodesis. Foot Ankle Surg 2008; 14:1–10.
5. Bonasia DE, Dettoni F, Femino JE, et al. Total ankle replacement: why, when and how? Iowa Orthop J 2010;30:119–30.
6. Giannini S, Leardini A, O'Connor JJ. Total ankle replacement: review of the design and of the current status. Foot Ankle Surg 2000;6:77–88.
7. Gougoulias NE, Khanna A, Maffulli N. History and evolution in total ankle arthroplasty. Br Med Bull 2009;89:111–51.
8. Henne TD, Anderson JG. Total ankle arthroplasty: a historical perspective. Foot Ankle Clin 2002;7:695–702.
9. van den Heuvel A, Van Bouwel S, Dereymaeker G. Total ankle replacement. Design evolution and results. Acta Orthop Belg 2010;76:150–61.
10. Lord G, Marotte JH. Total ankle prosthesis. Technic and 1st results. Apropos of 12 cases. Rev Chir Orthop Reparatrice Appar Mot 1973;59:139–51 [in French].
11. Muir DC, Amendola A, Saltzman CL. Forty-year outcome of ankle "cup" arthroplasty for post-traumatic arthritis. Iowa Orthop J 2002;22:99–102.
12. Hintermann B. History of total ankle arthroplasty. In: Hintermann B, editor. Total ankle arthroplasty: historical overview, current concepts and future perspectives. 1st edition. Wien (NY): Springer; 2005. p. 43–57.
13. Hintermann B, Valderrabano V. Total ankle replacement. Foot Ankle Clin 2003;8: 375–405.
14. Evanski PH, Waugh TR. Management of arthritis of the ankle. An alternative of arthrodesis. Clin Orthop Relat Res 1977;122:110–5.
15. Hamblen DL. Can the ankle joint be replaced? J Bone Joint Surg Br 1985;67: 689–90.
16. Alvine FG. The Agility ankle replacement: the good and the bad. Foot Ankle Clin 2002;7:737–53.
17. Cerrato R, Myerson MS. Total ankle replacement: the Agility LP prosthesis. Foot Ankle Clin 2008;13:485–94.
18. Vickerstaff JA, Miles AW, Cunningham JL. A brief history of total ankle replacement and a review of the current status. Med Eng Phys 2007;29:1056–64.
19. Kofoed H. Scandinavian Total Ankle Replacement (STAR). Clin Orthop Relat Res 2004;424:73–9.
20. Rippstein PF. Clinical experiences with three different designs of ankle prostheses. Foot Ankle Clin 2002;7:817–31.
21. Saltzman CL. Perspective on total ankle replacement. Foot Ankle Clin 2000;5: 761–75.
22. Barg A, Hintermann B. Implantate und Biomechanik des oberen Sprunggelenks. In: Neumann W, editor. AE-Manual der Endoprothetik: Sprunggelenk und Fuss. 1st edition. Heidelberg (Germany): Springer; 2012. p. 29–45.
23. Hintermann B. Current designs of total ankle prostheses. In: Hintermann B, editor. Total ankle arthroplasty. Historical overview, current concepts and future perspectives. 1st edition. Wien (New York): Springer; 2004. p. 69–100.
24. Younger A, Penner M, Wing K. Mobile-bearing total ankle arthroplasty. Foot Ankle Clin 2008;13:495–504.
25. Marx RC, Mizel MS. What's new in foot and ankle surgery. J Bone Joint Surg Am 2010;92:512–23.
26. Marx RC, Mizel MS. What's new in foot and ankle surgery. J Bone Joint Surg Am 2011;93:405–14.

27. Valderrabano V, Hintermann B, Nigg BM, et al. Kinematic changes after fusion and total replacement of the ankle: part 1: range of motion. Foot Ankle Int 2003;24:881–7.
28. Valderrabano V, Hintermann B, Nigg BM, et al. Kinematic changes after fusion and total replacement of the ankle: part 2: movement transfer. Foot Ankle Int 2003;24:888–96.
29. Valderrabano V, Hintermann B, Nigg BM, et al. Kinematic changes after fusion and total replacement of the ankle: part 3: Talar movement. Foot Ankle Int 2003;24:897–900.
30. Komistek RD, Stiehl JB, Buechel FF, et al. A determination of ankle kinematics using fluoroscopy. Foot Ankle Int 2000;21:343–50.
31. Detrembleur C, Leemrijse T. The effects of total ankle replacement on gait disability: analysis of energetic and mechanical variables. Gait Posture 2009; 29:270–4.
32. Valderrabano V, Nigg BM, von Tscharner V, et al. Gait analysis in ankle osteoarthritis and total ankle replacement. Clin Biomech (Bristol, Avon) 2007;22:894–904.
33. Valderrabano V, von Tscharner V, Nigg BM, et al. Lower leg muscle atrophy in ankle osteoarthritis. J Orthop Res 2006;24:2159–69.
34. Valderrabano V, Nigg BM, von Tscharner V, et al. J. Leonard Goldner Award 2006. Total ankle replacement in ankle osteoarthritis: an analysis of muscle rehabilitation. Foot Ankle Int 2007;28:281–91.
35. Lundberg A, Svensson OK, Nemeth G, et al. The axis of rotation of the ankle joint. J Bone Joint Surg Br 1989;71:94–9.
36. Lee KB, Cho SG, Hur CI, et al. Perioperative complications of HINTEGRA total ankle replacement: our initial 50 cases. Foot Ankle Int 2008;29:978–84.
37. Schuberth JM, Patel S, Zarutsky E. Perioperative complications of the Agility total ankle replacement in 50 initial, consecutive cases. J Foot Ankle Surg 2006;45:139–46.
38. Tochigi Y, Rudert MJ, Brown TD, et al. The effect of accuracy of implantation on range of movement of the Scandinavian Total Ankle Replacement. J Bone Joint Surg Br 2005;87:736–40.
39. Saltzman CL, Tochigi Y, Rudert MJ, et al. The effect of agility ankle prosthesis misalignment on the peri-ankle ligaments. Clin Orthop Relat Res 2004;424: 137–42.
40. Nicholson JJ, Parks BG, Stroud CC, et al. Joint contact characteristics in agility total ankle arthroplasty. Clin Orthop Relat Res 2004;424:125–9.
41. Fukuda T, Haddad SL, Ren Y, et al. Impact of talar component rotation on contact pressure after total ankle arthroplasty: a cadaveric study. Foot Ankle Int 2010;31:404–11.
42. Espinosa N, Walti M, Favre P, et al. Misalignment of total ankle components can induce high joint contact pressures. J Bone Joint Surg Am 2010;92:1179–87.
43. Espinosa N, Klammer G. Treatment of ankle osteoarthritis: arthrodesis versus total ankle replacement. Eur J Trauma Emerg Surg 2010;36:525–35.
44. Labek G, Klaus H, Schlichtherle R, et al. Revision rates after total ankle arthroplasty in sample-based clinical studies and national registries. Foot Ankle Int 2011;32:740–5.
45. Gougoulias N, Khanna A, Maffulli N. How successful are current ankle replacements?: a systematic review of the literature. Clin Orthop Relat Res 2010;468: 199–208.
46. Pyevich MT, Saltzman CL, Callaghan JJ, et al. Total ankle arthroplasty: a unique design. Two to twelve-year follow-up. J Bone Joint Surg Am 1998;80:1410–20.

47. Knecht SI, Estin M, Callaghan JJ, et al. The Agility total ankle arthroplasty. Seven to sixteen-year follow-up. J Bone Joint Surg Am 2004;86-A:1161–71.
48. Spirt AA, Assal M, Hansen ST Jr. Complications and failure after total ankle arthroplasty. J Bone Joint Surg Am 2004;86-A:1172–8.
49. Vienne P, Nothdurft P. OSG-Totalendoprothese Agility: Indikationen, Operationstechnik und Ergebnisse. Fuss Sprungg 2004;2:17–28.
50. Hurowitz EJ, Gould JS, Fleisig GS, et al. Outcome analysis of agility total ankle replacement with prior adjunctive procedures: two to six year followup. Foot Ankle Int 2007;28:308–12.
51. Schill S, Biehl C, Thabe H. Ankle prostheses. Mid-term results after Thompson-Richards and STAR prostheses. Orthopade 1998;27:183–7 [in German].
52. Fevang BT, Lie SA, Havelin LI, et al. 257 ankle arthroplasties performed in Norway between 1994 and 2005. Acta Orthop 2007;78:575–83.
53. Shinomiya F, Okada M, Hamada Y, et al. Indications of total ankle arthroplasty for rheumatoid arthritis: evaluation at 5 years or more after the operation. Mod Rheumatol 2003;13:153–9.
54. Nishikawa M, Tomita T, Fujii M, et al. Total ankle replacement in rheumatoid arthritis. Int Orthop 2004;28:123–6.
55. Takakura Y, Tanaka Y, Kumai T, et al. Ankle arthroplasty using three generations of metal and ceramic prostheses. Clin Orthop Relat Res 2004;424:130–6.
56. Buechel FF, Pappas MJ, Iorio LJ. New Jersey low contact stress total ankle replacement: biomechanical rationale and review of 23 cementless cases. Foot Ankle 1988;8:279–90.
57. Buechel FF Sr, Buechel FF Jr, Pappas MJ. Ten-year evaluation of cementless Buechel-Pappas meniscal bearing total ankle replacement. Foot Ankle Int 2003;24:462–72.
58. Buechel FF Sr, Buechel FF Jr, Pappas MJ. Twenty-year evaluation of cementless mobile-bearing total ankle replacements. Clin Orthop Relat Res 2004;424:19–26.
59. Doets HC, Brand R, Nelissen RG. Total ankle arthroplasty in inflammatory joint disease with use of two mobile-bearing designs. J Bone Joint Surg Am 2006; 88:1272–84.
60. Ali MS, Higgins GA, Mohamed M. Intermediate results of Buechel Pappas unconstrained uncemented total ankle replacement for osteoarthritis. J Foot Ankle Surg 2007;46:16–20.
61. van der Heide HJ, Schutte B, Louwerens JW, et al. Total ankle prostheses in rheumatoid arthropathy: outcome in 52 patients followed for 1-9 years. Acta Orthop 2009;80:440–4.
62. Wood PL, Sutton C, Mishra V, et al. A randomised, controlled trial of two mobile-bearing total ankle replacements. J Bone Joint Surg Br 2009;91:69–74.
63. Kofoed H. Cylindrical cemented ankle arthroplasty: a prospective series with long-term follow-up. Foot Ankle Int 1995;16:474–9.
64. Kofoed H, Sorensen TS. Ankle arthroplasty for rheumatoid arthritis and osteoarthritis: prospective long-term study of cemented replacements. J Bone Joint Surg Br 1998;80:328–32.
65. Anderson T, Montgomery F, Carlsson A. Uncemented STAR total ankle prostheses. Three to eight-year follow-up of fifty-one consecutive ankles. J Bone Joint Surg Am 2003;85-A:1321–9.
66. Hagena FW, Christ R, Kettrukat M. Die Endoprothese am oberen Sprunggelenk. Fuss Sprungg 2003;1:48–55.
67. Wood PL, Deakin S. Total ankle replacement. The results in 200 ankles. J Bone Joint Surg Br 2003;85:334–41.

68. Lodhi Y, McKenna J, Herron M, et al. Total ankle replacement. Ir Med J 2004;97: 104–5.
69. Valderrabano V, Hintermann B, Dick W. Scandinavian total ankle replacement: a 3.7-year average followup of 65 patients. Clin Orthop Relat Res 2004;424:47–56.
70. Murnaghan JM, Warnock DS, Henderson SA. Total ankle replacement. Early experiences with STAR prosthesis. Ulster Med J 2005;74:9–13.
71. Carlsson A. Single- and double-coated star total ankle replacements: a clinical and radiographic follow-up study of 109 cases. Orthopade 2006;35:527–32 [in German].
72. Kumar A, Dhar S. Total ankle replacement: early results during learning periods. Foot Ankle Surg 2007;13:19–23.
73. Schutte BG, Louwerens JW. Short-term results of our first 49 Scandinavian total ankle replacements (STAR). Foot Ankle Int 2008;29:124–7.
74. Wood PL, Prem H, Sutton C. Total ankle replacement: medium-term results in 200 Scandinavian total ankle replacements. J Bone Joint Surg Br 2008;90: 605–9.
75. Hobson SA, Karantana A, Dhar S. Total ankle replacement in patients with significant pre-operative deformity of the hindfoot. J Bone Joint Surg Br 2009;91: 481–6.
76. Skyttä ET, Koivu H, Eskelinen A, et al. Total ankle replacement: a population-based study of 515 cases from the Finnish Arthroplasty Register. Acta Orthop 2010;81:114–8.
77. Mann JA, Mann RA, Horton E. STAR ankle: long-term results. Foot Ankle Int 2011;32:473–84.
78. Nunley JA, Caputo AM, Easley ME, et al. Intermediate to long-term outcomes of the STAR Total Ankle Replacement: the patient perspective. J Bone Joint Surg Am 2012;94:43–8.
79. Patsalis T. Die AES-Sprunggelenksprothese: Indikation, Technik und erste Ergebnisse. Fuss Sprungg 2004;2:38–44.
80. Besse JL, Brito N, Lienhart C. Clinical evaluation and radiographic assessment of bone lysis of the AES total ankle replacement. Foot Ankle Int 2009;30:964–75.
81. Anders H, Kaj K, Johan J, et al. The AES total ankle replacement: a mid-term analysis of 93 cases. Foot Ankle Surg 2010;16:61–4.
82. Morgan SS, Brooke B, Harris NJ. Total ankle replacement by the Ankle Evolution System: medium-term outcome. J Bone Joint Surg Br 2010;92:61–5.
83. Bonnin M, Judet T, Colombier JA, et al. Midterm results of the Salto Total Ankle Prosthesis. Clin Orthop Relat Res 2004;424:6–18.
84. Weber M, Bonnin M, Columbier JA, et al. Erste Ergebnisse der SALTO-Sprunggelenkendoprothese: Eine französische Multizenterstudie mit 155 Implantaten. Fuss Sprungg 2004;2:29–37.
85. Bonnin M, Gaudot F, Laurent JR, et al. The Salto total ankle arthroplasty: survivorship and analysis of failures at 7 to 11 years. Clin Orthop Relat Res 2011;469: 225–36.
86. Hintermann B, Valderrabano V, Dereymaeker G, et al. The HINTEGRA ankle: rationale and short-term results of 122 consecutive ankles. Clin Orthop Relat Res 2004;424:57–68.
87. Valderrabano V, Pagenstert G, Horisberger M, et al. Sports and recreation activity of ankle arthritis patients before and after total ankle replacement. Am J Sports Med 2006;34:993–9.
88. Kim BS, Choi WJ, Kim YS, et al. Total ankle replacement in moderate to severe varus deformity of the ankle. J Bone Joint Surg Br 2009;91:1183–90.

89. Bai LB, Lee KB, Song EK, et al. Total ankle arthroplasty outcome comparison for post-traumatic and primary osteoarthritis. Foot Ankle Int 2010;31: 1048–56.
90. Kim BS, Knupp M, Zwicky L, et al. Total ankle replacement in association with hindfoot fusion: outcome and complications. J Bone Joint Surg Br 2010;92: 1540–7.
91. Barg A, Henninger HB, Knupp M, et al. Simultaneous bilateral total ankle replacement using a 3-component prosthesis: outcome in 26 patients followed for 2-10 years. Acta Orthop 2011;82:704–10.
92. Wood PL, Karski MT, Watmough P. Total ankle replacement: the results of 100 mobility total ankle replacements. J Bone Joint Surg Br 2010;92: 958–62.
93. Rippstein PF, Huber M, Coetzee JC, et al. Total ankle replacement with use of a new three-component implant. J Bone Joint Surg Am 2011;93: 1426–35.
94. Giannini S, Romagnoli M, O'Connor JJ, et al. Total ankle replacement compatible with ligament function produces mobility, good clinical scores, and low complication rates: an early clinical assessment. Clin Orthop Relat Res 2010; 468:2746–53.
95. Myerson MS, Mroczek K. Perioperative complications of total ankle arthroplasty. Foot Ankle Int 2003;24:17–21.
96. Saltzman CL, Amendola A, Anderson R, et al. Surgeon training and complications in total ankle arthroplasty. Foot Ankle Int 2003;24:514–8.
97. Henricson A, Skoog A, Carlsson A. The Swedish Ankle Arthroplasty Register: an analysis of 531 arthroplasties between 1993 and 2005. Acta Orthop 2007;78: 569–74.
98. Naal FD, Impellizzeri FM, Rippstein PF. Which are the most frequently used outcome instruments in studies on total ankle arthroplasty? Clin Orthop Relat Res 2010;468:815–26.
99. Pinsker E, Daniels TR. AOFAS position statement regarding the future of the AOFAS clinical rating systems. Foot Ankle Int 2011;32:841–2.
100. Hintermann B. Ankle osteoarthritis: five take-home points regarding total ankle arthroplasty in the rest of the world. Presented at the 26th Annual Summer Meeting, American Orthopaedic Foot & Ankle Society (AOFAS), National Harbor, Maryland, USA, July 7-10, 2010.
101. Saltzman CL. Ankle osteoarthritis: five take-home points regarding total ankle arthroplasty in USA. Presented at the 26th Annual Summer Meeting, American Orthopaedic Foot & Ankle Society (AOFAS), National Harbor, Maryland, USA, July 7-10, 2010.
102. Guyer AJ, Richardson G. Current concepts review: total ankle arthroplasty. Foot Ankle Int 2008;29:256–64.
103. Besse JL, Colombier JA, Asencio J, et al. Total ankle arthroplasty in France. Orthop Traumatol Surg Res 2010;96:291–303.
104. Goldberg AJ, Sharp RJ, Cooke P. Ankle replacement: current practice of foot & ankle surgeons in the United Kingdom. Foot Ankle Int 2009;30:950–4.
105. Hosman AH, Mason RB, Hobbs T, et al. A New Zealand national joint registry review of 202 total ankle replacements followed for up to 6 years. Acta Orthop 2007;78:584–91.
106. Koivu H, Kohonen I, Sipola E, et al. Severe periprosthetic osteolytic lesions after the Ankle Evolutive System total ankle replacement. J Bone Joint Surg Br 2009; 91:907–14.

107. Kokkonen A, Ikavalko M, Tiihonen R, et al. High rate of osteolytic lesions in medium-term followup after the AES total ankle replacement. Foot Ankle Int 2011;32:168–75.
108. San Giovanni TP, Keblish DJ, Thomas WH, et al. Eight-year results of a minimally constrained total ankle arthroplasty. Foot Ankle Int 2006;27:418–26.
109. Wood PL, Crawford LA, Suneja R, et al. Total ankle replacement for rheumatoid ankle arthritis. Foot Ankle Clin 2007;12:497–508.

Techniques and Pitfalls with the Salto Prosthesis

Our Experience of the First 15 Years

J.A. Colombier, MD[a,*], Th. Judet, MD, PhD[b], M. Bonnin, MD[c], F. Gaudot, MD[b]

KEYWORDS

• Salto • Total • Ankle • Replacement • Technique • Pitfalls

KEY POINTS

- The Salto prosthesis is a third-generation total ankle replacement.
- Good clinical and radiographic results can be obtained when implanting a Salto total ankle replacement.
- Precise indications and preoperative planning lead to success.

INTRODUCTION

The development of ankle prosthesis began in the 1970s. After several different biomechanical approaches and numerous modifications in their design, they now represent a reliable alternative to arthrodesis for the treatment of ankle arthrosis. The Salto prosthesis is designed to replace the tibiotalar and talomalleolar joints as first-line treatment or revision surgery for patients whose tibiotalar joint is damaged by a severe form of rheumatoid arthritis, posttraumatic arthrosis, or degenerative arthrosis.

Long-term follow-up of the results in most cases shows good functional results. Analysis of the current surgical techniques allows optimization of these results.[1,2]

The authors have used the Salto prosthesis (Tornier) for more than 15 years, and this article discusses this treatment and its limitations.

The Salto ankle prosthesis comes in 2 versions: A fixed bearing and a mobile bearing version (**Figs. 1** and **2**). A revision implant is being evaluated.

Conflict of interest: J.A. Colombier, Th. Judet, and M. Bonnin are the designers of the Salto prosthesis. One or more authors (MB, JAC, and TJ) received royalties from Tornier SA, Montbonnot, France. Each author certifies that his or her institution approved the human protocol for this investigation, and that all investigations were conducted in conformity with ethical principles of research.

[a] Clinique de l'Union, bd de Ratalens, Saint Jean 31240, France; [b] Centre Hospitalier Raymond Poincaré, 104 Boulevard Raymond Poincaré, Garches 92380, France; [c] Centre Orthopédique Santy, 24 Avenue Paul Santy, Lyon 69008, France

* Corresponding author.

E-mail address: j-a.colombier@clinique-union.fr

Foot Ankle Clin N Am 17 (2012) 587–605
http://dx.doi.org/10.1016/j.fcl.2012.08.012
1083-7515/12/$ – see front matter

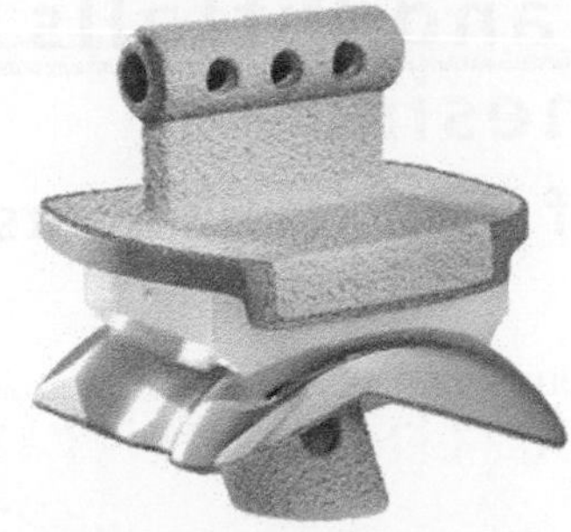

Fig. 1. The Salto total ankle replacement (TAR) system. The prosthesis consists of a tibial component with a central fin/stem and a talar component. A mobile bearing polyethylene inlay is placed between the tibial and talar components.

HISTORY AND DEVELOPMENT OF THE SALTO

When the prosthesis was conceived in 1995, the challenge was to answer 3 questions:

Why an Ankle Prosthesis?

Surgical treatment of tibiotarsal arthrosis normally takes place after exhaustion of medical and functional treatment. The most commonly accepted treatment remains arthrodesis. However, outcomes of arthrodesis may be good at the pain level but cannot be considered a gold standard because:

- It does not allow conservation of the locomotor program of the ankle (adaptability, shock absorption, and propulsion)
- It deteriorates over time because of arthrosic decompensation of the overlying and underlying joints

However, the development of joint prostheses is advancing in orthopedics at the level of each joint, which has been a difficult process requiring abandonment of arthrodesis in favor of implantation of joint prostheses. The tibiotarsal joint does not escape this rule.

Why a New Prosthesis?

The available prostheses were not anatomic, only allowing a flexion-extension movement, leading to elevated constraints at interfaces and ligamentous structures

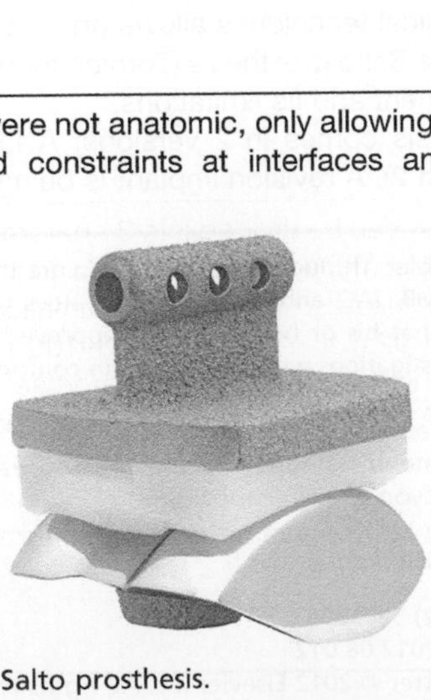

Fig. 2. Close-up view of the Salto prosthesis.

despite the mobile gliding effect. This assessment led us to develop an anatomic implant, with a conical shaft rotational surface, incorporating talar curves allowing pronosupination.

Morphology of the joint surfaces and kinematics

Tibial component Designed to receive the superior gliding surface of the polyethylene insert, the smooth and flat tibial component permits adaptation in translation and rotation for the insert. Epiphyseal covering is optimized by the anatomic design. A 3-mm medial flange prevents a conflicting interaction between the medial malleolus and the polyethylene insert. An anchoring block allows a strong primary stability.

Talar component The talar component imitates the anatomy of the talar dome, which as the shape of a truncated rotational surface; the width is greater at the front than at the back and the radius of curvature of the lateral condyle is greater than that of the medial condyle. As a result, the flexion-extension axis of the talar prosthesis beneath the insert imitates the physiologic axis (ie, oblique from the outside in, from the back to the front, and from the base to the top, with an incline of 10° to the horizontal). The external dome of the talus is covered by the prosthesis, which connects with the lateral malleolus.

The intermediate component The intermediate component is made from ultrahigh-molecular-weight polyethylene, a high-density polyethylene. It is mobile beneath the tibia with which it articulates via its upper surface.

Via its lower surface, it articulates with the talar component in a congruent manner in the flexion-extension plane and with a varus/valgus tolerance range of 4° in the frontal plane, avoiding edge-loading effects.

Why a Mobile Bearing?

The reduction in constraint caused by near-normal tibiotalar kinetics and the potential problems of the mobile bearing sliding core (increased wear, overhanging, conflicting mediolateral interactions) have led to a fixed bearing in the Salto Talaris, thus creating a third-generation anatomic prosthesis with a fixed bearing.

Its use is possible in most cases, and is providing encouraging results (article in preparation).

STANDARD SURGICAL TECHNIQUE

In general, this is a resurfacing prosthesis, meaning that bone resection must be minimal (subcortical compact bone remains, and facilitates revision surgeries, if necessary, and bone stock conservation).

In most cases it is not recommended misalignement by reorientating the cuts.

Bone cuts must be made after prior correction of such deformities if they are present (deviations in the frontal or sagittal planes). The positioning and initial stability depend on the accuracy of the bone cuts guided by the ancillary and the design of the anchoring surfaces. Secondary anchoring is ensured by bone ingrowth into the coated surface: titanium plasma coating in the Salto mobile bearing with a second hydroxyapatite (HA) plasma spray. Initial anchoring at the tibia is ensured by epiphyseal adaptation reinforced with a keel and an anteroposterior cylindroconical fixation peg.

At the talus, stability is provided by 3 bone cuts (anterior, posterior, and lateral) completed by a hollow 11-mm diameter plug press fitted into the body of the talus.

Planning

Preoperative planning includes a standard radiological assessement comprising 3 weight bearing views: anteroposterior, lateral, and 30° medially rotated anterioposterior to see the talo and tibio-fibular joints.

This assessement report should be comparative.

In most cases additional views may be required, especially CT scan to assess the joint status in several planes (malunions) or to identify preexisting bone cysts.

This planning helps to predict the size of the implant, to assess the joint line level, to evaluate anterior osteophytes and the bone volume that will have to be removed, and to check the talar dome shape.

Instrumentation

Instrumentation was designed and regularly improved to obtain optimal reproducibility while still adapting to diverse anatomic conditions occurring in post-traumatic, degenerative, neurological or congenital conditions.

Approach

The ankle is exposed through a wide, anterior longitudinal approach. This approach facilitates anterior joint dissection and allows broad arthrolysis with resection of all the osteophytes (see **Fig. 1**). The apex of the dome as well as the contours between the pilon and each of the malleoli stand out as a result of this approach. In the same way, dissection of the malleolar processes is performed if lateral and/or medial release is necessary. Therefore, if realignment is necessary, it can only be performed by ligamental dissection, performed in a gradual manner, during which the bone cuts improve access to the collateral planes.

The Surgery Then Progresses Step by Step

The goal is to carry out bone cuts fulfilling several requirements:

- Being sufficiently precise to guarantee initial stability for the implants
- Being oriented in such a way that the final position of the sole of the food is neutral
- Having, at the level of the tibia and talus, a relative position allowing accurate superposition of the prosthetic parts, with no risk of anteroposterior overhang or, in case of a mobile bearing, no risk of lateral overhang, and with no risk of excess tangential constraint in case of a fixed bearing

Surgery starts with placement of a tibial alignment guide, which is the most important instrument for all of the bone cuts. Guide placement is ensured by the following steps:

- Adjustment of the alignment guide in the frontal and sagittal planes
- Definitive adjustment of the section height, the rotation (guide should be aligned on the bisecting line of the angle formed by lateral and medial gutters), and the lateral positioning
- Implementation of tibial cuts
- Talar cutting guide setting and posterior talar cut over guide pins
- Implementation of anterior talar chamfer, which determines anteroposterior positioning of the talar implant beneath the tibial implant
- Talar plug drilling and lateral talar cut
- Trial implant placement and dynamic testing

At this stage, correct positioning of the implant can be checked with the image intensifier in both frontal and lateral views while performing flexion and extension movements of the ankle to check the joint kinematics. The tibial trial will automatically find an optimal position in all planes.

- Drilling of the tibial plug
- Positioning of final implants
- After careful washing of the joint, all the orifices should be filled with cancellous grafts removed from the sectioned bone to avoid any circulation of joint fluid in the bone
- Layer-by-layer closure over a subcutaneous drain

Surgical Follow-up

A plaster cast is set in place either immediately after the operation or shortly after a 48-hour delay for performing physiotherapeutic drainage and passive mobilization on a motorized splint.

The aim of this immobilization is to protect the healing process of the skin and ligaments.

Weight bearing is often allowed with the support of crutches.

This immobilization is withdrawn after 2 to 6 weeks depending on associated procedures, then rehabilitation is started to recover joint amplitude and muscular strength.

THE ADDITIONAL PROCEDURES

The ideal situation is implantation of a total ankle prosthesis in a normally aligned ankle with little or no impairment in the overall anatomy: surgery is then simplified. It is in these cases that the outcomes have a chance of being uncomplicated, predicting a good result.

In numerous cases, anatomic changes of various causes can necessitate, in addition to the prosthesis, additional procedures.

These changes may be:

- Defects in skin coverage, of traumatic cause
- Bone malalignment following trauma or caused by wear to a greater or lesser extent associated with ligamental retraction and distension
- Major stiffness with or without periarticular osteophyte production
- Muscular instability, paralytic sequelae, or musculotendinous lesions
- Deformations of the calcaneopedal block or abnormality associated with the neighboring joints

All these individual or combined changes require specific actions. The necessity for such additional procedures must always be considered at the time of examination of an ankle being considered for prosthesis. Planning of such procedures must be carefully considered, to choose an intervention at the same time as or before implantation of the prosthesis: all associated actions intensify the procedure and can have an impact on the outcome, and a previous intervention can sufficiently improve the functional state to allow extensive delay of joint replacement.

Ankle Coverage Defects

Ankle coverage defects are not exceptional in posttrauma disorders. Any skin adhesion at or close to the joint is a contraindication for prosthetic replacement and justifies a preceding phase of plastic surgery. Although sometimes simple (excision and direct suture), it is often necessary to anticipate the surgery using free covering flaps. It is then wise to wait a period of 3 months for the prosthesis.

Major Malalignments

Malalignment from bone deformities should be distinguished from progressive malalignment caused by wear at the joint line level whether or not it is associated with ligamental retraction or distension.

Bone deformities

Bone deformities can include malunions of the leg skeleton, generally the tibial pilon or lower part of the leg, with associated instability at the bimalleolar process. In all cases, correction of the deformation by an osteotomy is essential before total ankle replacement. Planning is performed in 2 phases, by diaphyseal or, more often, supramalleolar osteotomy. It is possible to perform this correction at the same time as the prosthetic implantation. There are 2 reasons to advise their separation: the sequelae of a combined intervention are more severe, and, in a large number of cases, simple axial correction can provide functional improvement even in the presence of advanced arthrotic lesions.

Malalignments caused by wear

Malalignments caused by wear are frequently observed, mostly in cases of varus deformity within a context of chronic instability (**Fig. 3**). The malleolar structure is retained, bone wear is always predominantly on the tibial pilon, and the medial ligamentous plane is always retracted, whereas the lateral plane is inconsistently

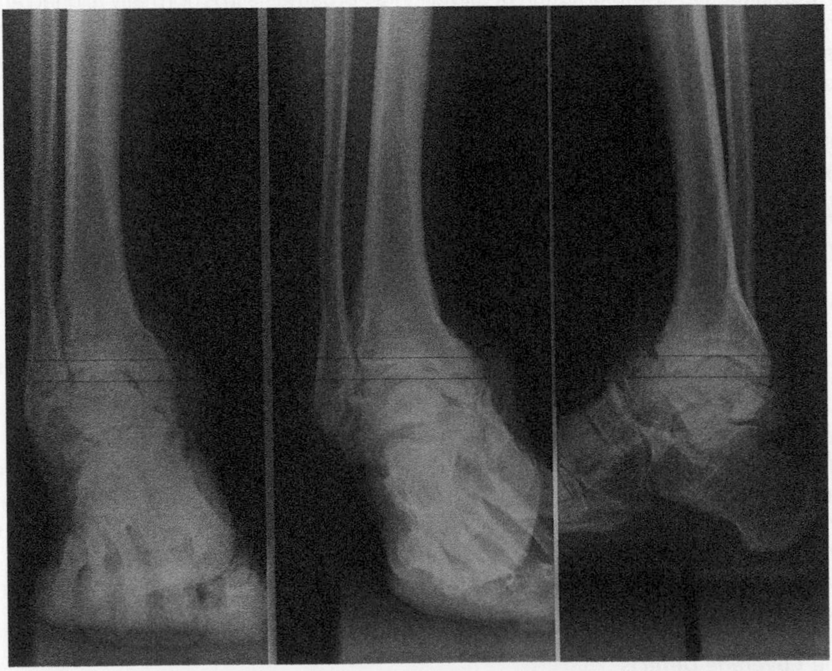

Fig. 3. Severe posttraumatic varus deformity of the hindfoot. The talus is maximally tilted, indicating gross instability of the ankle joint. Note the malformation of the medial malleolus. The patient suffered not only from ankle arthritis but also from degenerative changes within the subtalar and talonavicular joints.

distended. The deformation limit for placement of prosthesis is variable.[3,4] It seems to us that this limit can be pushed far out by careful and complete dissection of the medial plane, taking into account adaptive deformations of the forefoot.

Dissection of the medial plane is started after the tibial cut and will be completed after the posterior cut of the talus, which improves the view and access for the deep surface of the ligamentous layer. Tensioning of this layer with a joint distractor facilitates dissection, which is performed gradually with the tip of a fine knife. It is preceded by a resection of the medial, malleolar, and talar osteophytes that is as complete as possible. Beginning with distal disinsertion of the ligamentous layer, it must proceed in the posterior direction up to the point of the posterointernal angle and the deep portion of the posterior tibial sheath taking care not to cause injury to it. Beyond this, the posterior capsule must be resected. At this stage, if restabilization is not obtained, sagittal osteotomy is suggested to lower the medial malleolus. To avoid drawbacks to this procedure, because lowering of the malleolar projection can cause difficulties with footwear and with consolidation, we prefer to complete the procedure solely on the soft tissues by high-level delamination of the ligamental layer remaining, with the tip of knife blade at the level of the medial surface of the malleolus, thus maintaining continuity with the tibial periosteum.

Given such extensive dissection combined with thickness oversizing of the poly insert by 1 or 2 mm, ligamental stability is generally attained and repair of the lateral plane is not necessary.

If the option of repair of this lateral plane is chosen, it is performed through an independent approach and with the aid of all or part of the peroneus brevis tendon, being aware of the small increase in risk of skin complications induced by this intervention.[1]

In all cases, the ankle is immobilized in a boot cast and its mobilization is postponed by 3 to 4 weeks.

For major varus deformities, following correction, it is necessary to evaluate pronation of the forefoot as revealed by realignment of the hindfoot, which must be corrected, generally by osteotomy of the base of the first metatarsal, at the risk of repercussions caused by intraprosthetic recurrence of the varus deformity.

Sagittal malalignments

Arthrosis with anterior or, more rarely, posterior subluxation of the talus, as a classic contraindication for total ankle arthroplasty (**Fig. 4**), can receive a prosthesis under 2

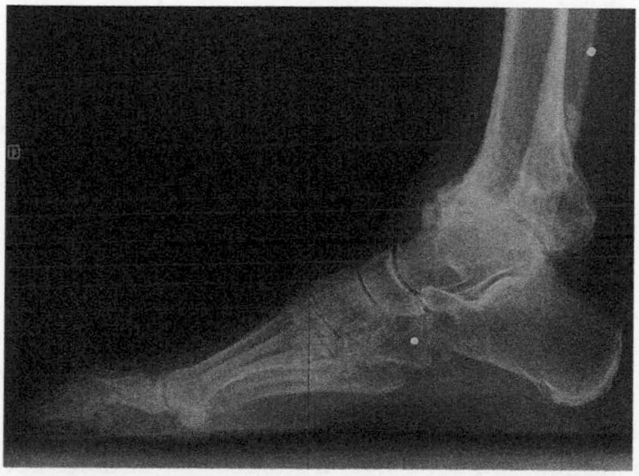

Fig. 4. An anterior subluxation of the foot in relation to the tibia. This subluxation is the sequel to an intraarticular step at the anterior part of the distal tibia, as is frequently caused by trauma (eg, pilon fracture).

conditions: to perform a broad medial and lateral dissection, and to implant a fixed bearing prosthesis to avoid the major risk of polyethylene insert overhang beneath the tibial component.

Severe Stiffness

In these cases, 3 forms of problems can arise: those affecting the capsule, bone, and tendons.

- Capsular problems must always be treated by collateral dissection, medial as described earlier, or lateral in the same manner, but there is never an indication in this situation to perform bipolar dissection. Total posterior capsulectomy is always performed: with obvious caution, it is performed using the tip of a fine knife blade.
- Periarticular ossifications must be treated with the greatest care because of residual conflicting factors. Submalleolar calcifications must be excised at the same time as the lateral dissection. Contact via osteophytic malleolar or talar hypertrophy persisting despite reestablishment of the height by implantation of trial components must be regulated using a rongeur, if not by resection with the oscillating saw. In the same way, osteophytic hypertrophy of the posterior process of the talus, which is likely to cause a conflicting posterior interaction and limitations in plantar flexion, must be corrected using a chisel or a bur to avoid a large bone step at the posterior edge of the talar component.
- Retraction of the Achilles tendon is only evaluated at the end of the dissection, once all the preceding procedures have been performed. It is only in the case of zero dorsal flexion or flexion barely extending beyond the right angle that an extension tenotomy will be performed through 2 percutaneous hemisections, 4 to 5 cm apart (**Fig. 5**). If the immediate result is spectacular, the aftereffects are severe: a loss of range of motion despite early rehabilitation and slightly painful loss of strength are sometimes observed over an extended period. Our indications for Achilles tendon lengthening were initially frequent, but have become rarer.[2]

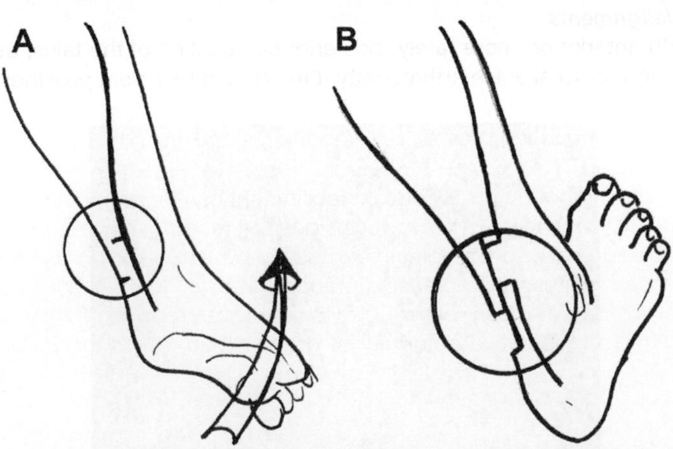

Fig. 5. (*A*) When Achilles tendon lengthening is needed this can be done percutaneously. Short and small stab incisions are done with a scalpel. The distance between the stab incisions averages 3 cm. (*B*) The ankle is gently moved dorsally. One hand feels the Achilles tendon until the fibers start to separate. Care is needed not to force the ankle in too much dorsiflexion because this could result in Achilles tendon rupture.

Muscular Instability

In general, neurologic oot disease is a contraindication to total ankle replacement.[5] However in some cases of peripheral palsy, TAR may be considerd on the condition that an assoiciated tendon tranfer or arthrodesis can restore satisfactory muscular balance in the coronal and sagittal planes.

Deformities of the Calcaneopedal Block and Disorders of the Hindfoot

We have seen the need for correcting residual pronation of the forefoot in varus arthrosis. In a few similar cases, corrective frontal calcaneal osteotomy may be indicated at the same time as the prosthesis. Arthrosis of 1 or several joints of the midtarsal joint line have to be managed in a variable manner.

- When a major deformity exists, necessitating extensive interventions involving dissection, repositioning, and fusion, correction located in the midtarsal joint is an essential prerequisite to the arthroplasty. Prosthetic implantation is a second step, and it is likely that the delay will have to be extended because of the possible risk of talar necrosis (the prosthesis failure factor).
- In the presence of an arthropathy focused torque joint combined with the affliction of the ankle, its contribution to the functional discomfort is called into question. The clinical examination can be assisted by infiltration tests guided radiologically to decide on the initial action.
- A localized and symptomatic affliction of the torque joint can lead to a simultaneous intervention being proposed: talonavicular arthrodesis is easy and is performed by simple extension of the approach, whereas talocalcaneal arthrodesis necessitates an additional, preferably limited, approach, centered on the sinus tarsi. In the 2 cases, strong fixation is recommended to allow, if not weight bearing, at least rehabilitation of the ankle that is not overly delayed.

RESULTS

Implantation of the Salto prosthesis has been performed since 1997. Its advantages are well known but it also has limitations and areas for improvement. Our patients are being followed up regularly, and data collection is performed prospectively in a database dedicated for this purpose.

Survival Curve

Case studies published on the Salto implant are rare because, as in all case studies of ankle prostheses, the low annual number of implants delays publication of the results. Multicentre studies are required, which we undertook in the 3 centers of the implant designers (M. Bonnin, Lyon; J.A. Colombier, Toulouse; Th. Judet, Garches) with publications on a cohort of 98 prostheses and their medium-term then long-term outcomes.[2,6]

The meta-analyses give a good general overview but mix several types of implants: Haddad and colleagues,[7] in a meta-analysis of 852 prostheses, show a survival rate of 77% at 10 years (95% confidence interval [CI] 69–90.8), with 7% of revisions. Gougouglias and colleagues[8] colligated 1105 prostheses from 13 studies and showed large disparities in the survival curves, with survival rates ranging from 67% at 6 years to 95% at 12 years.[9–15]

The data in the registries are of interest because of their exhaustiveness: the Swedish registry [16] reports a survival rate of 62% at 10 years, including all revisions.

The New Zealand registry[17] reports a survival rate of 86% at 5 years. However, the data from the registries is so heterogeneous that their analysis is difficult.

Our initial series, including the first implantations of the Salto prosthesis, shows a survival rate at 10 years of 85% (95% CI 75–95).[2] Schenk and colleagues[18] report a study of 218 Salto (Tornier) prostheses. Survival rate was 86.6% at 5 years (95% CI 82.2–91.1).

From our data, we extracted a more homogenous series, temporally distanced from the first implantations to exclude the learning curve effect. In 1 unpublished continuous series of Salto prostheses implanted at Garches Hospital from November 2001 to September 2003, we included 33 prostheses. At nearly 9 years (114 months), overall survivorship according to Kaplan-Meier is 90.7% with a 5% confidence interval (CI5%) from 80.7 to 100%. Three patients had their implants removed: 2 mobilizations of the talar component caused by secondary talar necrosis and 1 subtalar degradation with cysts. Eight revision surgeries were performed: 5 grafts of cysts, 2 material (osteosynthesis) removals, and 1 arthrolysis. The significance of the learning curve was shown by the Swedish registry[16]: the survival rate at 5 years went from 70% for the first 30 surgeries to 86% for the subsequent patients. With experience, we have fewer revisions for pain associated with malleolar afflictions and 3-mm thick poly inserts are no longer used because they were producing fractures. Current doubts are linked to the occurrence of cysts, which are addressed in another chapter (complications) of this article, and talar necroses. In this last case, we avoid performing subtalar arthrodesis of the joint close to or at the same time as the arthroplasty, to preserve the talar vascularization (**Fig. 6**).

The disparities between the series from the reference centers and the series from less active centers or national registries may be explained by numerous factors: disparities in the results criteria, inclusion criteria, and level of experience of the surgeons. Labek and colleagues[19] state that this type of difference between the clinical series and the registries is also found in the studies of hip and knee prostheses, with differences of up to 300%.

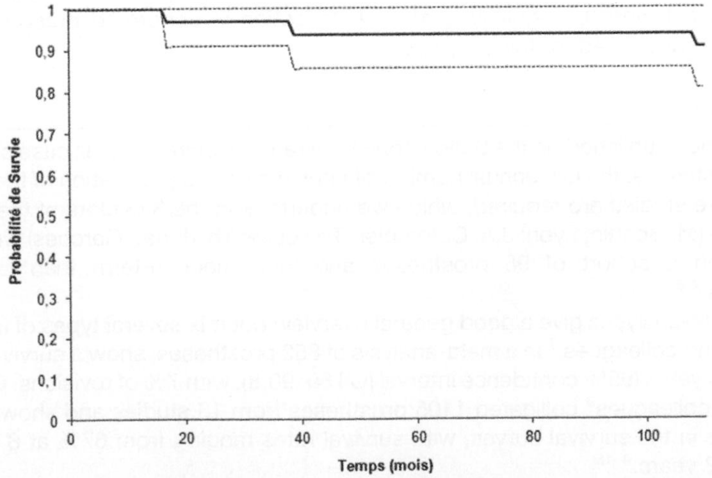

Fig. 6. Kaplan-Meier survival estimate with ablation of the Salto total ankle arthroplasty as the end point, at 109 months: 90.7% (CI 5%: 80.7 to 100).

Clinical Outcome

We evaluate clinical results using the American Orthopaedic Foot and Ankle Score (AOFAS) of the hindfoot.[20] The improvement in the score and in pain is always significant in our series. In our cohort,[2] the score at the mean follow-up of 8.9 years is 79 points. In the Garches study, more recently, this score at a mean follow-up of 7.4 years was 86 points.

Bonnin and colleagues[21] studied the patient activity in a study of 179 Salto prostheses at 53 months of follow-up. The quality of life after an ankle arthroplasty is considered normal in 15.2% of cases, almost normal for 61%, abnormal for 20%, and very abnormal in 4% of cases. Fifty-three percent were able to resume a sport, most frequently men (68.4% vs 53%) and in posttraumatic arthrosis indications. As in the other types of arthroplasties, resumption of activities is more frequent in nonimpact sports (hiking, cycling, swimming, and golf). Impact sports are not advised (jogging, racing, mountain biking, jumps).

Concerning overall mobility, our initial cohort presented at 8.9 years' average follow-up, an average dorsal flexion of 9°, and plantar flexion of 18°. The increase in flexion/extension range of movement (ROM) was also found to be significant by Schenk and colleagues[18]: it improves from 25.2° to 33.1°.

Analysis of Walking

After implantation of a total ankle prosthesis, baropodometry shows normalization of phases and weight pressure while taking steps. Step symmetry returns.[22] The kinematics of the ankle during gait analysis was studied in the gait analysis laboratory of Garches Hospital.[23] Three groups of patients were studied: healthy volunteers, a group of patients with Salto prosthesis, and a group of patients who had undergone ankle fusion. In the group with prostheses, movement of the knee and the hip had improved; in the group that had undergone fusion, movement of the knee at the time of walking was significantly increased. The duration of weight bearing normalizes as well as the rhythm. Step length remains less than the norms. The prosthesis allows gain in gait stability, fluidity, and symmetry.

COMPLICATIONS

Long-term follow-up of ankle prostheses brings to light a number of complications that are specific or difficult to correct depending on the implant and the joint concerned. The total ankle prosthesis does not escape this rule and, apart from minor complications (some considered major), can lead to failure of the implant, necessitating revision.

Among the nonspecific complications this article mentions only alignment faults, infections, and periprosthetic ossifications to elaborate on 3 more specific complications:

Ruptures of the Polyethylene Insert

Ruptures of the polyethylene insert have been observed with 3-mm thick inserts (**Fig. 7**). They are reported more rarely in series from the literature: 8 cases out of 530 in the Swedish registry[16] and no cases in the New Zealand registry.[17] These problems are of normal or premature wear caused by abnormal constraints. Their therapeutic treatment is theoretically simple (change the mobile bearing) but it should be ensured that there are no placement errors inducing mediolateral, rotational, or anterolateral hyperconstraints with problems of overhanging. In some cases exchange and

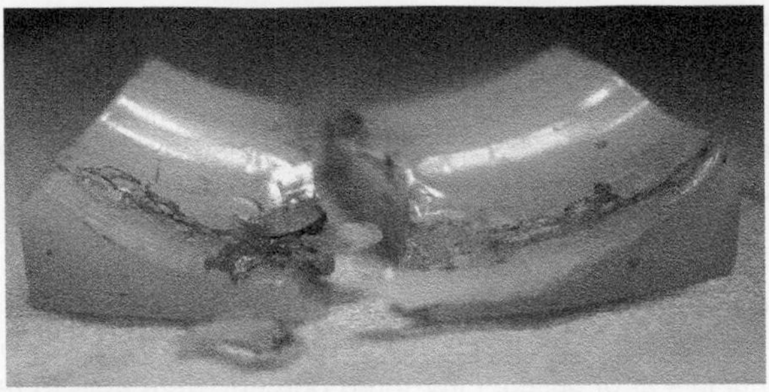

Fig. 7. A fractured polyethylene inlay.

repositioning of 1 or several components of the prosthesis is necessary to avoid a recurrence of the problem.

Unexplained Pain After Total Ankle Arthroplasty

Unexplained pain after total ankle arthroplasty is difficult to analyze. These cases involve painful ankles, with correct articular ROM and with no radiographic abnormalities. They necessitate an additional checkup, primarily a computed tomography (CT) scan to search for talar or tibial cysts, intraarticular bone fragments, conflicting talomalleolar interactions, malrotation, or loosening. Bone scintigraphy with technetium is difficult to interpret because of frequent fixation to the implant. Single-photon emission CT allows more precise location of a zone of hyperactivity. A low-grade infection can likewise be a cause of chronic pain and must be eliminated by a biologic checkup, scintigraphy, and sometimes puncture or a biopsy.

Analysis of this pain is even more complicated because the tibiotalar joint prosthesis functions in synergy with a complex articular chain integrating the subtalar joint and midfoot. In addition, it is surrounded by multiple anatomic structures. Any dysfunction in this articular chain or surrounding structures can be the cause of this pain, making evaluation and treatment difficult.

Osteolytic Cysts

Osteolytic cysts represent the most frequently encountered complication. This phenomenon was reported by Pyevich[24] in 1998 with the Agility prosthesis, describing cases of ballooning osteolysis. Knecht[19] clarified this phenomenon in 2004 with the Agility prosthesis and distinguished 2 types of osteolysis:

Mechanical osteolyses occur in the first months after prosthesis implantation. They reflect micromovements of the tibial implant (associated with a delay in fusion of the tibioperoneal syndesmosis in the case of the Agility prosthesis) and stabilize or regress with time.

Expansive osteolyses appear later, are not always in contact with prosthetic components, and are associated with a reaction to wear particles. Knecht[9] reports 49% mechanical lysis, only 14% of which are progressive, and 15% expansile lysis, 22% of which were progressive over time.

In a study of 200 STAR (Scandinavian Total Ankle Replacement) prostheses, Wood and Deakin[25] described 7 cases of tibial cysts in 2003, then 25 (12.5%), 10 of which were asymptomatic, among the 143 patients evaluated in 2008.[15] Koivu and colleagues[26] recently reported a rate of osteolysis cysts of 31% (cysts $\geq$2 mm) and 21% (cysts $\geq$10 mm) in a study of 130 Ankle Evolutive System (AES) prostheses at 31 months of follow-up. These osteolyses led to 16 revisions among the 27 affected patients. In a study of 50 AES prostheses reviewed at 40 months of follow-up, Besse and colleagues[27] reported 62% of tibial cysts and 43% of talar cysts more than 5 mm in diameter.[27,28]

In our initial cohort of 98 patients, 19 patients presented with 1 or several tibial and/or talar cysts greater than or equal to 5 mm in diameter. Among these patients, 8 received revision surgery for a graft and did not progress and 3 required removal of the prosthesis and fusion. Eight other patients have radiological cysts but are asymptomatic (**Fig. 8**).

The cause of these cysts is still poorly explained and is probably multifactorial.

Small, nonprogressive cysts seem to have a mechanical origin, compared with phenomena of stress shielding or bone remodeling of the distal tibia.[9]

Large cysts seem to be linked to chemical phenomena associated with release of particles caused by wear. Three sources of particles can theoretically be implicated: polyethylene, titanium, and hydroxyapatite.

Release of polyethylene particles following total ankle replacement was authenticated by Kobayashi[29] and Valderrabano[14] who described polyethylene debris in the periarticular tissue in 3 cases of osteolysis. The concentration ($1.02 \pm 0.43 \times 107$/mL) and the average size of wear particles (0.81 ± 0.09 dm) are nevertheless close to those observed in total knee prostheses, which are rarely sources of osteolysis.[20] For Koivu and colleagues,[26] the early stage of osteolyses combined with no significant wear noted on polyethylene explants rules out polyethylene as a possible cause.[26] In our study, a traditional anatomopathologic analysis was performed on products of curettage, and has shown, in a variable manner, birefringent foreign bodies or metallic particles within an inflammatory macrophage reaction. Volumetric wear is not observed in mobile inserts.

In the study of Koivu and colleagues,[26] the level of osteolysis increased after modification of the coating of the AES prosthesis. The risk is multiplied by 3.1 for prostheses with a dual coating (HA and titanium) compared with those with single HA coating on cobalt chrome ($P = .001$).[26] The role of titanium particles is thus discussed by the investigators. The conclusions of Koivu and colleagues[26] nonetheless conflict with those of Wood,[15–25] who reports an improvement in outcomes with the titanium and HA dual coating compared with HA alone, at least in terms of fixation of the prosthetic components.

Titanium particles also present the problem of quality of fixation of the titanium plasma spray onto the cobalt chrome. The criteria and quality of fixation of the titanium

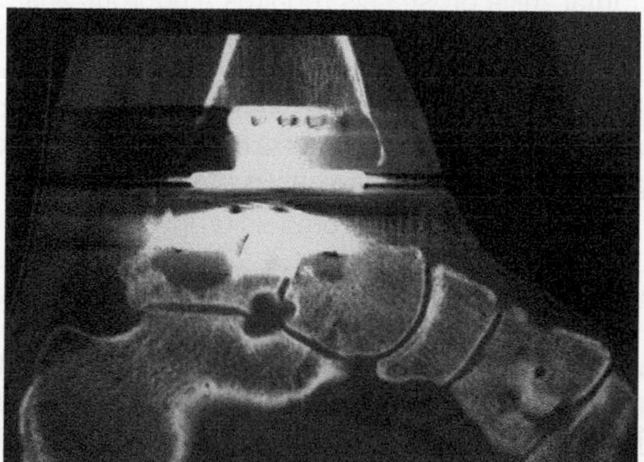

Fig. 8. Example of talar and tibial bone cyst.

layer can vary from manufacturer to manufacturer. The US Food and Drug Administration imposes strict fixation criteria.[30] In Europe, fixation of the calcium hydroxyapatite layer alone is subject to a normative requirement.

The role of hydroxyapatite can likewise be discussed. This type of coating has been successfully used for many years for femoral stems of total hip prostheses[31,32] without osteolysis phenomena having been reported. In contrast, some have reported an increase in the rate of acetabular osteolyses[33,34] and polyethylene wear[35] following the use of implants coated with HA. Resorption of the hydroxyapatite coating can be a source of particle release, generating inflammatory reactions and wear phenomena. This release of particles can be linked to an osteoclastic resorption at the contact with the bone,[33] delamination phenomena with separation from metal, dissolution in the joint fluid at neutral pH, and abrasion in the case of insufficient primary fixation of the implants. The role of the joint fluid is of particular importance. We observed phenomena of osteolysis preferentially in the zones accessible to joint fluid and thus to the debris from wear. Our observation corroborates the concept of the effective joint space, developed by Schmalzried.[36] To isolate the Salto implant keel from the joint fluids, we adapted our surgical technique and, since 2003, we have been systematically closing the anterior tibial window with a bone graft, following impaction of the tibial component.

A large proportion of our failures could be eliminated by our technical improvements (disappearance of stiffness, bone fragments, and unexplained pain), through the use of thicker polyethylene inserts (polyethylene fractures), through better selection of patients (contraindication in the case of bad condition of the skin, cautious indications in the case of doubt concerning the viability of the talus), and through systematic filling with grafts of the anterior cortical tibial window (tibial cysts). A CT scan is now part of our systematic preoperative checkup before total ankle arthroplasty, to precisely localize the osteophytes and/or bone fragments. In addition, meticulous cleaning of the talomalleolar grooves is performed at the time of the intervention to avoid conflicting interactions at this level.

INDICATIONS AND CONTRAINDICATIONS

Total ankle arthroplasty calls for radical treatment of advanced tibiotalar arthrosis, which implies that all the conservative methods are surpassed (osteotomies of joint malunion, supramalleolar osteotomies to correct mortise orientation, arthrolysis, synovectomy).

The indication for total ankle prosthesis requires a rigorous analysis not only of the functional state of the ankle but also of the surrounding joints. Due consideration of the situation and the expectations of the patient is paramount. If the indication either for a prosthesis or arthrodesis can be firmly delayed, on other occasions 1 or the other can be envisaged and it will be necessary to take greater account of patient opinion, duly informed of the advantages and drawbacks of each option.

Decision Tree

Planning ankle arthroplasty is performed in 3 steps that must always be performed sequentially.

The first step consists of confirming the diagnosis of advanced tibiotalar arthrosis and checking that the symptoms are properly linked to this arthrosis. This point may be obvious in the sequelae of an isolated fracture of the tibial pilon, but more delicate where there is damage at several levels, such as fractures of talar body or inflammatory arthropathies. In this case, we carry out invasive diagnostics with Xylocaine for an arthrographic examination. Arthrographic examination enables verification that there is no diffusion of the product into other joints.

The second step consists of verifying that there is no contraindication for the prosthesis. It could be formal and final (advanced osteonecrosis) or just formal and temporary (tendon imbalance awaiting possible transposition). In the case of definitive contraindication, the only therapeutic solution is fusion.

These 2 points being fulfilled, there is an indication for ankle arthroplasty. However, the advantages and disadvantages of this choice should be discussed as the third point.

Confirmation of the Diagnosis of Advanced Tibiotalar Arthrosis

Functional impairment must be major, affecting day-to-day activities within the context of a sedentary lifestyle. For this purpose, we use the AOFAS (Kitaoka and colleagues[20]) of the hindfoot. The causes of joint affliction are classic and can be either of the arthrotic degenerative type or of the inflammatory rheumatic type.

The cause is of interest in technical implementation of the ankle arthroplasty. Arthroses caused by chronic instability necessitate equilibration of the ankle by substantial internal arthrolysis and possibly ligamentoplasty. Arthroses after malunions of the tibia, the pilon, or the malleolus necessitate discussing initial correction of the malunion. The sequelae of a fracture of the talus often include arthrotic subtalar damage. Subtalar fusion before the arthroplasty can be discussed. The same applies with inflammatory arthropathies. Primary correction of a valgus of subtalar origin by arthrodesis of the midtarsal joint or correction of a spontaneous fusion must always precede implantation of ankle prosthesis.

1. Posttraumatic arthrosis: this is the most frequent.
   - i. Fracture affecting the joint (malleolar fracture, fracture of the tibial pilon, fracture of the talus).
   - ii. Ligamental trauma (chronic laxity leading to varus arthrosis). At this stage, the lateral laxity is often compensated and retraction of the medial ligaments occurs.
   - iii. Extra-articular fracture: fracture of the leg with frontal and/or rotational malalignment. In this context, the arthrosis occurs late after the fracture.
2. Inflammatory arthritis (psoriatic rheumatoid arthritis, lupus, scleroderma, hemochromatosis).
3. Idiopathic arthrosis.
4. Partial talar necrosis.
5. Ankle disorders resulting from malformation or from early childhood.

Search for a Contraindication

Given formal indication for surgery of the ankle, it must be verified that there is no absolute contraindication to the prosthesis.

1. Definitive formal contraindications to the ankle prosthesis.
   - a. Contraindications associated with the local state of the ankle.
     - i. Neuropathic joint (Charcot) and major loss of bone stock.
     - ii. Severe avascular necrosis of the talus: as soon as they become significant, necroses of the talar dome give rise to the problem of quality of bone anchorage of the talar component. Small osteochondral lesions are not a contraindication, but in this case must be accompanied by arthrosis.
     - iii. Active or recent infection: prior histories of infection are a contraindication unless they are old and have not shown any recurrence for several years.

iv. Insufficient skin and soft tissue envelope. The skin covering must be satisfactory or restored by prior coverage surgery to allow mobilizing surgery.
v. Relevant unbalanced spastic and neurologic foot contraindications.
vi. Patient unlikely to commit in long-term follow-up.
vii. Peripheral vascular problems.

2. Formal and temporary contraindications to the ankle prosthesis.
   a. Contraindications associated with biomechanical implantation conditions.
      i. Severe, uncorrected axis malalignment: arthroses on deformations of the hindfoot (in the subtalar or calcaneal region) first necessitate a corrective intervention for realignment, most often by arthrodesis. The same applies to major malalignments of the tibia or knee, which should be corrected beforehand.
      ii. For the paralytic foot linked to peripheral nerves, an indication must be raised with caution on the condition that the muscular balance equilibrium in the frontal and sagittal plane are respected or reestablished by a palliative surgery (arthrodesis of the hindfoot or tendon transfer).
      iii. Severe, uncorrected instability of the ligaments of the ankle or hindfoot, especially instability of the medial ligaments.

Third Phase

The relative advantages and disadvantages between arthroplasty and arthrodesis are discussed.

Patient age

Patient age is a controversial subject. There are several opinions: the advantages of a prosthesis in a young patient are that it protects against degradation of the underlying joints, which are well shown in long-term outcomes of arthrodesis. Knowing the risk of wear of the prosthesis, the prosthesis thus serves as an intermediate measure with the aim of postponing arthrodesis as long as possible. In making the decision, it must be considered that, in the case of failure, withdrawal of the prosthesis through arthrodesis, at the cost of a meticulous technique, yields results similar to those of primary arthrodesis. By contrast, a prosthesis can be envisaged in which arthrodesis is poorly tolerated and not susceptible to another intervention to improve the situation, but the technique is delicate and the results are uncertain, and often mediocre.

In contrast, older patients have less intense functional requirements. They put fewer constraints on the prosthesis, further increasing its lifespan. In this context, prosthesis implantation is a definitive treatment.

Stiffness of the other joints

Stiffness of the other joints is a strong argument in favor of the prosthesis. Subtalar and metatarsal disorders, a morphologic cavus foot, or disorders associated with the forefoot (hallux rigidus or anterior metatarsalgia) raise fears concerning poor tolerance of ankle fusion and favor total ankle replacement. Disorders of the overlying knee, or even the lumbar spine, can become decompensated because of disruption of the posterior gait induced by the arthrodesis. The same applies to bilateral lesions, because of the frequent poor functional tolerance of bilateral ankle fusions.

In cases in which the 2 alternatives are equivalent, the opinion of the patient is a determining factor, after the benefits, risks, and uncertainties of each technique have been explained.

Unrealistic expectations of the patient must be identified to properly define the therapeutic management and prevent the patient from being disappointed. The desire to resume sport, in particular impact sport, is not an argument because none of the techniques for prosthesis or arthrodesis can guarantee this. On a more general level, there is the difficulty of responding to patients who present with real discomfort that is objectively compatible with a normal active sedentary life. Neither arthrodesis, which is conceptually imperfect, with functional tolerance that is not always optimal, nor the prosthesis with its brilliant but inconsistent results and its future long-term uncertainties, provides patients with a perfect solution. These cases again point to small remedies, such as improvement in footwear; weight normalization; adaptation of physical and, where possible, professional activities; and therapeutic analgesics.

They illustrate the current limits of the surgery and justify pursuit of studies to improve prosthetic surgery of the ankle.

SUMMARY

Ankle arthroplasty remains a difficult operation in its indication (15%–20% of results remain inadequate in the medium term) and in its implementation, with a considerable learning curve for the surgeon to obtain reproducibility of results. These difficulties are also associated with the ankle environment and situation: tendons, ligaments, subtalar joint, tibial deformities, prior surgery, and causes. The prosthesis constitutes a valuable alternative to arthrodesis, and nowadays it is the therapeutic solution of choice in the treatment of arthrosis of the ankle. With more than 15 years of follow-up, revisions are less frequent, more often allowing conservation of the implant: cyst grafts, poly insert exchange, more or less extended synovectomy, or arthrolyses. In the case of failure, it is reversible and it is easy to move to ankle fusion.

All these factors must encourage the continued replacement of the tibiotalar joint when it is destroyed because the benefits for the symptoms are significant, allowing disabled patients to return to the life of an active sedentary person, if not reasonable sports activity.

Resumption of activity must not be excessive.

Nevertheless, questions remain:

- Concerning anatomoclinical comparison, there is not always a perfect correlation between the radiographic images and the quality of the results obtained.
- Concerning projected aspects in the light of ankle arthrosis to evaluate the quality of the result that can be expected, it is still difficult to draw up a precise profile of the ideal patient for ankle arthroplasty.
- On the aspect of radiographic development, the appearance over time of modifications to the bone-prosthesis interface with formation of tibial, but also talar, cysts suggest numerous questions regarding the long-term survival of these implants. Their determination, frequency, and ability to evolve are the subject of ongoing studies.

This type of surgery is still young, with few evaluations being available beyond 10 years. In contrast with the knee or the hip, ankle arthroplasty it is still immature and justifies evaluation studies and research as much on the concepts as on the materials.

Constant development of new biomaterials would also have to be applied logically in total ankle arthroplasty. This joint is particularly constrained and presents particular challenges in fixation of implants and ability to support wear. Progress toward polyethylene or stronger implant sliding surfaces that are more resistant to wear will be welcome once they are duly validated. This burdened environment can also give rise to development of implants that are more intimately integrated into the bone tissue, at the attachment level and at the level of load transmission, as soon as the emerging technologies for the materials and manufacturing techniques become accessible to the medical domain.

For the ankle, the planning, orientation, and precision of bone cuts require significant technical competency with conventional tools. Developments in this field are keys to a broader dissemination of the total ankle arthroplasty.

The accumulated follow-up of ankle prostheses should also give rise to the development of specific revision solutions.

REFERENCES

1. Besse JL, Colombier JA, Asencio J, et al, l'AFCP. Total ankle arthroplasty in France [review article]. Orthop Traumatol Surg Res 2010;96(3):291–303.
2. Bonnin M, Gaudot F, Laurent JR, et al. The Salto total ankle arthroplasty: survivorship and analysis of failures at 7 to 11 years. Clin Orthop Relat Res 2011;469(1): 225–36.
3. Trincat S, Kouyoumdjian P, Asencio G. Total ankle arthroplasty and coronal plane deformities. Orthop Traumatol Surg Res 2012;98(1):75–84.
4. Ryssman D, Myerson MS. Surgical strategies: the management of varus ankle deformity with joint replacement. Foot Ankle Int 2011;32(2):217–24.
5. Thermann H, Gavriilidis I, Longo UG, et al. Total ankle arthroplasty and tibialis posterior tendon transfer for ankle osteoarthritis and drop foot deformity. Foot Ankle Surg 2011;17(3):203–6.
6. Bonnin M, Judet T, Colombier JA, et al. Midterm results of the Salto total ankle prosthesis. Clin Orthop Relat Res 2004;424:6–18.
7. Haddad SL, Coetzee JC, Estok R, et al. Intermediate and long-term outcomes of total ankle arthroplasty and ankle arthrodesis: a systematic review of the literature. J Bone Joint Surg Am 2007;89:1899–905.
8. Gougoulias N, Khanna A, Maffulli N. How successful are current ankle replacements?: a systematic review of the literature. Clin Orthop Relat Res 2010;468: 199–208.
9. Knecht SI, Estin M, Callaghan JJ, et al. The Agility total ankle arthroplasty: seven to sixteen-year follow-up. J Bone Joint Surg Am 2004;86:1161–71.
10. Hurowitz B, Anderson T, Montgomery F, et al. Uncemented STAR total ankle prostheses: three to eight-year follow-up of fifty-one consecutive ankles. J Bone Joint Surg Am 2003;85:1321–9.
11. Buechel FF Sr, Buechel FF Jr, Pappas MJ. Twenty-year evaluation of cementless mobile-bearing total ankle replacements. Clin Orthop Relat Res 2004;424:19–26.
12. Kofoed H. Scandinavian total ankle replacement (STAR). Clin Orthop Relat Res 2004;424:73–9.
13. San Giovanni TP, Keblish DJ, Thomas WH, et al. Eight-year results of a minimally constrained total ankle arthroplasty. Foot Ankle Int 2006;27:418–26, 31.
14. Valderrabano V, Hintermann B, Dick W. Scandinavian total ankle replacement: a 3.7-year average followup of 65 patients. Clin Orthop Relat Res 2004;424: 47–56, 32.
15. Wood PL, Prem H, Sutton C. Total ankle replacement: medium-term results in 200 Scandinavian total ankle replacements. J Bone Joint Surg Br 2008;90:605–9.

16. Henricson A, Skoog A, Carlsson A. The Swedish ankle arthroplasty register: an analysis of 531 arthroplasties between 1993 and 2005. Acta Orthop 2007; 78(5):569–74.
17. Hosman AH, Mason RB, Hobbs T, et al. A New Zealand National Joint Registry review of 202 total ankle replacements followed for up to 6 years. Acta Orthop 2007;78(5):584–91.
18. Schenk K, Lieske S, John M, et al. Prospective study of a cementless, mobile-bearing, third generation total ankle prosthesis. Foot Ankle Int 2011;32(8):755–63.
19. Labek G, Klaus H, Schlichtherle R, et al. Revision rates after total ankle arthroplasty in sample-based clinical studies and national registries. Foot Ankle Int 2011;32(8):740–5.
20. Kitaoka HB, Alexander IJ, Adelaar RS, et al. Clinical rating systems for the ankle-hindfoot, midfoot, hallux, and lesser toes. Foot Ankle Int 1994;15(7):349–53.
21. Bonnin MP, Laurent JR, Casillas M. Ankle function and sports activity after total ankle arthroplasty. Foot Ankle Int 2009;30(10):933–44.
22. Zerahn B, Kofoed H. Bone mineral density, gait analysis, and patient satisfaction, before and after ankle arthroplasty. Foot Ankle Int 2004;25(4):208–14.
23. Piriou P, Culpan P, Mullins M, et al. Ankle replacement versus arthrodesis: a comparative gait analysis study. Foot Ankle Int 2008;29(1):3–9.
24. Pyevich MT, Saltzman CL, Callaghan JJ, et al. Total ankle arthroplasty: a unique design. Two to twelve-year follow-up. J Bone Joint Surg Am 1998;80:1410–20.
25. Wood PL, Deakin S. Total ankle replacement. The results in 200 ankles. J Bone Joint Surg Br 2003;85(3):334–41.
26. Koivu H, Kohonen I, Sipola E, et al. Severe periprosthetic osteolytic lesions after the ankle evolutive system total ankle replacement. J Bone Joint Surg Br 2009; 91(7):907–14.
27. Besse JL, Brito N, Lienhart C. Clinical evaluation and radiographic assessment of bone lysis of the AES total ankle replacement. Foot Ankle Int 2009;10:964–75.
28. Hanna RS, Haddad SL, Lazarus ML. Evaluation of periprosthetic lucency after total ankle arthroplasty: helical CT versus conventional radiography. Foot Ankle Int 2007;28:921–6.
29. Kobayashi A, Minoda Y, Kadoya Y, et al. Ankle arthroplasties generate wear particles similar to knee arthroplasties. Clin Orthop Relat Res 2004;424:69–72.
30. Food and Drug Administration. Available at: http://www.fda.gov/downloads/MedicalDevices/DeviceRegulationandGuidance/GuidanceDocuments/ucm107699.pdf.
31. Froimson MI, Garino J, Machenaud A, et al. Minimum 10-year results of a tapered, titanium, hydroxyapatite-coated hip stem: an independent review. J Arthroplasty 2007;22(1):1–7.
32. Reikerås O, Gunderson RB. Excellent results of HA coating on a grit-blasted stem: 245 patients followed for 8-12 years. Acta Orthop Scand 2003;74(2):140–5.
33. Bauer TW. Severe osteolysis after third-body wear due to hydroxyapatite particles from acetabular cup coating. J Bone Joint Surg Br 1998;80(4):745.
34. Duffy P, Sher JL, Partington PF. Premature wear and osteolysis in an HA-coated, uncemented total hip arthroplasty. J Bone Joint Surg Br 2004;86(1):34–8.
35. Røkkum M, Reigstad A, Johansson CB. HA particles can be released from well-fixed HA-coated stems: histopathology of biopsies from 20 hips 2-8 years after implantation. Acta Orthop Scand 2002;73(3):298–306.
36. Schmalzried TP, Jasty M, Harris WH. Periprosthetic bone loss in total hip arthroplasty. Polyethylene wear debris and the concept of the effective joint space. J Bone Joint Surg Am 1992;74:849–63.

Total Ankle Replacement Using HINTEGRA, an Unconstrained, Three-Component System

Surgical Technique and Pitfalls

Alexej Barg, MD[a,b,*], Markus Knupp, MD[a], Heath B. Henninger, PhD[b], Lukas Zwicky, MSc[a], Beat Hintermann, MD[a]

KEYWORDS

- Total ankle replacement • Three-component total ankle prosthesis
- HINTEGRA prosthesis • Valgus osteoarthritic ankle • Varus osteoarthritic ankle
- Functional outcome

KEY POINTS

- Total ankle replacement (TAR) has become a valuable treatment option in patients with end-stage ankle osteoarthritis (OA).
- One popular 3-component system, the HINTEGRA TAR, is an unconstrained system that provides inversion-eversion stability.
- Both primary (degenerative) and posttraumatic OA are important indicators for TAR, but the ankle joint is rarely affected by primary OA.

INDICATIONS FOR TOTAL ANKLE REPLACEMENT

Both primary (degenerative) and posttraumatic osteoarthritis (OA) are important indicators for total ankle replacement (TAR), but the ankle joint is rarely affected by primary OA. Clinical and epidemiologic studies revealed that previous trauma is the most common origin of ankle OA (**Fig. 1**).[1–19] Although rotational ankle fractures with consecutive cartilage damage were identified as the most common reason for

One or more of the authors (B.H.) has received royalties from Integra. All royalties that the senior author (B.H.) received were given to the research fund at the institution were the work was performed (Kantonsspital Liestal, Switzerland).
[a] Clinic of Orthopaedic Surgery, Kantonsspital Liestal, Rheinstrasse 26, Liestal CH-4410, Switzerland; [b] Harold K. Dunn Orthopaedic Research Laboratory, University Orthopaedic Center, University of Utah, 590 Wakara Way, Salt Lake City, UT 84108, USA
* Corresponding author.
E-mail address: alexejbarg@mail.ru

Foot Ankle Clin N Am 17 (2012) 607–635
http://dx.doi.org/10.1016/j.fcl.2012.08.006

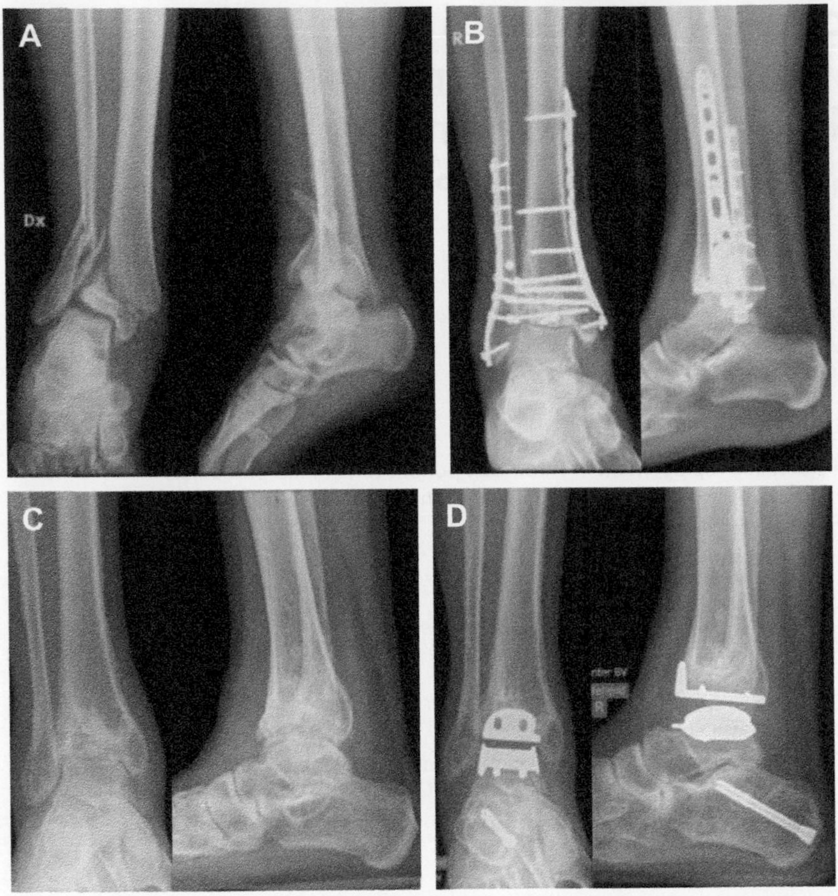

Fig. 1. (*A*) Anteroposterior and lateral radiographs of a 24-year-old man with displaced lower leg fracture sustained from a fall down stairs. (*B*) Weight-bearing radiographs show complete fracture healing after open reduction and internal fixation 10 months postoperatively. (*C*) Hardware was removed 23 months postoperatively. Despite the anatomic reduction and uneventful healing of the fracture, significant degenerative changes of the tibiotalar joint are visible. (*D*) All conservative treatment attempts were unsuccessful, and therefore 32 months after the accident, TAR using HINTEGRA was performed.

posttraumatic ankle OA,[19] repetitive ligament injuries may play a crucial role in joint degeneration (ligamentous posttraumatic ankle OA).[20] Other common indications for TAR are systemic (rheumatoid) arthritis[21–23] and secondary OA. Secondary OA has been found to be associated with underlying diseases such as hemophilia,[24] hereditary hemochromatosis,[25] gout,[26] postinfectious arthritis, and avascular talar necrosis.

Patients with bilateral ankle OA are good candidates for TAR because bilateral ankle fusion may not be optimal in this patient cohort, given its detrimental influence on gait and functional results.[27–29]

TAR has additional indications, like the salvage of failed primary procedures. Regarding the salvage of failed primary TAR, 1 critical issue is the quality and amount of remaining bone stock to ensure long-term stability of revision components.[30] If the residual bone stock is not sufficient, ankle fusion should be performed.[31–35] Another special indication for TAR is the salvage of nonunion or malunion of previous ankle fusion.[36–38] Taking down an ankle fusion, and its conversion to TAR, is a technically demanding procedure, which should be performed only if bone stock is sufficient and soft tissue conditions are appropriate.[39] If performed by an experienced foot and ankle surgeon, this procedure shows promising midterm results with low intraoperative and postoperative complication rates.[38]

CONTRAINDICATIONS FOR TAR

The absolute contraindications for TAR are the following[8,40,41]: acute or chronic infections, avascular necrosis of more than one-third of the talus, neuromuscular disorders, neuroarthropathy (Charcot arthropathy of the midfoot or hindfoot), and diabetic syndrome with polyneuropathy. Patients with unmanageable instability or malalignment, which cannot be sufficiently addressed by additional procedures (eg, corrective osteotomies[42]), should not be considered for TAR. High demand for physical activities (eg, contact sports, jumping) is also a contraindication. Suspected or documented metal allergy/intolerance is rare; however, these patients should be excluded preoperatively.

The relative contraindications for TAR are the following[8,40,41]: severe osteoporosis, immunosuppressive therapy, and diabetic syndrome without polyneuropathy. Patients with increased demands for physical activities (eg, jogging, tennis, downhill skiing) should be informed about possible prosthesis failure because of increased wear and potential for a higher rate of aseptic loosening.[43,44]

IDEAL CANDIDATE FOR TAR

Based on our clinical experience, the ideal candidate for TAR

- is middle-aged or older
- is reasonably mobile
- has no significant comorbidities
- has low demands for physical activities (eg, hiking, swimming, biking, golfing)
- is not obese/overweight (normal or low body mass index, calculated as weight in kilograms divided by the square of height in meters; however, obesity is not a contraindication for TAR[45])
- has good bone stock
- has well-aligned and stable hindfoot
- has good soft tissue condition (eg, no previous surgeries of the foot/ankle)
- has no neurovascular impairment of the lower extremity

PREOPERATIVE PLANNING

Clinical Examination

First, all previous medical (surgery) reports and imaging data are collected and carefully analyzed. Second, careful assessment of the patient's history is performed, with specific address of the following aspects: pain, limitations in daily activities, sports activities, and current and previous treatments. Patients with any contraindications are excluded. If necessary, a consultation in neurology or internal medicine is performed before planning of surgery.

The routine physical examination includes careful inspection of the foot and ankle while walking and standing, with special attention given to obvious deformities and the skin and soft tissue condition. Hindfoot stability is assessed manually with the patient sitting. Ankle alignment is assessed with the patient standing.

Ankle range of motion is determined with a goniometer placed along the lateral border of the leg and foot.[3,46] All goniometer measurements are performed in the weight-bearing position, comparable with the method described by Lindsjö and colleagues.[47]

Radiographic Evaluation

Radiographic evaluation of affected ankles is performed using weight-bearing radiographs, including anteroposterior views of the foot and ankle and a lateral view of the foot. Only weight-bearing radiographs should be used for evaluation of foot and ankle alignment because nonweight-bearing radiographs are often misleading.[48–50] Furthermore, the standing position standardizes the radiograph technique, allowing more reliable comparison between preoperative and postoperative radiographs. The supramalleolar ankle alignment (**Fig. 2**) should be assessed in coronal and sagittal planes by measurement of the medial distal tibial angle and anterior distal tibial angle (**Fig. 3**), respectively.[51,52] The medial distal tibial angle has been measured to be 92.4 $\pm$ 3.1° (range 88–100°) in a radiographic study[51] and 93.3 $\pm$ 3.2° (range 88–100°) in a cadaver study.[51,53] The measurement of the medial distal tibial angle depends on radiograph technique; it is not the same on whole leg images and mortise views of the ankle.[54] The anterior distal tibial angle has been measured to be 83.0 $\pm$ 3.6° (range 76–97°).[52] The Saltzman view should be used to assess the inframalleolar alignment.[55] In patients with degenerative changes of the adjacent joints, single-photon emission computed tomography (SPECT) may help to evaluate the morphologic changes and their biological activities.[56,57] We do not recommend the routine use of magnetic resonance imaging (MRI) in patients with ankle OA. However, MRI may be helpful to assess injuries or morphologic changes of ligament structures and tendons, and to evaluate the localization and degree of avascular necrosis of talus or tibia.[58]

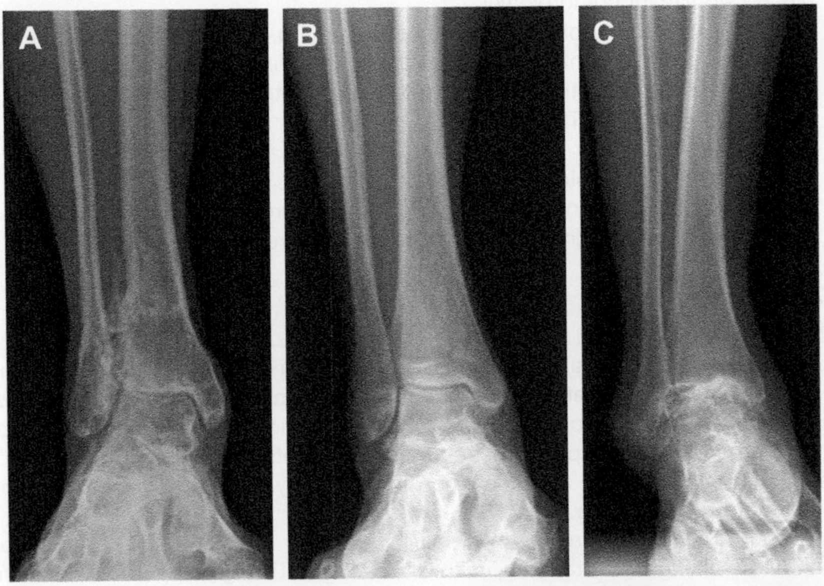

Fig. 2. Weight-bearing anteroposterior ankle radiographs showing (*A*) valgus alignment, (*B*) normal alignment, and (*C*) varus alignment in the coronal plane.

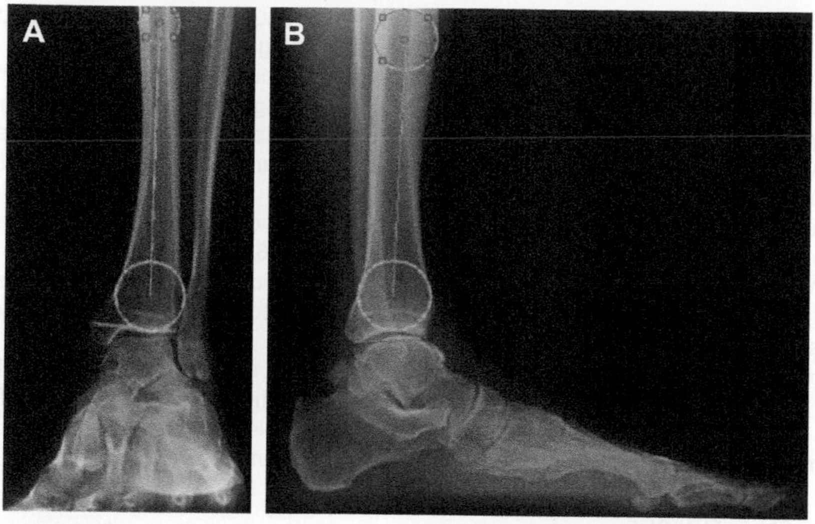

Fig. 3. Weight-bearing (*A*) anteroposterior and (*B*) lateral views of the ankle of a 51-year-old man showing the measurement of the medial distal tibial angle[54] (in this case 87°) and the measurement of anterior distal tibial angle[52] (in this case 84°).

HINTEGRA TOTAL ANKLE PROSTHESIS

The HINTEGRA total ankle prosthesis was designed and developed in 2000 by Dr B. Hintermann (Basel, Switzerland), Dr G. Dereymaeker (Pellenberg, Belgium), Dr R. Viladot (Barcelona, Spain), and Dr P. Diebold (Maxeville, France).[59] The HINTEGRA prosthesis is an unconstrained, 3-component system that provides high inversion/eversion stability.[3,40,59] Since its introduction in 2000, there have been 3 prosthesis generations (**Fig. 4**): (1) first-generation with single hydroxyapatite coating (May 2000–April 2001); (2) second-generation with 200 μm porous cobalt-chromium

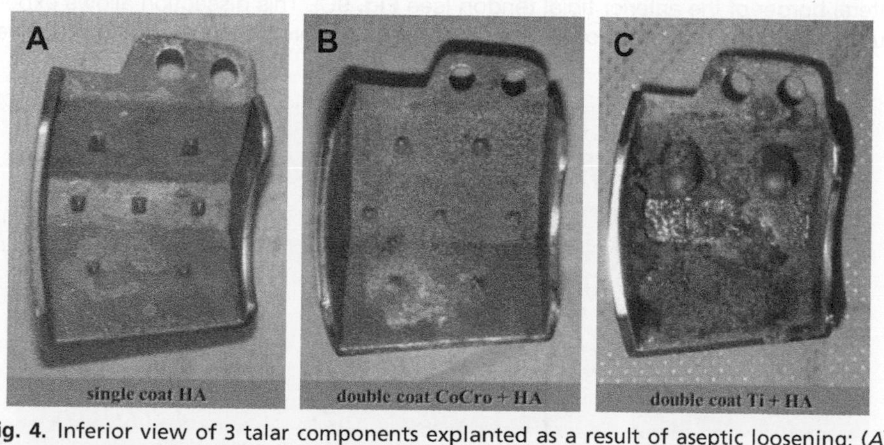

Fig. 4. Inferior view of 3 talar components explanted as a result of aseptic loosening: (*A*) first-generation with single hydroxyapatite coating; (*B*) second-generation with 200 μm porous cobalt-chromium with double hydroxyapatite coating; (*C*) third-generation with 200 μm titanium with double hydroxyapatite coating.

with double hydroxyapatite coating (May 2001–May 2003); and (3) third-generation with 200 μm titanium with double hydroxyapatite coating (since May 2003).

In the current (third) generation, the tibial component consists of a flat, 4-mm-thick loading plate, with 6 pyramidal peaks against the tibia (**Fig. 5**). It has an anterior shield for appropriate contact with anterior border of the distal tibia, including 2 oval holes for screw fixation (in most cases, screw fixation is not required). The anatomically sized surfaces ensure optimal bone-prosthesis contact and require only minimal bone resection of 2 to 3 mm. The talar component is anatomically shaped, with a conical form, with a smaller radius medially than laterally (**Fig. 6**A, B). It has 2 2.5-mm rims on the medial and lateral sides, which ensure stable position of the polyethylene insert. Two pegs (see **Fig. 6**A) facilitate the insertion of the talar component and provide additional stability.

The polyethylene insert (ultrahigh molecular weight) has a flat surface on the tibial side and a concave surface that perfectly matches the talar prosthesis surface (**Fig. 7**). It has a minimum thickness of 5 mm and is available in different sizes. The insert position aligns well with the longitudinal tibial axis and remains stable over time.[60]

SURGICAL TECHNIQUE

Anesthesia and Patient Positioning

General or regional anesthesia can be used for TAR. The patient is placed in a supine position with the feet on the edge of the table (**Fig. 8**). The ipsilateral back of the patient is lifted until a strictly upward position of the whole lower extremity is obtained. A pneumatic tourniquet is applied on the ipsilateral thigh. In most cases, a pressure of 320 mm Hg is sufficient, and total tourniquet time of 2 hours should not be exceeded. If significant deformity is to be corrected, the unaffected lower extremity should also be draped.

Surgical Approach

A standard anterior ankle approach is used for TAR (**Fig. 9**A, B).[3,8] An anterior longitudinal incision (10–14 cm) is made to expose the retinaculum, which is thickening of the deep fascia above the ankle, running from tibia to fibula.[61,62] After the anterior tibial tendon is identified, sharp dissection of the retinaculum is performed along the lateral border of the anterior tibial tendon (see **Fig. 9**C). This dissection allows exposure of the anterior aspect of the distal tibia. During preparation of the soft tissue

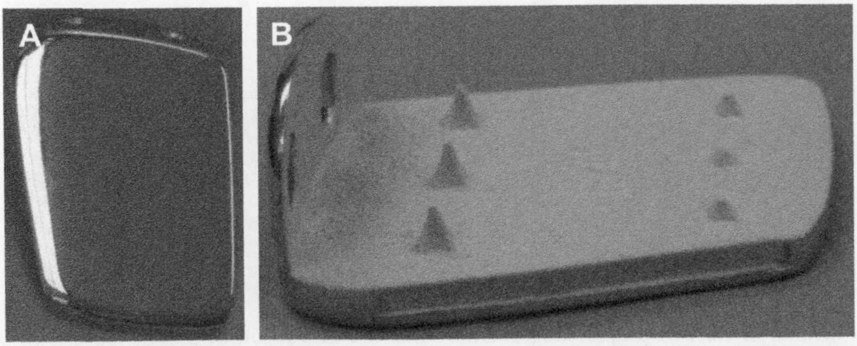

Fig. 5. (*A*) Inferior and (*B*) lateral-superior view of the tibial component of HINTEGRA total ankle prosthesis. The tibial component is anatomically shaped, with 6 pyramidal peaks on the flat surface, double-coated with hydroxyapatite.

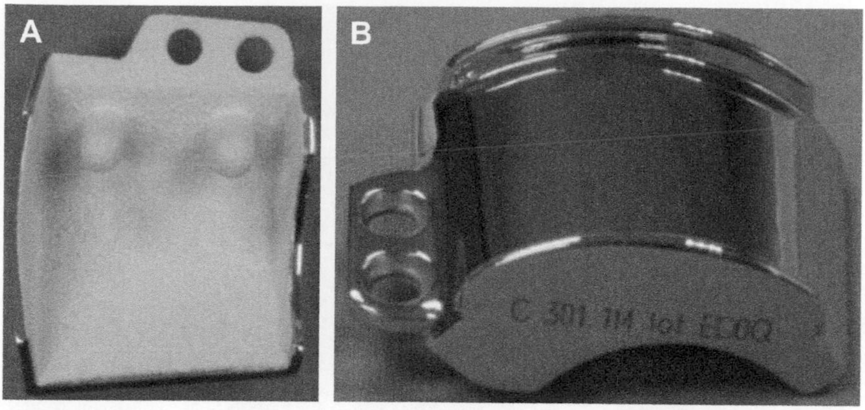

Fig. 6. (*A*) Inferior and (*B*) lateral-superior view of the talar component of HINTEGRA total ankle prosthesis. The talar component is conical, with 2 pegs on the inferior surface, and double-coated with hydroxyapatite.

mantle, special attention is paid to the tibialis anterior vascular bundle, which is localized behind the extensor hallucis longus or between the extensor hallucis longus and the extensor digitorum longus.[63] After the ankle joint is sufficiently exposed, capsulotomy and capsulectomy are performed (**Fig. 10**A). A self-retaining retractor is applied to control the soft tissue mantle; skin hooks should not be used so as not to disturb wound healing. Osteophytes on the tibia (especially on the anterolateral aspect) and on the talar neck should be removed; however, the bone cortex should not be destroyed (see **Fig. 10**B, C).

Tibial Preparation

First, the tibial cutting block should be aligned using the following anatomic landmarks: the tibial tuberosity (or the anterior iliac crest in patients with significant lower leg deformities) as the proximal reference and the middle of the anterior border of the tibiotalar joint as the distal reference (**Fig. 11**). The natural slope of the tibial plafond,

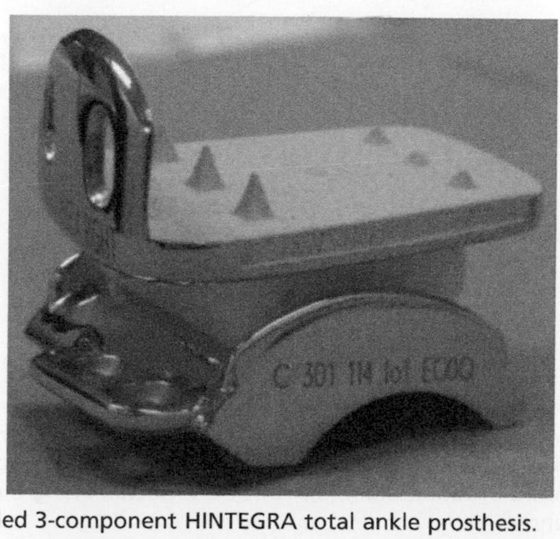

Fig. 7. The assembled 3-component HINTEGRA total ankle prosthesis.

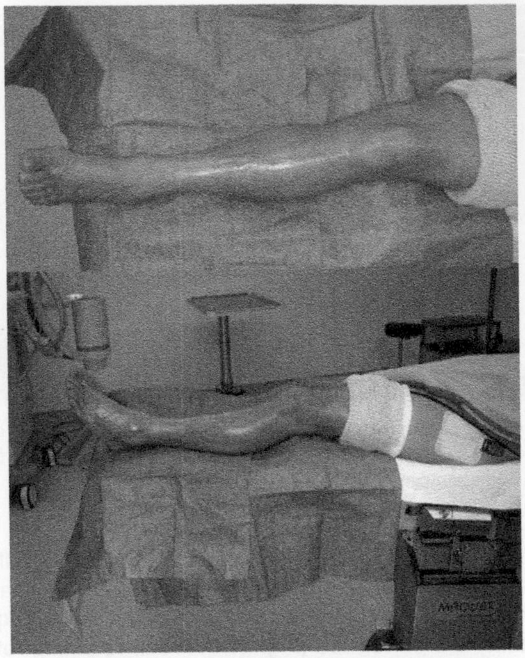

Fig. 8. Patient in supine position with the feet on the edge of the table.

approximately 2° to 4°, should be considered. After final adjustments in sagittal and frontal planes are made, the proximal part of the tibial cutting block should be fixed by 2 pins. Then, resection height should be adjusted; usually no more than 2 to 3 mm of the tibial plafond should be resected. In ankles with varus deformity, more tibial resection should be performed, whereas in patients with valgus deformity or significant ligamental laxity, less bone resection is advised. Regarding rotational adjustment, the medial surface of the tibial resection block should be parallel to the medial surface of the talus. This position may help to avoid intraoperative malleolar

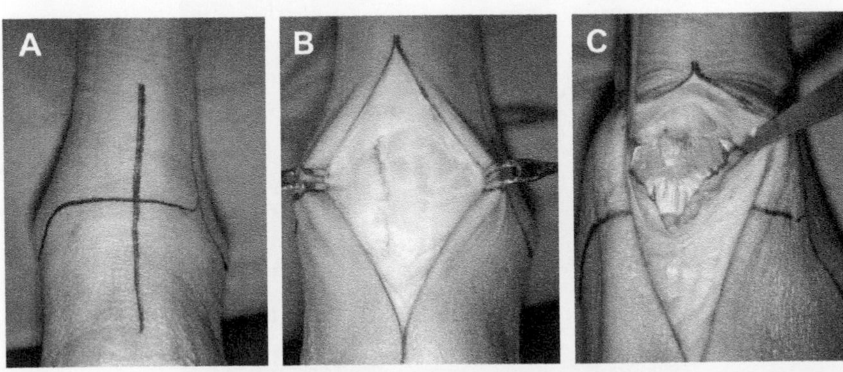

Fig. 9. Standard anterior ankle approach for TAR. (*A*) Landmarks for planning of approach: medial and lateral malleoli and tibiotalar joint line. (*B*) Anterior longitudinal incision up to 12 cm long for exposure of retinaculum (*C*), which is dissected along the lateral border of the anterior tibial tendon.

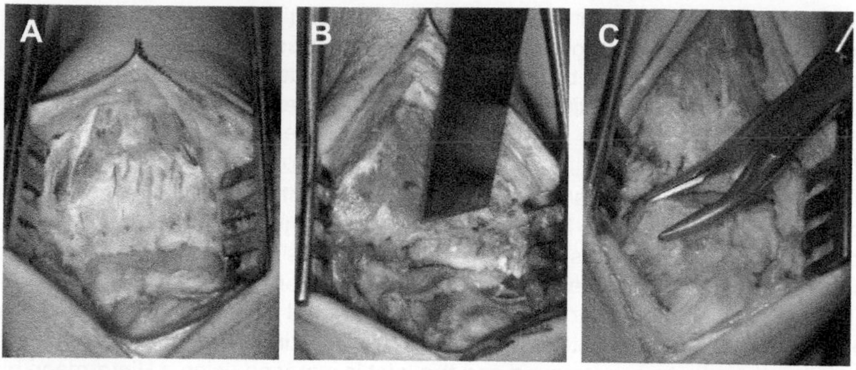

Fig. 10. (*A*) Ankle joint is exposed and capsulotomy/capsulectomy is performed and a self-retaining retractor is applied to protect the soft tissues. Osteophytes (*B*) on the tibia and (*C*) on the talar neck are removed.

fractures caused by the oscillating saw blade. After the position of the tibial resection block is adjusted and fixed, the tibial cutting guide is placed into the cutting block. The cut is performed through the cutting slot and attention is paid to avoid any injuries to the malleoli. Malleolar fractures have been reported as a common intraoperative complication, with a prevalence as high as 10%.[64–66] We suggest prophylactic pinning of the malleoli. After the tibial cut is performed, a reciprocating saw should be used to finalize the cuts, particularly for the vertical cut on the medial side. Careful

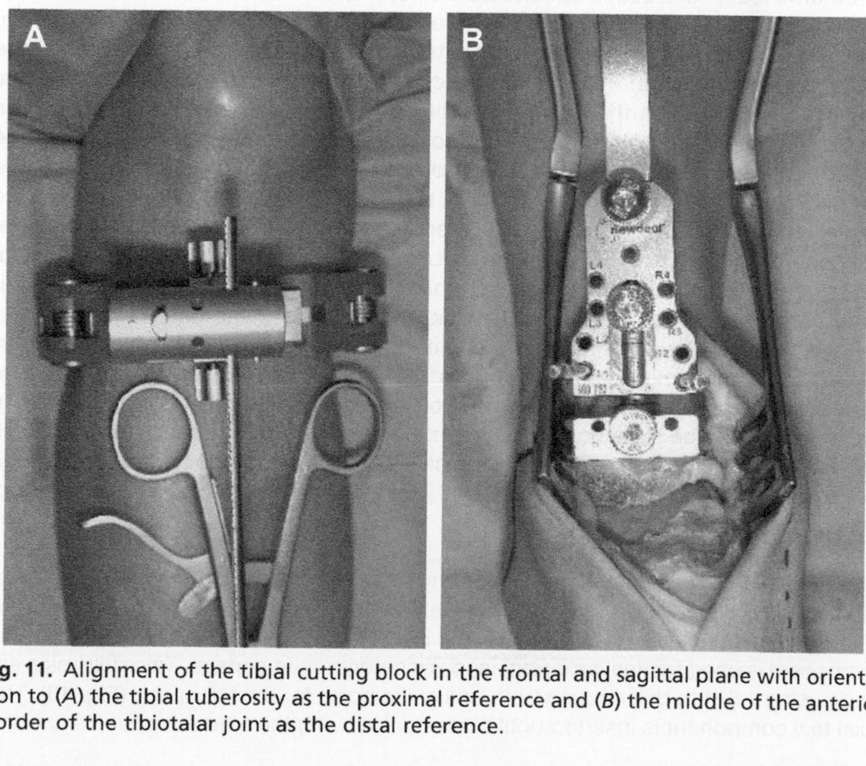

Fig. 11. Alignment of the tibial cutting block in the frontal and sagittal plane with orientation to (*A*) the tibial tuberosity as the proximal reference and (*B*) the middle of the anterior border of the tibiotalar joint as the distal reference.

debridement of the posterior capsule is performed and ossifications are removed if necessary. A measuring gauge is used to determine the size of the tibial component. In cases in which the anterior border of the tibia is projected between 2 markers on the gauge, the bigger size should be selected to avoid undersizing the tibial component.

Talar Preparation

The talar resection block is placed into the tibial cutting block. To achieve the proper tension of collateral ligaments of the ankle, the talar resection should be moved distally as much as possible. All distractors and spreaders should be removed to avoid any influence on foot/ankle position. Once the foot is held in a neutral position, the talar resection block is fixed by 2 pins. First, the talar dome is cut through the cutting slot using an oscillating saw. Both the tibial and talar resection blocks are removed and the joint is exposed using a Hintermann distractor. In order to achieve physiologic range of motion (especially dorsiflexion), posterior debridement is performed until fatty tissue and tendon structures are visible. The 12-mm-thick spacer is inserted into the joint. This measurement corresponds to the thickness of the tibial and talar prosthesis components and the insert with minimum thickness of 5 mm. The foot and ankle should be held in a neutral position and the following aspects should be checked: (1) whether an appropriate amount of bone has been removed; (2) whether the hindfoot alignment; and (3) whether stability is appropriate. When the spacer cannot be inserted properly without pressure, contracture of the remaining posterior capsule should be checked and if necessary addressed by careful debridement. Otherwise, additional bony resection should be performed (mostly on the tibial side using the tibial resection block). If hindfoot alignment is not appropriate, the origin of deformity should be determined. A corrective cut should be performed only in cases in which associated deformities (eg, valgus or varus heel position) can be excluded. A corrective cut can be performed on the tibial side after angular position is corrected. In cases with obvious ligamental instability, a thicker inlay may be used to increase the intrinsic stability. When the desired stability cannot be achieved, a release of the contralateral ligament, or ligament reconstruction on the affected side, should be performed. The ligament reconstruction procedure should be performed after the insertion of the definitive implants (and only if the instability still persists). The medial side of the talus is used as the reference for determining the size of the talar resection block: approximately 2 mm of bone is removed from the medial side of the talus. The size of the talar component should not be different from the previously determined tibial component by more than 1 size. The final talar resection block is fixed by short pins (**Fig. 12**). First, posterior resection of the talus is performed using an oscillating saw, followed by medial and lateral resections of the talus. The anterior slot of the talar resection block is used for the anterior resection of the talus. After the resection block is removed, all cuts are finalized using a chisel. The medial and lateral gutters should be cleaned using a rongeur and, if necessary, the remaining ossifications and posterior joint capsule removed.

Final Surface Preparation

Tibial and talar surfaces are checked for any cysts, which must be carefully removed, debrided, and filled with cancellous bone left over from previous bone cuts. The sclerotic areas of the prepared surfaces should be drilled with a 2.0-mm drill. The talar trial component is used for final preparation of the anterior talar surface. Two drill holes are made using 4.5-mm drill through both drill guide holes for the talar pegs (**Fig. 13**). The tibial trial component is inserted until close contact with the medial malleolus and the

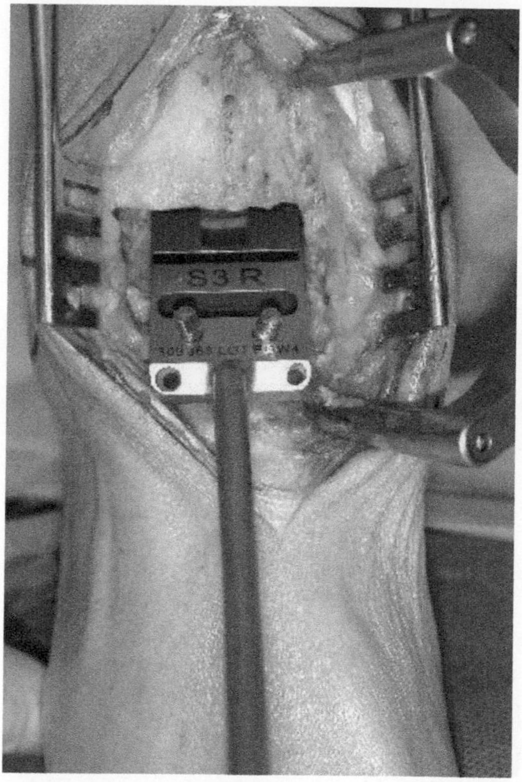

Fig. 12. Pin fixation of the talar resection block.

anterior surface of tibia is achieved. If necessary, the anterior border of the tibia should be smoothed with an oscillating saw or rongeur. After both metallic trial components are inserted, the 5-mm trial inlay is placed and all distractors are released. Soft tissue tension can be checked and if necessary a thicker trial inlay (7-mm or 9-mm inlay) is inserted. With all 3 components in place, fluoroscopy is then used to verify the component position with regard to proper fit and alignment (eg, anteroposterior offset ratio[46,60]) of prosthesis components to the prepared joint surfaces.

Insertion of Final Prosthesis Components

The talar component is inserted by placing the 2 pegs into the 2 drilled holes on the talar side. Talar insertion is performed with a press-fit technique using a hammer and special impactor. Then the tibial component is inserted along the medial malleolus until the proper contact between the component shield and anterior border of the tibia is achieved. The inlay with the same size as the talar component is inserted (**Fig. 14**). All distractors are removed, and the stability and motion of the ankle are checked (**Fig. 15**). We typically do not recommend screw fixation on the tibial or talar side if the initial stability of the prosthesis is sufficient. The position of the prosthesis is checked and documented using fluoroscopy. If any remaining bony fragments or osteophytes are visible, they should be removed to avoid future pain or range-of-motion restriction. Wound closure is performed sequentially (**Fig. 16**). We use drainage without suction. Soft wound dressing is used to avoid any pressure so as not to compromise wound healing (**Fig. 17**). A splint is used to keep the foot in a neutral position (**Fig. 18**).

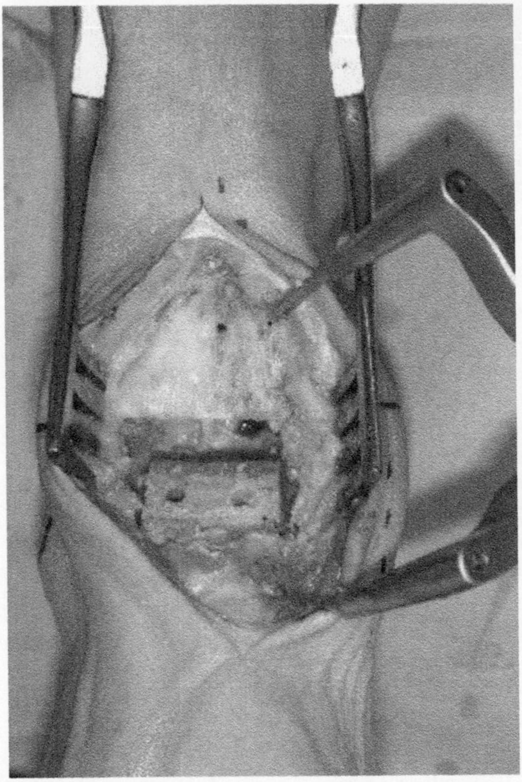

Fig. 13. Final preparation of bone surfaces before insertion of final prosthesis components. Two drill holes are made using 4.5-mm drill for the pegs of the talar prosthesis component. All ossifications are removed and the posterior joint capsule is debrided.

AFTERCARE

The dressing and splint are removed and changed at the second postoperative day. Physiotherapy with lymphatic drainage and active motion is begun. A pneumatic foot cuff (with intermittent pressure up to 130 mm Hg) may be used to reduce postoperative swelling (**Fig. 19**). Active dorsal extension should be avoided in the first 4 weeks postoperatively to ensure the proper healing of the extensor tendon retinaculum. Active and passive mobilization in the first metatarsophalangeal joint may increase venous blood flow, which has an antiedema and thromboprophylactic effect (**Fig. 20**).[67] All patients receive thromboprophylaxis with subcutaneous low-molecular-weight heparin (Fragmin, 5000 IU; Pfizer AG, Zürich, Switzerland), starting 12 hours preoperatively and continuing daily for 6 weeks postoperatively.[68] When the wound conditions are appropriate (dry wound, no secretion), the foot is placed in a stabilizing walker or cast for 6 to 8 weeks (**Fig. 21**): in patients with additional procedures (eg, fusion of adjacent joint or corrective osteotomies), the immobilization is longer. Weight-bearing is allowed as tolerated with the exception of patients who underwent additional corrective osteotomies.[42,69,70] After the cast or walker is removed, a rehabilitation program is continued, including active and passive ankle motion, stretching and strengthening of the triceps surae, and proprioceptive exercises. In patients with persistent swelling, we recommend compression stockings. A

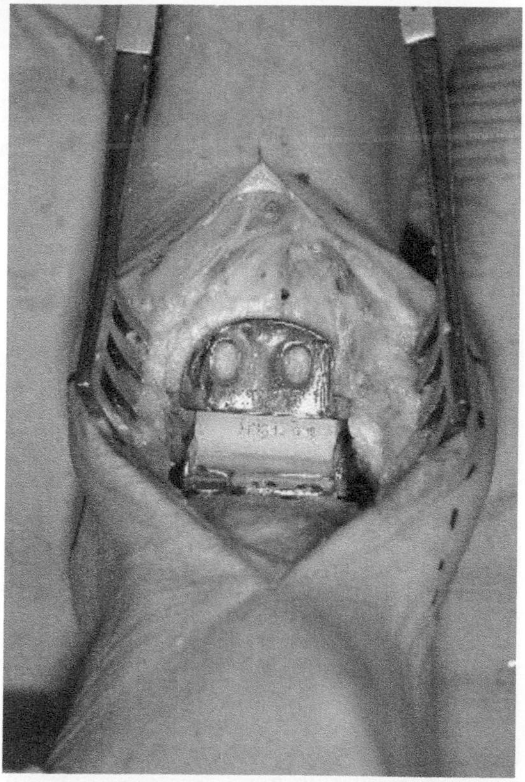

Fig. 14. Final surgery situs with inserted prosthesis components and inlay.

low level (eg, hiking, swimming, biking, golfing) and a normal level (eg, jogging, tennis, downhill skiing) of sports activities are recommended and allowed. Contact sports or activities involving jumping should be avoided.[44]

CLINICAL AND RADIOGRAPHIC FOLLOW-UP

The first clinical and radiographic follow-up is made at 6 to 8 weeks to check the healing of soft tissues including skin and osteointegration/position of the prosthesis components. The next clinical and radiographic follow-ups are performed at 4 months, 1 year, and then annually thereafter.

For appropriate analysis of the clinical outcome, the following parameters/scores are used. We measure the range of motion clinically with a goniometer along the lateral border of the leg and foot.[3,46] To assess the postoperative pain relief, all patients rate their pain on a visual analogue scale (VAS) of 0 points (no pain) to 10 points (maximal pain).[71] The American Orthopedic Foot and Ankle Society (AOFAS) hindfoot score is calculated.[72] The AOFAS score has been shown to have the discriminatory capacity to assess the postoperative improvement in patients with TAR.[73] However, this score is not validated and the research committee of the AOFAS recently published a statement recommending against its use.[74] SF-36 questionnaires are used to assess the quality of life.[75] Patients indicate their satisfaction with the procedure using a modified Coughlin rating for category scale: very satisfied, satisfied, partially satisfied, and not

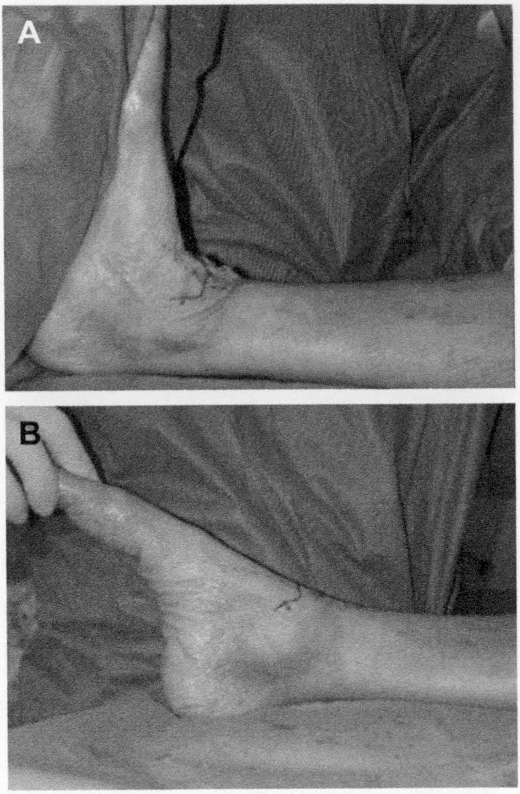

Fig. 15. Motion of the replaced ankle is checked clinically: (*A*) dorsiflexion and (*B*) plantar flexion.

satisfied.[76] Sports activity level is documented using a Valderrabano score: grade 0, none; grade 1, moderate; grade 2, normal; grade 3, high; and grade 4, elite.[44] Gait is observed clinically and then analyzed using pedobarography.[77]

Radiographic assessment is performed using weight-bearing radiographs with fluoroscopy. The postoperative hindfoot alignment is assessed using a Saltzman view.[55,78] The following angular values are used for standardized assessment of prosthesis components: α-angles, β-angles, and γ-angles (**Fig. 22**).[3,28,79] α-Angles and β-angles are used for assessment of the tibial component and measured between the longitudinal axis of the tibia and the articular surface of the tibial component in the anteroposterior and lateral views, respectively.[3,79] γ-Angle is used for assessment of the talar component and measured between a line drawn through the anterior shield and the posterior edge of the talar component and a line drawn along the center of the talar neck on the lateral view.[64] All radiographs are analyzed regarding the localization and degree of heterotopic ossifications. Heterotopic ossifications are described according to the Brooker classification[80] as modified by Lee and colleagues[81] and Choi and Lee[82]: 0, no heterotopic ossifications; I, islands of bone within the soft tissues about the ankle: II and III, bone spurs from the tibial or talus, reducing the posterior joint space by less than 50% or 50% or greater, respectively; and IV, bridging bone continuous between the tibia and the talus. Change in position of the flat base of the tibial

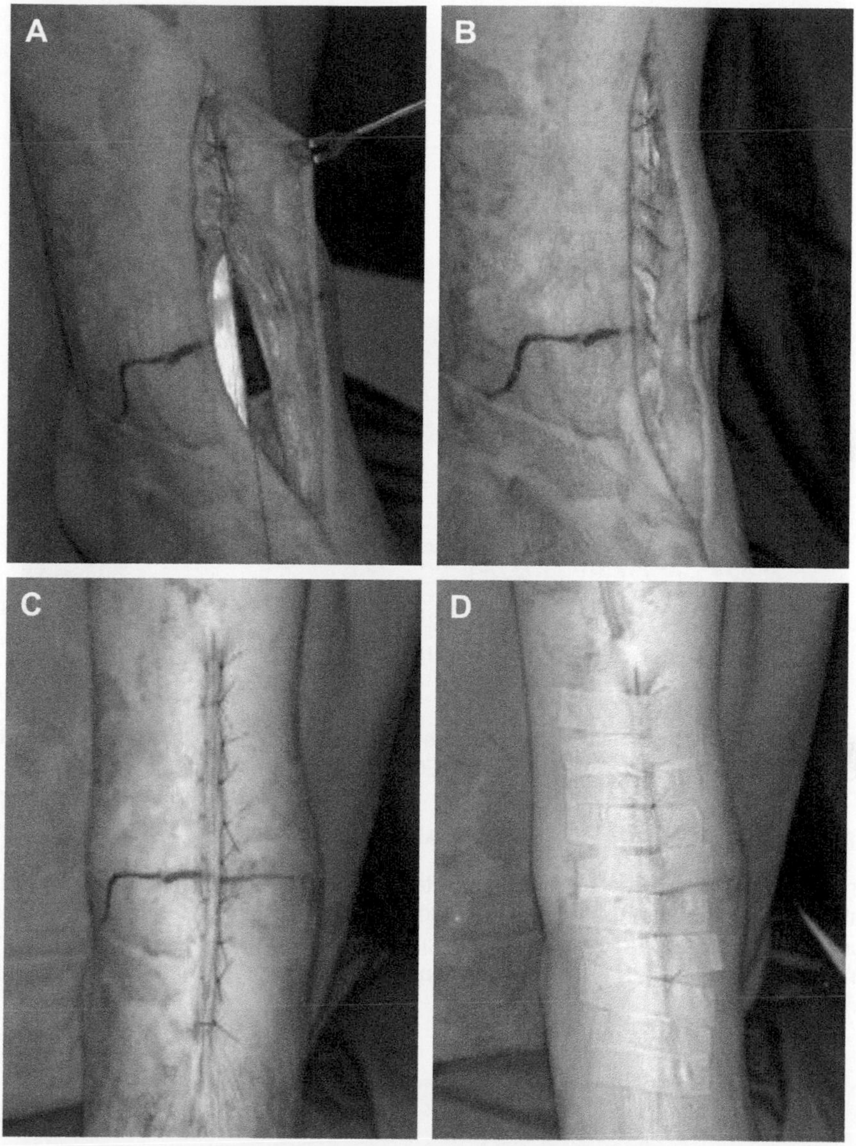

Fig. 16. Wound closure after insertion of the final prosthesis components. (*A*, *B*) Extensor retinaculum is closed using resorbable fibers (eg, Dexon 0; Covidien, Mansfield, MA). (*C*) Skin is closed using Donati technique with nonresorbable fibers (eg, Prolene 3-0; Ethicon, Johnson & Johnson Medical GmbH, Nordersted, Germany). (*D*) Steri-Strips (3M, Neuss, Germany) are used to protect the skin stitches.

component by more than 2° relative to the longitudinal axis of the tibia, or progressive radiolucency greater than 2 mm on the anteroposterior or lateral radiographs, is defined as loosening of the tibial component.[3,79] Subsidence of the talar component by more than 5 mm or a position change of greater than 5° relative to a line drawn from the top of the talonavicular joint to the tuberosity of the calcaneus is defined as loosening of the talar component.[3,79,83] Because of prosthesis design, it is difficult to assess the

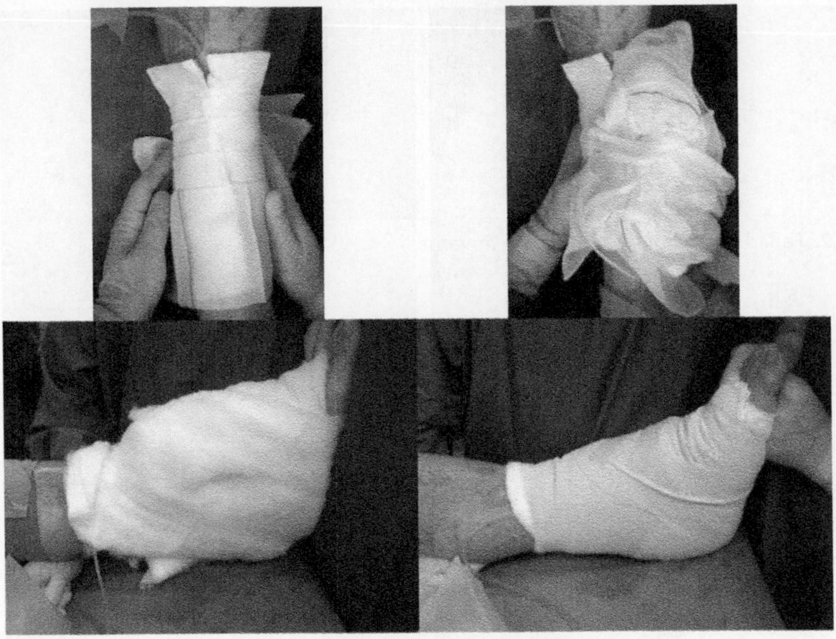

Fig. 17. Soft wound dress without any pressure on the surgery wounds.

position changes of the talar component, so in cases with suspicion of loosening or subsidence, computed tomography or SPECT should be performed.[56,57]

TAR IN VARUS/VALGUS OSTEOARTHRITIC ANKLE

In more than 60% of all patients with end-stage ankle OA, a significant varus or valgus malalignment of the hindfoot is observed.[19] Because of significantly altered ankle/hindfoot biomechanics, the asymmetric load consecutively leads to asymmetric joint wear and generative changes. The varus/valgus osteoarthritic ankle is often combined with significant joint instability.[84,85]

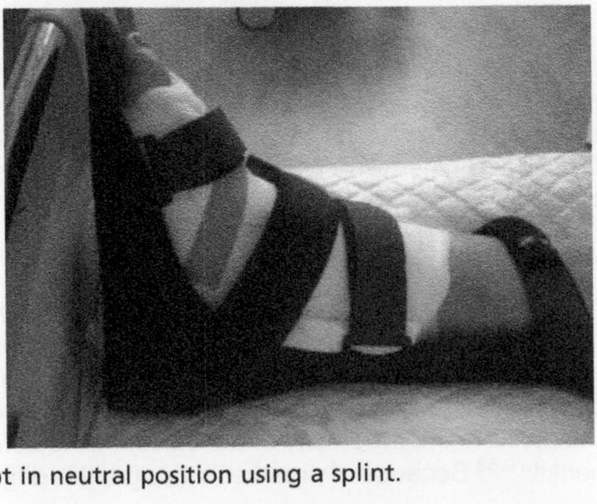

Fig. 18. Foot is kept in neutral position using a splint.

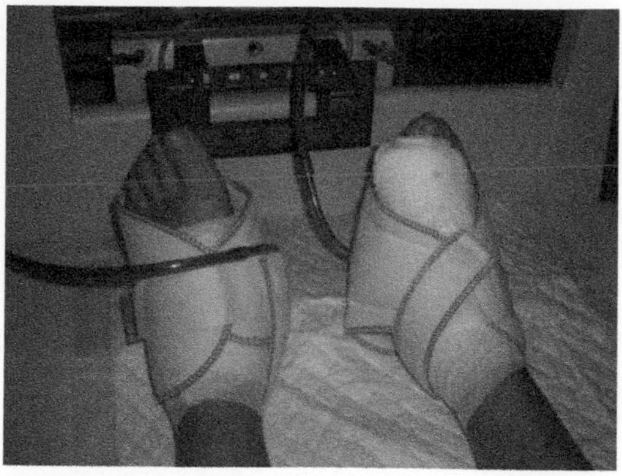

Fig. 19. Pneumatic foot pump (with intermittent pressure up to 130 mm Hg) may be used to reduce postoperative swelling of the foot and ankle.

Varus Osteoarthritic Ankle

In patients with significant varus malalignment, the medial malleolus retains the talus because of the significant talar tilting to the lateral side (**Fig. 23**). We often observe a functional conjunction between the medial malleolus and the talus: so-called neoarthros. Increased pressure on the medial tallus pushes the talus to the lateral side, resulting in development of large osteophytes on the lateral side. Because of asymmetric loading in the talocrural joint, the medial ligaments are contracted, whereas the lateral ligaments are elongated and insufficient. The patients often present with a tight posterior tibial tendon, whereas the tendon of the musculus peroneus brevis is elongated with insufficient tendon pull at the side of the base of the fifth metatarsal bone. This situation leads to plantar flexion of the first metatarsal bone. The significant ligamental and muscular imbalance causes the anterior-ventral tilting of the talus in the mortise view, resulting in an increased inner rotation position.

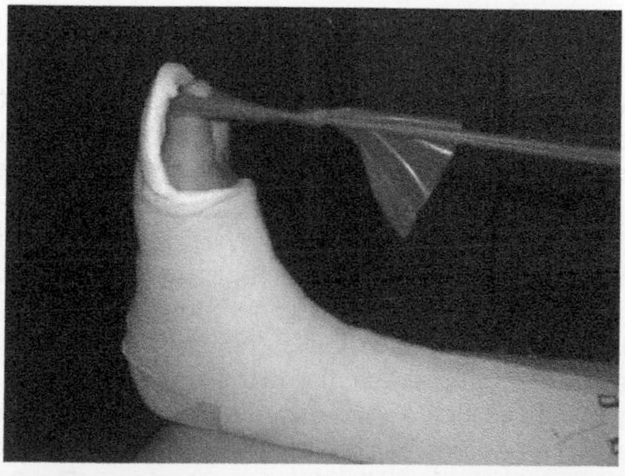

Fig. 20. The active and passive mobilization in the first metatarsophalangeal joint increases venous blood flow with antiedema and thromboprophylactic effect. (*Data from* Elsner A, Schiffer G, Jubel A, et al. The venous pump of the first metatarsophalangeal joint: clinical implications. Foot Ankle Int 2007;28:902–9.)

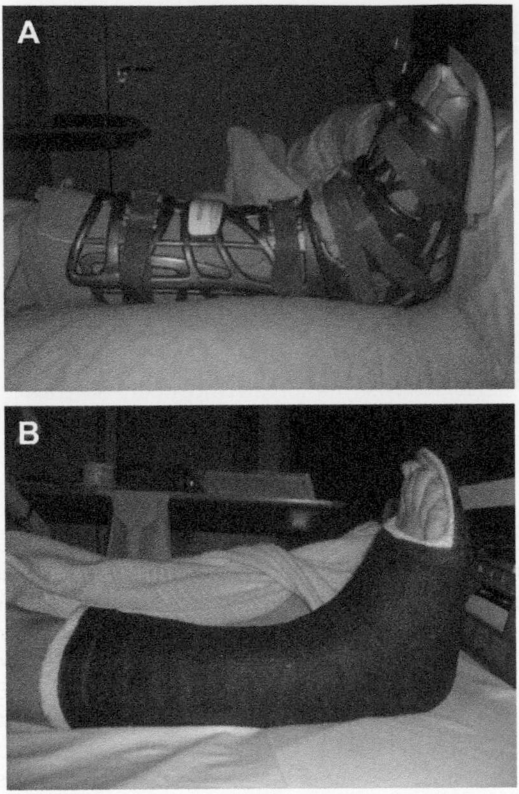

Fig. 21. Postoperatively, a (*A*) walker or (*B*) stabilizing cast is used for immobilization for 6 to 8 weeks.

TAR in Varus Osteoarthritic Ankle

We use a standard anterior approach for implantation of the total ankle, as described earlier.

In patients with a congruent tibiotalar joint, the varus deformity of less than 10° may be corrected by modification of the tibial resection. However, the more proximal tibial resection may result in consecutive instability of the replaced ankle; therefore a thicker inlay should be used to achieve ligamental tension. In patients with varus deformity of more than 10°, a medial open-wedge supramalleolar osteotomy is used, which can be performed using the same anterior approach with some extension proximally.[42,69,70,86–88] The supramalleolar osteotomy is fixed by a ventral plate, which should be placed more proximally to avoid contact between the distal end of the plate and the anterior shield of the tibial prosthesis component.

In patients with incongruent tibiotalar joints, the joint contracture at the medial side should be addressed by osteophyte resection of the medial malleolus. If medial contracture persists, a surgical release of the deltoid ligament should be performed.[85,89] In some cases, the lengthening osteotomy of the medial malleolus may resolve the medial contracture.[90] We recommend a so-called flipping osteotomy (**Fig. 24**). The medial malleolus is osteotomized using the main anterior approach for TAR.

After the proximal varus correction is performed, the hindfoot alignment should be verified clinically using fluoroscopy. In patients with a remaining varus position of the

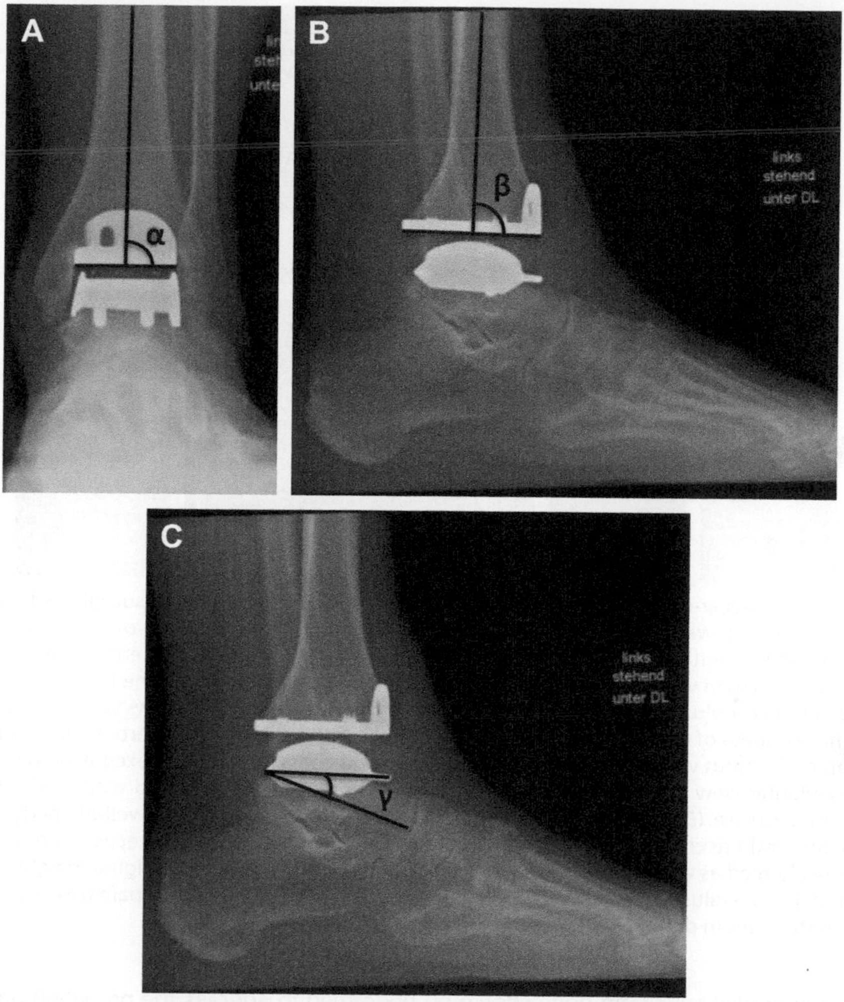

Fig. 22. Angular measurements of prosthesis component using anteroposterior and lateral ankle weight-bearing radiographs. (*A*) α-Angle, in this case 89.5° (normal values 90 ± 2°), (*B*) β-angle, in this case 90.5° (normal value 85 ± 2°), and (*C*) γ-angle, in this case 19° (normal values 20 ± 2°).

heel, the deformity may be corrected by Dwyer osteotomy[91–93] or Z-osteotomy of the calcaneus.[94] In patients with progressive degenerative changes of the subtalar joint, a subtalar arthrodesis should be performed.[95]

In patients with lateral ligamental instability, anatomic repair of the lateral ligament complex using suture anchors should be performed.[96,97] In patients with insufficient ligament tissues, an augmentation with a free plantaris tendon graft is preferred for reconstruction of the anterior fibulotalar ligament and calcaneofibular ligament.[98] Furthermore, the peroneus longus to peroneus brevis tendon transfer may provide reliable soft tissue stabilization and reduce the inversion moment arm of the first ray.[99]

After hindfoot correction and stabilization of the ankle complex in patients with a remaining plantar flexed first ray, a dorsiflexion osteotomy of the first metatarsal

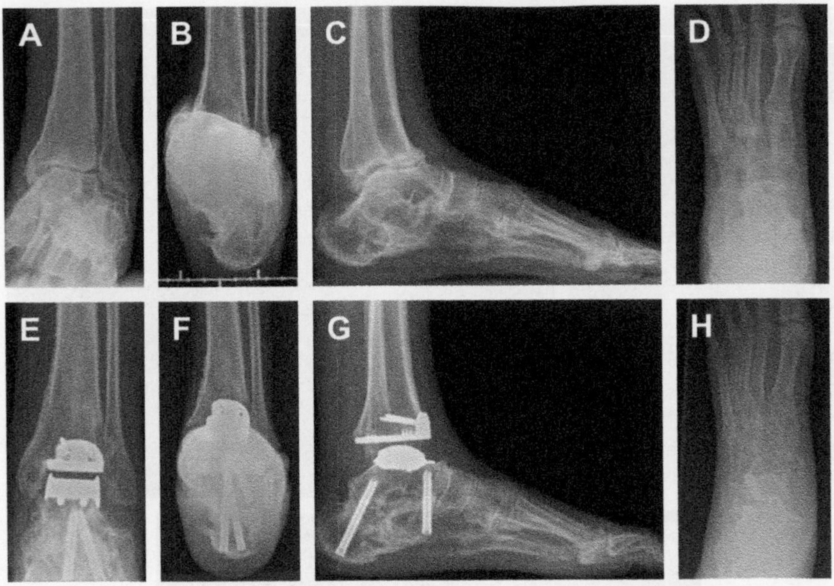

Fig. 23. A 41-year-old woman with painful ankle OA and malunion after subtalar arthrodesis.[119] The pain was localized ventral and subfibular and the preoperative range of motion was measured with 0°/25° (dorsiflexion/plantar flexion). (*A*) Anteroposterior radiograph shows the talus in varus malpositions, with well-preserved congruency of the tibiotalar joint and peritalar subluxation with lateral calcaneus tilt. (*B*) Saltzman view shows valgus position of the calcaneus of more than 1.5 cm. (*C*) Lateral radiograph shows the posteromedial subluxation of the talus with some posterior subsidence and consecutive dorsiflexed position. (*D*) Dorsoplantar view of the foot shows the lateral position of the talar head with medial tilt of the naviculare. (*E–H*) Postoperative radiographs (5 years follow-up) show well-aligned position of prosthesis components, with good osseous integration. Peritalar corrective osteotomy was performed as a 1-stage procedure with allograft interposition. The original height and position of the talus is restored, with a well-aligned hindfoot. The patient is pain free without any restrictions in daily activities and low-demand physical activities.

bone or medial cuneiform bone should be performed to address the pronation position.[100] In patients with varus malalignment of the hindfoot an equinus contracture is often observed, leading to limited ankle dorsiflexion. Depending on the results of the 2-joint muscle test or the Silfverskiold test,[101,102] percutaneous Achilles tendon lengthening or gastrocnemius resection should be performed. We recommend a percutaneous Achilles tendon lengthening by triple hemisection, with 2 incisions on the medial side and 1 incision on the lateral side.[103,104] Surgeons should avoid the failure of triple hemisection at the ankle mobilization.[105]

Valgus Osteoarthritic Ankle

In patients with valgus malalignment of the hindfoot, 2 different morphologic types of deformity are observed.[84] In the first type, the insufficiency of the medial ligaments results in valgus tilting of the talus (**Fig. 25**). The patients present with asymmetric joint loading and incongruence of the tibiotalar joint, especially on the lateral side. The joint load increasingly occurs over the fibula, which may result in stress fractures. Because of the lateralization of the heel, the excentric pull of the musculus triceps surae increases the valgus malalignment of the hindfoot and causes foot eversion.[106] In

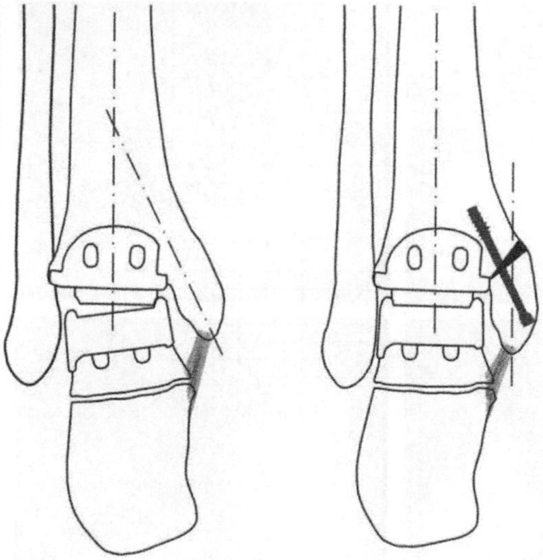

Fig. 24. Flipping osteotomy of the medial osteotomy to restore the incongruence of the tibiotalar joint. (*Data from* Knupp M, Bolliger L, Barg A, et al. Total ankle replacement for varus deformity. Orthopade 2011;40:964–70 [in German].)

the second type of valgus malalignment, impaction of the talus into the lateral part of tibial plafond is observed (**Fig. 26**). The tibiotalar joint shows no incongruence with sufficient medial ligaments. However, the ankle mortise is exposed to increased loading pressures, leading to insufficiency of the ankle syndesmosis. Also in this type of deformity, lateralization of the heel is often observed as a result of excentric pull of the Achilles tendon.[106]

TAR in Valgus Osteoarthritic Ankle

We use the standard anterior approach for implantation of the total ankle, as described earlier.

In patients with valgus malalignment of the distal tibia of more than 5°, we suggest a supramalleolar correcting osteotomy.[42,69,70,87,107] The malunion of the distal fibula may hinder the realignment of the talus within the ankle mortise, and therefore an additional fibula osteotomy should be performed.[108]

After the supramalleolar correction, the heel position should be verified clinically and using fluoroscopy. In patients with a remaining inframalleolar valgus deformity, a medial displacement osteotomy of the calcaneus should be performed, with the aim of the neutral alignment of the heel (0–5° of valgus).[109] In patients with significant subtalar contracture or degenerative changes of the subtalar joint, a subtalar arthrodesis should be performed. In patients with significant ligamental instability, medial or lateral ligament reconstruction should be performed.

PITFALLS

In patients with insufficiently addressed hindfoot misalignment, pain may persist postoperatively. In most cases, the pain is localized on the medial side, and considered medial pain syndrome.[110] We established the following classification of the medial pain syndrome: type I, medial impingement/contracture of medial ligaments; type II, valgus deformity; type III, varus deformity; type IV, combined varus-valgus deformity.[110]

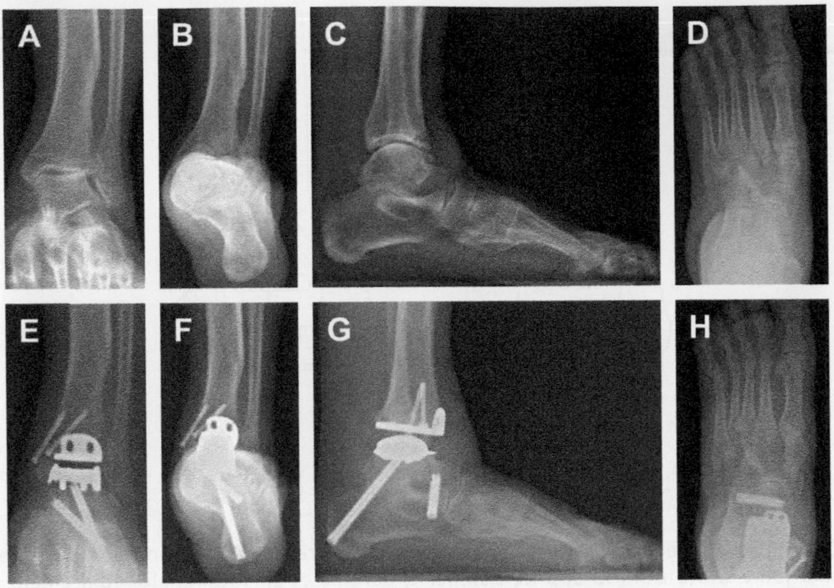

Fig. 25. A 63-year-old man with degenerative changes of the tibiotalar joint 34 years after conservatively treated lower leg fracture.[119] The pains were localized subfibular and in the area of the distal syndesmosis. The subtalar joint is rigid and painful. (*A*) Anteroposterior radiograph shows the varus of the distal tibia of approximately 12°, with inner rotation malposition. The talus shows valgus tilting, with widening of the medial tibiotalar joint space caused by insufficiency of the medial ligaments. (*B*) Saltzman view shows severe valgus malposition of the heel. (*C*) Lateral radiograph shows degenerative changes of the subtalar joint. (*D*) Dorsoplantar view of the foot shows normal articulations of the midfoot. (*E–H*) The patient declined the supramalleolar osteotomy, and therefore corrective arthrodesis of the subtalar joint has been performed. After implantation of ankle prosthesis, a lengthening osteotomy (flipping osteotomy) of the medial osteotomy was performed to restore the ankle mortise. At 3-year follow-up, the patient presented with good outcomes of the replaced ankle; however, medial pain syndrome was observed. Medial displacement osteotomy of the calcaneus was performed, which resolved the medial pain syndrome (radiographic follow-up will be performed).

In patients with significant remaining valgus deformity of the hindfoot, the following problems may occur postoperatively: medial ankle instability, asymmetric wear/dislocation of insert, and type II medial pain syndrome. In patients with insufficiently addressed varus deformity of the hindfoot, the following problems are observed postoperatively: lateral ankle instability, asymmetric wear/dislocation of insert, and type III/IV medial pain syndrome.

RESULTS

A total of 301 consecutive patients (150 men, 151 women, mean age 60.7 years, range 25.3–90.0 years) with 311 primary TAR had a minimum follow-up of 4 years. Preoperative diagnosis was posttraumatic OA (243), primary OA (28), and systemic OA (38). All patients were clinically and radiologically assessed after 59.5 (48–108) months. Twenty-three ankles had to be revised (18 revision TAR and 5 ankle fusions) at a mean of 2.8 (0.5–7.1) years. Revision was typically performed in

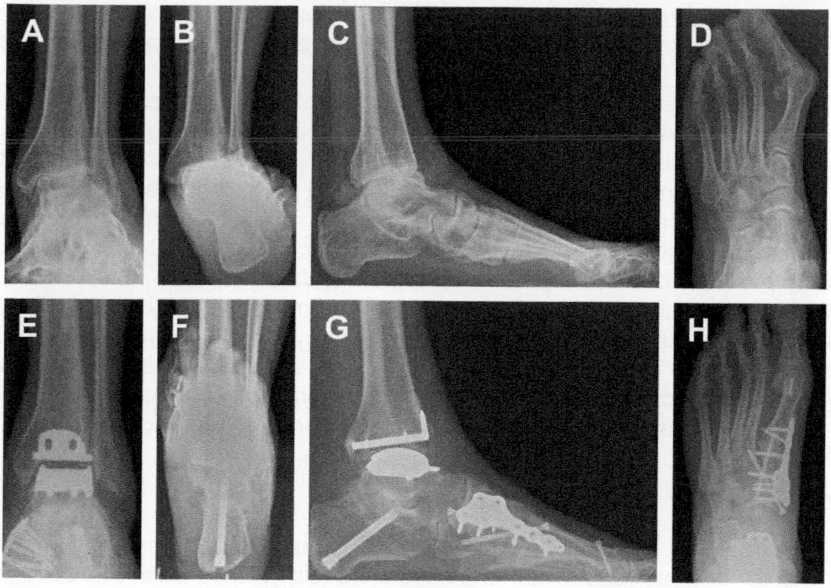

Fig. 26. A 61-year-old man with valgus osteoarthritic ankle.[119] The patient presented with painful instability of the first ray and hallux valgus with painful bunion at the first metatarsophalangeal joint. (*A*) Anteroposterior radiograph shows valgus impaction of the talus into the lateral part of the tibial plafond. (*B*) Saltzman view shows severe valgus malposition of the heel. (*C*) Lateral radiograph shows slight breakdown at the naviculocuneiform joint, with incongruence of the first tarsometatarsal joint (plantar widening of joint space). (*D*) Dorsoplantar view of the foot shows normal articulation of the Chopart joint and the midfoot, and varus position of the first metatarsal and halgus valgus. (*E–H*) Postoperative radiographs (4 years follow-up) show well-aligned position of prosthesis components, with good osseous integration. The following additional procedures were performed as 1-stage procedures: medial displacement osteotomy of the calcaneus, fusion of the naviculocuneiform joint, and chevron osteotomy. The patient is pain free without any restrictions in daily activities.

patients with first-generation prostheses with a single coating of hydroxyapatite (11), rather than in patients with second-generation (9) or third-generation (3) prostheses. Revision was performed for loosening of 1 or both components (15), subsidence of talar component (6), cyst formation (1), deep infection (1), unmanageable instability (1), and painful arthrofibrosis (2). Of the remaining 288 ankles, radiolucency was seen in 11 ankles; however, none of these showed progression of lucency over time.

The VAS pain score significantly decreased from 6.7 preoperatively to 1.8 ($P<.001$). The AOFAS score significantly increased from 41.7 preoperatively to 73.7 ($P<.001$). The mean range of motion at latest follow-up was 33.1° (preoperative 24.0°, $P<.001$).

SUMMARY

Approximately 1% of the world's adult population is affected by ankle OA, with pain, dysfunction, and impaired mobility.[19,111] The mental and physical disability associated with end-stage ankle OA is at least as severe as that associated with end-stage hip OA.[111] Clinical and epidemiologic studies have identified previous trauma as the most common origin for ankle OA, showing that patients with posttraumatic OA are younger than patients with primary OA.[18,19,112–115] Furthermore, more than half of all patients with posttraumatic OA have valgus or varus malalignment of the arthritic ankle.[19,116]

In the last 2 decades, TAR has evolved to become a valuable treatment option in patients with end-stage ankle OA, and therefore ankle fusion is no longer the gold standard.[117] However, one of the requirements for good long-term results is the appropriate position of prosthesis components[46] and physiologic osseous balancing of the hindfoot complex.[118] Therefore, TAR is not only a resurfacing procedure addressing the degenerative changes of the tibiotalar joint but has become a reconstruction procedure addressing deformities and instabilities.[42,84,85,118]

We observed encouraging results in patients who underwent TAR using HINTEGRA prostheses, with survivorship comparable with other recently published series. Our data suggest that TAR in patients with end-stage ankle OA produces significant pain relief and functional improvement. Overall favorable results support the belief that TAR has become a viable and superior alternative to ankle fusion.

REFERENCES

1. Gougoulias N, Khanna A, Maffulli N. How successful are current ankle replacements?: a systematic review of the literature. Clin Orthop Relat Res 2010;468: 199–208.
2. Mann JA, Mann RA, Horton E. STAR ankle: long-term results. Foot Ankle Int 2011;32:473–84.
3. Hintermann B, Valderrabano V, Dereymaeker G, et al. The HINTEGRA ankle: rationale and short-term results of 122 consecutive ankles. Clin Orthop Relat Res 2004;424:57–68.
4. Valderrabano V, Hintermann B, Nigg BM, et al. Kinematic changes after fusion and total replacement of the ankle: part 3: talar movement. Foot Ankle Int 2003;24:897–900.
5. Valderrabano V, Hintermann B, Nigg BM, et al. Kinematic changes after fusion and total replacement of the ankle: part 1: range of motion. Foot Ankle Int 2003;24:881–7.
6. Valderrabano V, Hintermann B, Nigg BM, et al. Kinematic changes after fusion and total replacement of the ankle: part 2: movement transfer. Foot Ankle Int 2003;24:888–96.
7. Hintermann B. Surgical techniques. In: Hintermann B, editor. Total ankle arthroplasty: historical overview, current concepts and future perspectives. 1st edition. Vienna: Springer; 2005. p. 105–26.
8. Hintermann B, Barg A. The HINTEGRA total ankle arthroplasty. In: Wiesel SW, editor. Operative techniques in orthopaedic surgery. 1st edition. Philadelphia: Lippincott Williams & Wilkins; 2010. p. 4022–31.
9. Valderrabano V, Pagenstert GI, Hintermann B. Total ankle replacement–three-component prosthesis. Techniques in Foot & Ankle Surgery 2005;2:84–90.
10. Besse JL, Colombier JA, Asencio J, et al. Total ankle arthroplasty in France. Orthop Traumatol Surg Res 2010;96:291–303.
11. Goldberg AJ, Sharp RJ, Cooke P. Ankle replacement: current practice of foot & ankle surgeons in the United Kingdom. Foot Ankle Int 2009;30:950–4.
12. Gougoulias NE, Khanna A, Maffulli N. History and evolution in total ankle arthroplasty. Br Med Bull 2009;89:111–51.
13. Kim BS, Choi WJ, Kim YS, et al. Total ankle replacement in moderate to severe varus deformity of the ankle. J Bone Joint Surg Br 2009;91:1183–90.

14. Skytta ET, Koivu H, Eskelinen A, et al. Total ankle replacement: a population-based study of 515 cases from the Finnish Arthroplasty Register. Acta Orthop 2010;81:114–8.
15. Henricson A, Skoog A, Carlsson A. The Swedish Ankle Arthroplasty Register: an analysis of 531 arthroplasties between 1993 and 2005. Acta Orthop 2007;78:569–74.
16. Fevang BT, Lie SA, Havelin LI, et al. 257 ankle arthroplasties performed in Norway between 1994 and 2005. Acta Orthop 2007;78:575–83.
17. Hosman AH, Mason RB, Hobbs T, et al. A New Zealand national joint registry review of 202 total ankle replacements followed for up to 6 years. Acta Orthop 2007;78:584–91.
18. Saltzman CL, Salamon ML, Blanchard GM, et al. Epidemiology of ankle arthritis: report of a consecutive series of 639 patients from a tertiary orthopaedic center. Iowa Orthop J 2005;25:44–6.
19. Valderrabano V, Horisberger M, Russell I, et al. Etiology of ankle osteoarthritis. Clin Orthop Relat Res 2009;467:1800–6.
20. Valderrabano V, Hintermann B, Horisberger M, et al. Ligamentous posttraumatic ankle osteoarthritis. Am J Sports Med 2006;34:612–20.
21. Rippstein PF, Naal FD. Total ankle replacement in rheumatoid arthritis. Orthopade 2011;40:984–90 [in German].
22. Rippstein PF, Huber M, Coetzee JC, et al. Total ankle replacement with use of a new three-component implant. J Bone Joint Surg Am 2011;93:1426–35.
23. Wood PL, Crawford LA, Suneja R, et al. Total ankle replacement for rheumatoid ankle arthritis. Foot Ankle Clin 2007;12:497–508.
24. Barg A, Elsner A, Hefti D, et al. Haemophilic arthropathy of the ankle treated by total ankle replacement: a case series. Haemophilia 2010;16:647–55.
25. Barg A, Elsner A, Hefti D, et al. Total ankle arthroplasty in patients with hereditary hemochromatosis. Clin Orthop Relat Res 2011;469:1427–35.
26. Barg A, Knupp M, Kapron AL, et al. Total ankle replacement in patients with gouty arthritis. J Bone Joint Surg Am 2011;93:357–66.
27. Barg A, Knupp M, Hintermann B. Simultaneous bilateral versus unilateral total ankle replacement: a patient-based comparison of pain relief, quality of life and functional outcome. J Bone Joint Surg Br 2010;92:1659–63.
28. Barg A, Henninger HB, Knupp M, et al. Simultaneous bilateral total ankle replacement using a 3-component prosthesis: outcome in 26 patients followed for 2–10 years. Acta Orthop 2011;82:704–10.
29. Karantana A, Martin GJ, Shandil M, et al. Simultaneous bilateral total ankle replacement using the S.T.A.R.: a case series. Foot Ankle Int 2010;31:86–9.
30. Hintermann B, Barg A, Knupp M. Revision arthroplasty of the ankle joint. Orthopade 2011;40:1000–7 [in German].
31. Espinosa N, Wirth SH, Jankauskas L. Ankle fusion after failed total ankle replacement. Techniques in Foot & Ankle Surgery 2010;9:199–204.
32. Espinosa N, Wirth SH. Ankle arthrodesis after failed total ankle replacement. Orthopade 2011;40:1008–17 [in German].
33. Hopgood P, Kumar R, Wood PL. Ankle arthrodesis for failed total ankle replacement. J Bone Joint Surg Br 2006;88:1032–8.
34. Kotnis R, Pasapula C, Anwar F, et al. The management of failed ankle replacement. J Bone Joint Surg Br 2006;88:1039–47.
35. Plaass C, Knupp M, Barg A, et al. Anterior double plating for rigid fixation of isolated tibiotalar arthrodesis. Foot Ankle Int 2009;30:631–9.

36. Barg A, Hintermann B. Takedown of painful ankle fusion and total ankle replacement using a 3-component ankle prosthesis. Techniques in Foot & Ankle Surgery 2010;9:190–8.
37. Greisberg J, Assal M, Flueckiger G, et al. Takedown of ankle fusion and conversion to total ankle replacement. Clin Orthop Relat Res 2004;424:80–8.
38. Hintermann B, Barg A, Knupp M, et al. Conversion of painful ankle arthrodesis to total ankle arthroplasty. J Bone Joint Surg Am 2009;91:850–8.
39. Hintermann B, Barg A, Knupp M, et al. Conversion of painful ankle arthrodesis to total ankle arthroplasty. Surgical technique. J Bone Joint Surg Am 2010; 92(Suppl 1 Pt 1):55–66.
40. Hintermann B, Valderrabano V. Total ankle replacement. Foot Ankle Clin 2003;8: 375–405.
41. Hintermann B. Total ankle arthroplasty: historical overview, current concepts and future perspectives. Vienna: Springer; 2004.
42. Knupp M, Stufkens SA, Bolliger L, et al. Total ankle replacement and supramalleolar osteotomies for malaligned osteoarthritis ankle. Techniques in Foot & Ankle Surgery 2010;9:175–81.
43. Naal FD, Impellizzeri FM, Loibl M, et al. Habitual physical activity and sports participation after total ankle arthroplasty. Am J Sports Med 2009;37: 95–102.
44. Valderrabano V, Pagenstert G, Horisberger M, et al. Sports and recreation activity of ankle arthritis patients before and after total ankle replacement. Am J Sports Med 2006;34:993–9.
45. Barg A, Knupp M, Anderson AE, et al. Total ankle replacement in obese patients: component stability, weight change, and functional outcome in 118 consecutive patients. Foot Ankle Int 2011;32:925–32.
46. Barg A, Elsner A, Anderson AE, et al. The effect of three-component total ankle replacement misalignment on clinical outcome: pain relief and functional outcome in 317 consecutive patients. J Bone Joint Surg Am 2011;93(21):1969–78.
47. Lindsjo U, Danckwardt-Lilliestrom G, Sahlstedt B. Measurement of the motion range in the loaded ankle. Clin Orthop Relat Res 1985;199:68–71.
48. Min W, Sanders R. The use of the mortise view of the ankle to determine hindfoot alignment: technique tip. Foot Ankle Int 2010;31:823–7.
49. Hunt MA, Birmingham TB, Jenkyn TR, et al. Measures of frontal plane lower limb alignment obtained from static radiographs and dynamic gait analysis. Gait Posture 2008;27:635–40.
50. Ellis SJ, Deyer T, Williams BR, et al. Assessment of lateral hindfoot pain in acquired flatfoot deformity using weightbearing multiplanar imaging. Foot Ankle Int 2010;31:361–71.
51. Knupp M, Ledermann H, Magerkurth O, et al. The surgical tibiotalar angle: a radiologic study. Foot Ankle Int 2005;26:713–6.
52. Magerkurth O, Knupp M, Ledermann H, et al. Evaluation of hindfoot dimensions: a radiological study. Foot Ankle Int 2006;27:612–6.
53. Inman VT. The joints of the ankle. Baltimore (MD): Williams & Wilkins; 1976.
54. Stufkens SA, Barg A, Bolliger L, et al. Measurement of the medial distal tibial angle. Foot Ankle Int 2011;32:288–93.
55. Saltzman CL, el Khoury GY. The hindfoot alignment view. Foot Ankle Int 1995;16: 572–6.
56. Knupp M, Pagenstert GI, Barg A, et al. SPECT-CT compared with conventional imaging modalities for the assessment of the varus and valgus malaligned hindfoot. J Orthop Res 2009;27:1461–6.

57. Pagenstert GI, Barg A, Leumann AG, et al. SPECT-CT imaging in degenerative joint disease of the foot and ankle. J Bone Joint Surg Br 2009;91:1191–6.
58. Hintermann B. What the orthopaedic foot and ankle surgeon wants to know from MR imaging. Semin Musculoskelet Radiol 2005;9:260–71.
59. Hintermann B. Current designs of total ankle prostheses. In: Hintermann B, editor. Total ankle arthroplasty. Historical overview, current concepts and future perspectives. 1st edition. Vienna: Springer; 2004. p. 69–100.
60. Barg A, Elsner A, Chuckpaiwong B, et al. Insert position in three-component total ankle replacement. Foot Ankle Int 2010;31:754–9.
61. Abu-Hijleh MF, Harris PF. Deep fascia on the dorsum of the ankle and foot: extensor retinacula revisited. Clin Anat 2007;20:186–95.
62. Numkarunarunrote N, Malik A, Aguiar RO, et al. Retinacula of the foot and ankle: MRI with anatomic correlation in cadavers. AJR Am J Roentgenol 2007;188: W348–54.
63. Solomon LB, Ferris L, Henneberg M. Anatomical study of the ankle with view to the anterior arthroscopic portals. ANZ J Surg 2006;76:932–6.
64. Lee KB, Cho SG, Hur CI, et al. Perioperative complications of HINTEGRA total ankle replacement: our initial 50 cases. Foot Ankle Int 2008;29:978–84.
65. Saltzman CL, Amendola A, Anderson R, et al. Surgeon training and complications in total ankle arthroplasty. Foot Ankle Int 2003;24:514–8.
66. Wood PL, Deakin S. Total ankle replacement. The results in 200 ankles. J Bone Joint Surg Br 2003;85:334–41.
67. Elsner A, Schiffer G, Jubel A, et al. The venous pump of the first metatarsophalangeal joint: clinical implications. Foot Ankle Int 2007;28:902–9.
68. Barg A, Henninger HB, Hintermann B. Risk factors for symptomatic deep-vein thrombosis in patients after total ankle replacement who received routine chemical thromboprophylaxis. J Bone Joint Surg Br 2011;93:921–7.
69. Hintermann B, Knupp M, Barg A. Osteotomies of the distal tibia and hindfoot for ankle realignment. Orthopade 2008;37:212–3 [in German].
70. Pagenstert GI, Hintermann B, Barg A, et al. Realignment surgery as alternative treatment of varus and valgus ankle osteoarthritis. Clin Orthop Relat Res 2007; 462:156–68.
71. Huskisson EC. Measurement of pain. Lancet 1974;2:1127–31.
72. Kitaoka HB, Alexander IJ, Adelaar RS, et al. Clinical rating systems for the ankle-hindfoot, midfoot, hallux, and lesser toes. Foot Ankle Int 1994;15:349–53.
73. Pena F, Agel J, Coetzee JC. Comparison of the MFA to the AOFAS outcome tool in a population undergoing total ankle replacement. Foot Ankle Int 2007;28:788–93.
74. Pinsker E, Daniels TR. AOFAS position statement regarding the future of the AOFAS clinical rating systems. Foot Ankle Int 2011;32:841–2.
75. Ware JE Jr, Sherbourne CD. The MOS 36-item short-form health survey (SF-36). I. Conceptual framework and item selection. Med Care 1992;30:473–83.
76. Coughlin MJ. Arthrodesis of the first metatarsophalangeal joint with mini-fragment plate fixation. Orthopedics 1990;13:1037–44.
77. Horisberger M, Hintermann B, Valderrabano V. Alterations of plantar pressure distribution in posttraumatic end-stage ankle osteoarthritis. Clin Biomech (Bristol, Avon) 2009;24:303–7.
78. Frigg A, Nigg B, Hinz L, et al. Clinical relevance of hindfoot alignment view in total ankle replacement. Foot Ankle Int 2010;31:871–9.
79. Valderrabano V, Hintermann B, Dick W. Scandinavian total ankle replacement: a 3.7-year average followup of 65 patients. Clin Orthop Relat Res 2004;424: 47–56.

80. Brooker AF, Bowerman JW, Robinson RA, et al. Ectopic ossification following total hip replacement. Incidence and a method of classification. J Bone Joint Surg Am 1973;55:1629–32.
81. Lee KB, Cho YJ, Park JK, et al. Heterotopic ossification after primary total ankle arthroplasty. J Bone Joint Surg Am 2011;93:751–8.
82. Choi WJ, Lee JW. Heterotopic ossification after total ankle arthroplasty. J Bone Joint Surg Br 2011;93:1508–12.
83. Knecht SI, Estin M, Callaghan JJ, et al. The Agility total ankle arthroplasty. Seven to sixteen-year follow-up. J Bone Joint Surg Am 2004;86:1161–71.
84. Brunner S, Knupp M, Hintermann B. Total ankle replacement for the valgus unstable osteoarthritic ankle. Techniques in Foot & Ankle Surgery 2010;9:174.
85. Kim BS, Lee JW. Total ankle replacement for the varus unstable osteoarthritic ankle. Techniques in Foot & Ankle Surgery 2010;9:157–67.
86. Knupp M, Stufkens SA, Pagenstert GI, et al. Supramalleolar osteotomy for tibiotalar varus malalignment. Techniques in Foot & Ankle Surgery 2009;8:17–23.
87. Knupp M, Stufkens SA, Bolliger L, et al. Classification and treatment of supramalleolar deformities. Foot Ankle Int 2011;32:1023–31.
88. Knupp M, Pagenstert G, Valderrabano V, et al. Osteotomies in varus malalignment of the ankle. Oper Orthop Traumatol 2008;20:262–73 [in German].
89. Bonnin M, Judet T, Colombier JA, et al. Midterm results of the Salto Total Ankle Prosthesis. Clin Orthop Relat Res 2004;424:6–18.
90. Doets HC, van der Plaat LW, Klein JP. Medial malleolar osteotomy for the correction of varus deformity during total ankle arthroplasty: results in 15 ankles. Foot Ankle Int 2008;29:171–7.
91. Dwyer FC. Osteotomy of the calcaneum for pes cavus. J Bone Joint Surg Br 1959;41:80–6.
92. Barenfeld PA, Weseley MS, Munters M. Dwyer calcaneal osteotomy. Clin Orthop Relat Res 1967;53:147–53.
93. Weseley MS, Barenfeld PA. Mechanism of the Dwyer calcaneal osteotomy. Clin Orthop Relat Res 1970;70:137–40.
94. Knupp M, Horisberger M, Hintermann B. A new z-shaped calcaneal osteotomy for 3-plane correction of severe varus deformity of the hindfoot. Techniques in Foot & Ankle Surgery 2008;7:90–5.
95. Tuijthof GJ, Beimers L, Kerkhoffs GM, et al. Overview of subtalar arthrodesis techniques: options, pitfalls and solutions. Foot Ankle Surg 2010;16:107–16.
96. Valderrabano V, Wiewiorski M, Frigg A, et al. Direct anatomic repair of the lateral ankle ligaments in chronic lateral ankle instability. Unfallchirurg 2007;110:701–4 [in German].
97. Valderrabano V, Wiewiorski M, Frigg A, et al. Chronic ankle instability. Unfallchirurg 2007;110:691–9 [in German].
98. Pagenstert GI, Valderrabano V, Hintermann B. Lateral ankle ligament reconstruction with free plantaris tendon graft. Techniques in Foot & Ankle Surgery 2005;4:104–12.
99. Kilger R, Knupp M, Hintermann B. Peroneus longus to peroneus brevis tendon transfer. Techniques in Foot & Ankle Surgery 2009;8:146–9.
100. Maskill MP, Maskill JD, Pomeroy GC. Surgical management and treatment algorithm for the subtle cavovarus foot. Foot Ankle Int 2010;31:1057–63.
101. Silfverskiold N. Reduction of the uncrossed two-joints muscles of the leg to one-joint muscles in spastic conditions. Acta Chir Scand 1924;56:315–28.

102. Mayich DJ, Younger A, Krause F. The reverse Silfverskiold test in Achilles tendon rupture. CJEM 2009;11:242–3.
103. Salamon ML, Pinney SJ, Van Bergeyk A, et al. Surgical anatomy and accuracy of percutaneous Achilles tendon lengthening. Foot Ankle Int 2006;27:411–3.
104. Lee WC, Ko HS. Achilles tendon lengthening by triple hemisection in adult. Foot Ankle Int 2005;26:1017–20.
105. Hoefnagels EM, Waites MD, Belkoff SM, et al. Percutaneous Achilles tendon lengthening: a cadaver-based study of failure of the triple hemisection technique. Acta Orthop 2007;78:808–12.
106. Arangio G, Rogman A, Reed JF III. Hindfoot alignment valgus moment arm increases in adult flatfoot with Achilles tendon contracture. Foot Ankle Int 2009;30:1078–82.
107. Pagenstert G, Knupp M, Valderrabano V, et al. Realignment surgery for valgus ankle osteoarthritis. Oper Orthop Traumatol 2009;21:77–87.
108. Hintermann B, Barg A, Knupp M. Corrective supramalleolar osteotomy for malunited pronation-external rotation fractures of the ankle. J Bone Joint Surg Br 2011;93:1367–72.
109. Stufkens SA, Knupp M, Hintermann B. Medial displacement calcaneal osteotomy. Techniques in Foot & Ankle Surgery 2009;8:85–90.
110. Barg A, Suter T, Zwicky L, et al. Medial pain syndrome in patients with total ankle replacement. Orthopade 2011;40:991–9 [in German].
111. Glazebrook M, Daniels T, Younger A, et al. Comparison of health-related quality of life between patients with end-stage ankle and hip arthrosis. J Bone Joint Surg Am 2008;90:499–505.
112. Thomas RH, Daniels TR. Ankle arthritis. J Bone Joint Surg Am 2003;85:923–36.
113. Saltzman CL. Ankle arthritis. In: Coughlin MJ, Mann RA, Saltzman CL, editors. Surgery of the foot and ankle. 8th edition. Philadelphia (PA): Mosby Elsevier; 2006. p. 923–84.
114. Hintermann B. Characteristics of the diseased ankle. In: Hintermann B, editor. Total ankle arthroplasty: historical overview, current concepts and future perspectives. 1st edition. Vienna: Springer; 2005. p. 5–9.
115. Daniels T, Thomas R. Etiology and biomechanics of ankle arthritis. Foot Ankle Clin 2008;13:341–52.
116. Horisberger M, Valderrabano V, Hintermann B. Posttraumatic ankle osteoarthritis after ankle-related fractures. J Orthop Trauma 2009;23:60–7.
117. Saltzman CL, Mann RA, Ahrens JE, et al. Prospective controlled trial of STAR total ankle replacement versus ankle fusion: initial results. Foot Ankle Int 2009; 30:579–96.
118. Hintermann B. Ankle joint prosthetics in Switzerland. Orthopade 2011;40:963 [in German].
119. Hintermann B, Barg A. Total ankle replacement in patients with osteoarthritis. Arthroskopie 2011;24:274–82 [in German].

The Mobility Total Ankle Replacement: Techniques and Pitfalls

Kyung Tai Lee, MD, PhD, Young Uk Park, MD, PhD*, Hyuk Jegal, MD

KEYWORDS

• Ankle arthritis • Total ankle replacement • Mobility • Surgical technique

KEY POINTS

- The Mobility total ankle replacement (DePuy, Leeds, United Kingdom) is an uncemented, three-component, mobile-bearing design.
- This article highlights the design rationale and explains the surgical technique with the Mobility implant, as well as offering technical tips and pitfalls gained through personal experiences and literature review.
- The tibial component has a flat articular surface and a conical intramedullary stem on the tibial side.

OVERVIEW

Although total ankle replacement (TAR) was almost abandoned because of the high failure rate associated with first-generation prostheses,[1–4] modern 3-component implants have demonstrated favorable clinical results and improved survivorship, with survival reported to exceed 90% at 10 years or longer.[5–7] The Mobility TAR (DePuy, Leeds, United Kingdom) is an uncemented, 3-component, mobile-bearing design. The tibial and talar components are made of a cobalt-chromium alloy and are porous coated. The insert is made of ultrahigh molecular weight polyethylene, with a deep sulcus on the talar component and a flat surface on the tibial side to minimize shear stresses.[8] This article highlights the design rationale and explains the surgical technique with the Mobility implant, as well as offering technical tips and pitfalls gained through personal experiences and literature review.

No benefits in any form have been received or will be received from a commercial party related directly or indirectly to the subject of this article.
No funds were received in support of this study.
Foot and Ankle Service, KT Lee's Orthopedic Hospital, Seoul, Korea
* Corresponding author. Foot and Ankle Service, KT Lee's Orthopedic Hospital, 111-13, Nonhyun 2-dong, Gangnam-Gu, Seoul 135-820, South Korea.
E-mail address: parkyounguk@gmail.com

Foot Ankle Clin N Am 17 (2012) 637–645
http://dx.doi.org/10.1016/j.fcl.2012.08.013 foot.theclinics.com
1083-7515/12/$ – see front matter

FEATURES OF THE MOBILITY DESIGN

The Mobility total ankle prosthesis is an unconstrained 3-component mobile-bearing system consisting of a tibial component, a talar component, and a mobile-bearing, highly cross-linked polyethylene inlay. The backsides of the tibial and the talar component are porous-coated titanium surfaces designed to provide good primary fixation and osseous ingrowth after press-fit implantation without cementation.

The tibial component has a flat articular surface and a conical intramedullary stem on the tibial side. The stem provides primary fixation into tibia and allows for lateral and medial adjustment and final rotational adjustment after placement of the tibial component through an anterior cortical window; additional stability can then be achieved by impacting the cancellous bone around the stem, if needed. The tibial plate is relatively long in the anteroposterior direction to allow for posterior overhang of posterior distal tibial cortex. It also prevents nonuniform loading of the distal tibia. The posterior aspect of the tibial plate is narrower and rounded to avoid posterior impingement with the fibula or the medial soft tissues.

The mobile-bearing polyethylene insert is made of an ultrahigh molecular weight polyethylene that allows unconstrained rotation and translation with the flat tibial plate and unconstrained dorsiflexion/plantarflexion and a small amount of inversion/eversion with the talar condyles. The surface of the tibial side of the polyethylene insert is smaller than the articular surface of the tibial component, to avoid protrusion of the polyethylene insert medially or laterally and to prevent edge loading. A fully conforming congruent surface with a profile of the talar component provides low- contact stress.

The talar component is designed to leave the malleolar surfaces intact. One advantage of retaining the articular surfaces of the malleoli, in addition to providing more physiologic ankle biomechanics, is that the intact medial and lateral cortices of the talar dome provide improved support for the talar component, reducing the risk of secondary subsidence or migration. Because the amount of bone resection is minimal, revision to an ankle fusion is facilitated in the case of a failure, the amount of limb shortening resulting from the fusion is minimized, and the bone graft used to fill the central defect is not required to provide as much support. The deep and doubly curved shape of the articular surface of the talar component stabilizes the polyethylene insert so as not to dislocate or subside unilaterally and enables articular congruency during eversion and inversion.

This shape also increases stability if the talar component has not been implanted perfectly parallel to the ground. Two anterior fins on the backside of the talar component increase the rotational stability, provide good primary press fit fixation, and create additional surface area for bone ingrowth. The interface between the implant and the bone can be visualized from the side during implantation, allowing intraoperative confirmation that the component is fully seated on the talar dome. The talar component is available in 6 sizes. Talar resections are the same for sizes 1 through 4 and for sizes 5 and 6. Thus, except in the case of a switch between sizes 4 and 5, no additional bone cut is necessary.

All 3 components narrow posteriorly to prevent impingement on the posterior neurovascular bundles, medial flexor tendons, and lateral posterior fibula. The instruments used for implantation allow centering of the tibial and the talar component with respect to each other in both the sagittal and the frontal plane.

SURGICAL PROCEDURE

The operation can be undertaken with the patient under general or epidural/spinal anesthesia. The patient is placed in a supine position, and a pneumatic tourniquet is applied. The anterior approach is used: the sheath of the extensor hallucis longus tendon is opened but that of the tibialis anterior is left intact. The neurovascular bundle is identified and retracted laterally. The incision is deepened posterior to tibialis anterior tendon to protect lateral neurovascular bundles. Once the joint is exposed, joint capsule is dissected to visualize the joint from the medial malleolus to the lateral malleolus. However, it caution is needed so as not to injure the anterior talofibular ligament. Anterior osteophytes and loose bodies are resected with an osteotome to see the exact joint shape and joint line. The distal tibial resection guide is then installed to facilitate a distal tibial resection that is oriented perpendicular to the weight-bearing axis in the frontal plane and has a posterior slope of 6° in the sagittal plane. The guide can be adjusted to control amount of posterior slope in case of severely eroded joint or sagittally malalignment leg. The transverse cut is made by a stiff and long saw to cut out sufficient bone to the posterior cortex. Because the fibula is positioned posterolateral to tibia, direction of transverse cut should be converged so as not to injure the fibula. The vertical medial malleolar cut is made with an oscillating saw or osteotome. Sufficient bone is resected to accommodate a 5-mm inlay. The cut can be repeated after adjusting the guide if there is insufficient space for a 5-mm inlay. The bone fragments that cut from the tibia are removed with a rongeur or a pituitary rongeur. The space should be cleaned to see the flexor hallucis longus tendon. The appropriate size of the tibial component is identified according to the width and depth of the implant. Even if the tibial implant is marginally overhung, this is not a concern because of a deep space of soft tissue and the Achilles tendon.

The long tibial plate design, which narrows posteriorly, provides some degree of posterior support. Therefore, the length of the component is a more important parameter than the width. The corresponding guide jig is used to mark and open the anterior tibial window. If the jig does not fit into the space properly, there should be unresected bone medial side in the space to be removed. The guide with the tibial template is placed over the middle of the talus dome and in line with the axis of the talus, following the orientation (rotation) of the talar body. The bone block is extracted using a cutting osteotome, and cancellous bone is impacted to the correct depth with a conical impactor to complete the tibial preparation. Overimpaction should be avoided to avoid a problem in press fit fixation.

The authors usually decorticate the anterior talar neck area with a rongeur or a saw blade before talar preparation, because it is not easy to make an anterior groove to the intact anterior cortex with large burrs during preparation of talus. The cutting shape of the talus was determined using a talar drill guide. The talar drill guide should fit into joint space with the foot held in a neutral position by the surgeon's belly. The drill guide is replaced with talar cutting block. The authors use a cutting block marked "0." Because it is a resurfacing implant, it should be cut as little as possible.

Sagittal and coronal alignment of the both components is adjusted using a centering device. The axis of the tibial component is transferred to a talar component relative to the center of the tibial component. The position of the talar component (frontal position and rotational orientation) is determined with a linked system that allows a central drill hole to be placed in the talus. The talar centering device is used to identify the correct position of the central drill hole in the sagittal plane. With the talar center guide and the talar flat cutting block in place, the end of the slot in the talar center guide indicates where the central point of the tibial component is located with respect to the talus. However, in such cases with an anterior subluxated talus, the talar center is not matched with the tibia, so it should be adjusted according to the amount of subluxation. If the anatomy of the joint is such that there is any anterior subluxation of the talus, the pin will be positioned more posteriorly. The center of the talar component as indicated by the central pin can be verified at this stage by using C-arm fluoroscopy. The talar preparation was completed by performing a superior, posterior, and anterior oblique resection and then contouring the resected talar surface to match the 2 pegs of the talar component.

Trial components are inserted, and the correct fit and alignment are verified with use of fluoroscopy before the definitive components are implanted. The size of the talar component must be the same as or smaller than the tibial component. The polyethylene bearing must match the talar component and must be the same size. The adequacy of the talar cut for implantation can be checked using the smallest talar trial. Because cutting surfaces are the same in any size and invisibility after trial of its own sized talar trial, if the fit is imperfect, the cut surface can be adjusted with a small osteotome. The porous-coated surfaces of the components usually provide excellent primary press-fit stability. Stability of the tibial component can be increased, if required, by impacting the cancellous bone chips around the tibial stem before reinserting the bone block to close the anterior tibial window. A slice of bone chip can be used to hold the graft securely in place. Following a trial and insertion of the final prosthesis, the capsule and extensor retinaculum should be repaired in layers over a wound drain and a well-padded cast is applied with a neutral ankle position.

POSTOPERATIVE MANAGEMENT

Postoperatively, the foot is elevated for 24 to 48 hours, after which the patient is fitted with a cast. The cast is removed 1 to 2 weeks postoperatively, and use of a removable walker boot and passive and active motion of the ankle are initiated, particularly aimed at regaining dorsiflexion. Patients are limited to partial weight-bearing with the use of crutches until 4 weeks postoperatively. Full weight-bearing, initially in the removable walker, is allowed after the clinical and radiographic evaluation 4 weeks after surgery, and therapy is adapted to include strengthening exercises. The boot is discarded 8 weeks after the operation.

TIPS AND PITFALLS

1. To avoid surgical infection

Infection is one of the most dreaded complications after total ankle arthroplasty. Treatment of infection may be associated with numerous challenges, including the need for multiple operations, longer hospitalization, higher incidence of morbidity and mortality, and increased cost. Therefore, surgeons have to use every available method to prevent surgical infection. Among them, the manageable intraoperative risk factor for infection in TAR is excessive surgical time. The surgeon should understand the system well and surgical assistants must also be well trained to perform this clean surgery.

2. Posterior slope of 6°

The distal tibial resection guide is used to facilitate a distal tibial resection that is oriented perpendicular to the weight-bearing axis in the frontal plane and has a posterior slope of 6° in the sagittal plane. Many surgeons prefer 0° of posterior slope. So, the guide can be adjusted to control the amount of posterior slope.

3. Tibial cut

Sufficient bone is removed to accommodate a 5-mm inlay. The cut can be repeated after adjusting the guide if there is not sufficient space for a 5-mm inlay. The bone fragments that cut from the tibia are removed with a rongeur or a pituitary rongeur. The space should be cleaned to view the flexor hallucis longus tendon. Caution is taken not to fracture the medial and lateral malleolus. Intraoperative fractures can occur during this procedure.[8–10] According to an earlier study,[9] malleolar fractures occurred more often using the Mobility model than with the Hintegra model (Newdeal SA, Lyon, France); the longer procedure and distraction time associated with more tibial procedures involving use of the Mobility system may have played a critical role.

4. Sizing

The appropriate size of the tibial component is identified according to the width and depth of the implant. Even if the tibial implant is marginally overhung, this will not be a concern because of a deep space of soft tissue and the Achilles tendon. The long tibial plate design, which narrows posteriorly, provides some degree of posterior support. At the least, the length of the tibial component should be longer than anteroposterior diameter of the tibia, even if it occurs with a slight posterior overhung. It is a more important parameter than the width. However, the width is a more important parameter for talar sizing. The size of the talar component must be the same as or smaller than the tibial component. The polyethylene bearing matches the talar component and must be the same size. One can check whether the talar cut is adequate for implantation using the smallest talar trial even at the end of the operation.

5. Balancing

Between 33% and 44% of arthritic ankles present with a coronal plane deformity exceeding 10°.[11–13] Wood and Deakin[14] identified deformities greater than 15° in 20% of cases. The difficulties of correction relate to the type of deformities. In these previous studies, associated procedures were necessary in all cases to correct ligament or hindfoot imbalances. Transfer of the peroneus longus onto the peroneus brevis for these incongruent varus ankles has been considered.[12,15] Congruent varus ankles also require numerous associated procedures including corrective malleolar osteotomies and hindfoot corrections. In many cases, these congruent varus ankles can be corrected by a tibial cut associated with deltoid ligament release.[12,16–18] Some authors preferred a medial malleolar lowering osteotomy.[19,20] Congruent valgus ankles are the simplest entity to correct with few associated procedures. Valgus instabilities are more complicated to discuss because of the small number of cases. They are rare in traumatic cases and are usually found in valgus pes planus.

6. Decortication of talar neck area

The authors usually decorticate anterior talar neck area before talar preparation, because it is not easy to make an anterior groove to the intact anterior cortex with large burrs during preparation of talus. More important, the talar cut should be in line with the anterior cortex of the distal tibial with neutral ankle position in cases with a sagittally malaligned ankle (**Fig. 1**). Centering of talus should be done with a free hand technique if it is not possible with a centering device. In cases with a flattened talus, a talar neck can be made to support talar drill guide in this procedure.

7. Centering of tibia and talar component

The position of the talar component (frontal position and rotational orientation) is determined by a linked system that allows a central drill hole to be placed in the talus. The talar centering device is used to identify the correct position of the central drill hole in the sagittal plane. However, in such cases with anterior subluxated talus, talar center is not matched with tibia, so it should be adjusted according to the amount

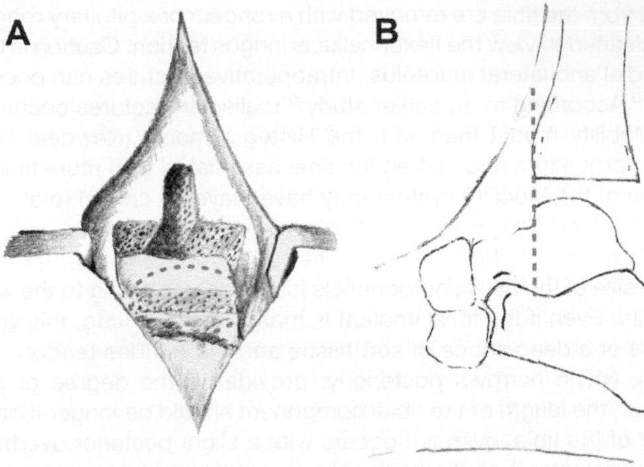

Fig. 1. The talar cut should be in line with the anterior cortex of the distal tibial with neutral ankle position.

of subluxation (**Fig. 2**). In such cases with severe coronal and sagittal malalignment, sometimes it is not possible to use a centering device. Therefore, the center of the talus should be created with a free hand technique and axial rotation of the talus to avoid posterior impingement.

8. Insertion of real implants

In cases for which insertion of real implants is difficult, insertion of the tibial implant might be delayed until the talar component is fitted and the polyethylene bearing is inserted. After press fit of talar implant and bearing, tibial implant is press fitted with

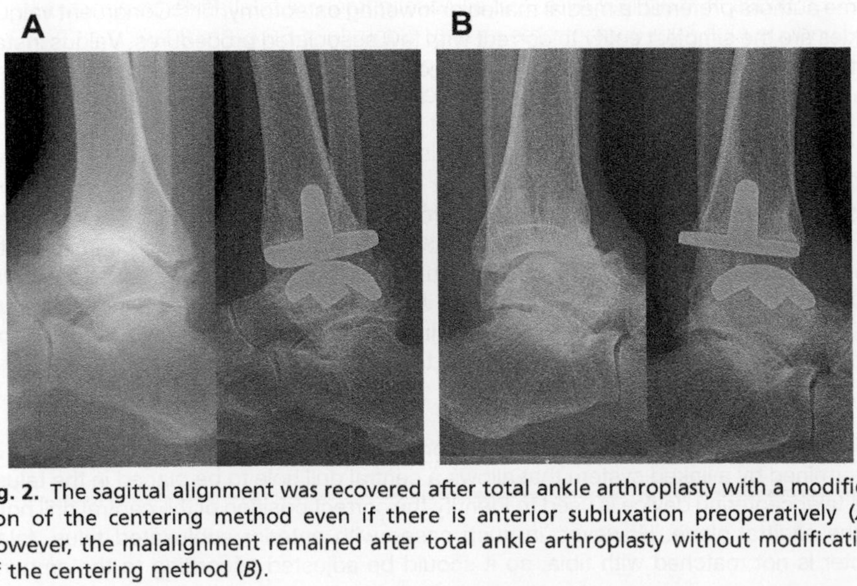

Fig. 2. The sagittal alignment was recovered after total ankle arthroplasty with a modification of the centering method even if there is anterior subluxation preoperatively (*A*). However, the malalignment remained after total ankle arthroplasty without modification of the centering method (*B*).

a blunt impactor. Caution should be taken not to scratch both components and bearing. One can check whether the talar cut is adequate for implantation using the smallest talar trial. Because cutting surfaces are the same in any size and invisibility after trial of its own sized talar trial, an imperfect fit can be corrected by adjusting the cut surface with a small osteotome.

9. Sealing tibial window

Stability of the tibial component can be increased, if required, by impacting the cancellous bone chips around the tibial stem before reinserting the bone block to close the anterior tibial window. A slice of bone chip can be used to hold the graft securely in place.

10. Learning curve

The incidence of complications is associated with the operator's experience; typically, the more experienced the surgeon, the fewer are the complications.[10,21] A new learning curve may affect the outcome of surgery when a newly designed implant is used for total ankle replacement arthroplasty.[9] A steep learning curve with the Hintegra total ankle prosthesis was also reported recently.[10,21]

COMPLICATIONS OF MOBILITY SYSTEM

There are many reports about the complications of total ankle arthroplasty.[3,5,8–10,15,16,21,22] The authors reported perioperative complications of the Mobility total ankle systemm[9] including medial malleolar fracture in 6 patients, lateral malleolar fracture in 1 patient, skin disorders in 2 patients, and varus deformity in 2 patients among 30 cases in the Mobility group. These fractures were developed during the operation; fixation was accomplished with cannulated screws or Kirschner wires during the operation, and no revision surgery was performed during the perioperative period (**Fig. 3**). However, there was no difference in the incidence of perioperative complications between the use of the Hintegra model and the Mobility model for total ankle replacement arthroplasty, although medial malleolar fracture was statistically increased with the use of Mobility.

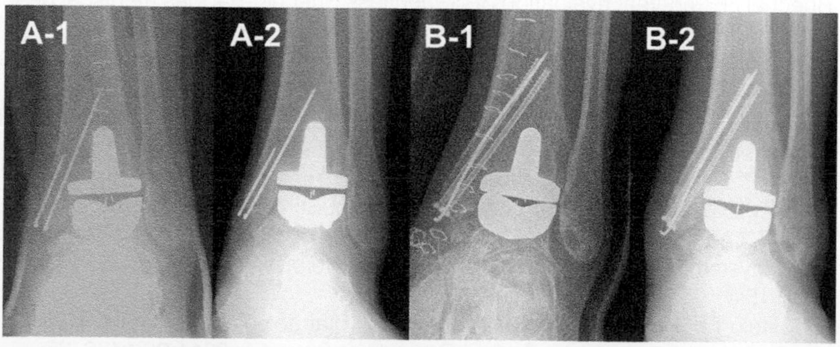

Fig. 3. Two examples of medial malleolar fracture. (*A-1*) Medial malleolar fracture was developed during preparation of medial gutter. The fracture was fixed with two K-wires. (*A-2*) It healed without difficulties. (*B-1*) Medial malleolar fracture was developed during impaction of tibial trial implant. This was fixed with 2 cannulated screws and K-wire. (*B-2*) It also healed without problems.

The Mobility model involves more procedures, particularly cutting of the distal tibia to match the height of the intramedullary post, conical shaping of the proximal portion inserting the post, and grafting of the cut bone, plus the longer distraction time required to maintain it. The thick tibial plate reduces the risk of plate failure as was reported with the early designs of the Buechel-Pappas ankle, but a thick tibial plate requires more distraction. More procedures and a longer distraction time make malleolar fracture more likely.

SUMMARY

The Mobility total ankle prosthesis is an unconstrained three-component mobile bearing system consisting of a tibial component, a talar component, and a mobile-bearing, highly cross-linked polyethylene inlay. The tibial component has a flat articular surface and a conical intramedullary stem on the tibial side. The mobile bearing polyethylene insert allows unconstrained rotation and translation with the flat tibial plate, and unconstrained dorsiflexion and plantarflexion and a small amount of inversion/eversion with the talar condyles. The talar component is designed to leave the malleolar surfaces intact. One advantage of retaining the articular surfaces of the malleoli, in addition to providing more physiological ankle biomechanics. The instruments used for implantation allow centering of the tibial and the talar component with respect to each other in both the sagittal and the frontal plane. The Mobility model involves more procedures. More procedures and a longer distraction time make malleolar fracture more likely.

REFERENCES

1. Bolton-Maggs B, Sudlow R, Freeman M. Total ankle arthroplasty. A long-term review of the London Hospital experience. J Bone Joint Surg Br 1985;67:785.
2. Harold BK, GARY LP. Clinical results of the Mayo total ankle arthroplasty. J Bone Joint Surg Am 1996;78:1658–64.
3. Helm R, Stevens J. Long-term results of total ankle replacement. J Arthroplasty 1986;1:271–7.
4. Newton S 3rd. Total ankle arthroplasty. Clinical study of fifty cases. J Bone Joint Surg Am 1982;64:104.
5. Buechel FF. Ten-year evaluation of cementless Buechel-Pappas meniscal bearing total ankle replacement. Foot Ankle Int 2003;24:462–72.
6. Buechel FF Sr, Buechel FF Jr, Pappas MJ. Twenty-year evaluation of cementless mobile-bearing total ankle replacements. Clin Orthop Relat Res 2004;424:19.
7. Kofoed H. Scandinavian total ankle replacement (star). Clin Orthop Relat Res 2004;424:73.
8. Wood P, Karski M, Watmough P. Total ankle replacement: the results of 100 Mobility total ankle replacements. J Bone Joint Surg Br 2010;92:958.
9. Lee KT, Lee YK, Young KW, et al. Perioperative complications of the Mobility total ankle system: comparison with the Hintegra total ankle system. J Orthop Sci 2010;15:317–22.
10. Rippstein PF, Huber M, Coetzee JC, et al. Total ankle replacement with use of a new three-component implant. J Bone Joint Surg Am 2011;93:1426–35.
11. Haskell A, Mann RA. Ankle arthroplasty with preoperative coronal plane deformity: short-term results. Clin Orthop Relat Res 2004;424:98.
12. Kim B, Choi W, Kim Y, et al. Total ankle replacement in moderate to severe varus deformity of the ankle. J Bone Joint Surg Br 2009;91:1183.

13. Wood P, Sutton C, Mishra V, et al. A randomised, controlled trial of two mobile-bearing total ankle replacements. J Bone Joint Surg Br 2009;91:69.
14. Wood P, Deakin S. Total ankle replacement. The results in 200 ankles. J Bone Joint Surg Br 2003;85:334.
15. Adrienne A, Mathieu A, Sigvard T. Complications and failure after total ankle arthroplasty. J Bone Joint Surg Am 2004;86:1172–8.
16. Bonnin M, Gaudot F, Laurent JR, et al. The Salto total ankle arthroplasty: survivorship and analysis of failures at 7 to 11 years. Clin Orthop Relat Res 2011;469:225–36.
17. Daniels TR, Cadden AR, Lim KK. Correction of varus talar deformities in ankle joint replacement. Operat Tech Orthop 2008;18:282–6.
18. Shock RP, Christensen JC, Schuberth JM. Total ankle replacement in the varus ankle. J Foot Ankle Surg 2011;50:5–10.
19. Comelis Doets H, van der Plaat LW, Klein JP. Medial malleolar osteotomy for the correction of varus deformity during total ankle arthroplasty: results in 15 ankles. Foot Ankle Int 2008;29:171–7.
20. Trincat S, Kouyoumdjian P, Asencio G. Total ankle arthroplasty and coronal plane deformities. Orthop Traumatol Surg Res 2012;98(1):75–84.
21. Lee KB, Cho SG, Hur CI, et al. Perioperative complications of Hintegra total ankle replacement: our initial 50 cases. Foot Ankle Int 2008;29:978.
22. Hintermann B, Valderrabano V, Dereymaeker G, et al. The Hintegra ankle: rationale and short-term results of 122 consecutive ankles. Clin Orthop Relat Res 2004;424:57.

14. Wood P, Sutton C, Mishra V, et al. A randomised, controlled trial of two mobile-bearing total ankle replacements. J Bone Joint Surg Br 2009;91:69.
15. Wood P, Deakin S. Total ankle replacement. The results in 200 ankles. J Bone Joint Surg Br 2003;85:334.
16. Accetone A, Mathieu A, Sigvard T. Complications and failure after total ankle arthroplasty. J Bone Joint Surg Am 2004;86:1172–8.
16. Bonnin M, Gaudot F, Laurent JR, et al. The Salto total ankle arthroplasty survivorship and analysis of failures at 7 to 11 years. Clin Orthop Relat Res 2011;469:225–36.
17. Daniels TR, Cadden AR, Lim KK. Correction of varus talar deformities in ankle joint replacement. Operat Tech Orthop 2008;18:282–6.
18. Shock RP, Christensen JC, Schuberth JM. Total ankle replacement in the varus ankle. J Foot Ankle Surg 2011;50:5–10.
19. Cornelis Doets H, van der Plaat LW, Klein JP. Medial malleolar osteotomy for the correction of varus deformity during total ankle arthroplasty: results in 15 ankles. Foot Ankle Int 2008;29:171–7.
20. Trincat S, Kouyoumdjian P, Asencio G. Total ankle arthroplasty and coronal plane deformities. Orthop Traumatol Surg Res 2012;98(1):75–84.
21. Lee KB, Cho SG, Hur CI, et al. Perioperative complications of Hintegra total ankle replacement: our initial 50 cases. Foot Ankle Int 2008;29:978.
22. Hintermann B, Valderrabano V, Dereymaeker G, et al. The Hintegra ankle: rationale and short-term results of 122 consecutive ankles. Clin Orthop Relat Res 2004;424:57.

Treatment of the Arthritic Valgus Ankle

Alexej Barg, MD[a,b,*], Geert I. Pagenstert, MD[a], André G. Leumann, MD[a], Andreas M. Müller, MD[a], Heath B. Henninger, PhD[b], Victor Valderrabano, MD, PhD[a,*]

KEYWORDS

- Total ankle replacement • Ankle alignment • Arthritic valgus ankle • Valgus deformity
- Realignment surgery for arthritic valgus ankle
- Total ankle replacement for arthritic valgus angle

KEY POINTS

- The ankle joint has highly congruent bony surfaces allowing for 3 articulations, and it is part of a biomechanical hindfoot complex.
- Ankle osteoarthritis (OA) is a growing problem; approximately 1% of the world's adult population is affected by pain, dysfunction, and impaired mobility.
- Trauma is the primary cause of ankle OA,[1,2] often resulting in varus or valgus deformities. Only 50% of all patients with end-stage ankle OA have normal hindfoot alignment.

ARTHRITIC VALGUS ANKLE

Ankle Alignment

The alignment of the hindfoot can be divided into 3 anatomic aspects: supramalleolar, tibiotalar (orientation of the line of the tibiotalar joint), and inframalleolar.[1–8] The medial distal tibial angle (MDTA) is used to quantify supramalleolar alignment. In a radiographic study[9] it measured 92.4 ± 3.1° (range 88–100°) and in a cadaver study it measured 93.3 ± 3.2° (range 88–100°).[10] The mortise view should be used for measurements of the MDTA because it depends on radiographic technique, specifically the length of the tibia visible in the radiograph.[11] In general, reliable assessment of the inframalleolar alignment is much more difficult. Visual inspection of the hindfoot and clinical measurements with a goniometer are inaccurate.[8,12–14] The mortise view

---

The authors have nothing to disclose.

[a] Orthopaedic Department, University Hospital of Basel, University of Basel, Spitalstrasse 21, Basel CH-4031, Switzerland; [b] Harold K. Dunn Orthopaedic Research Laboratory, University Orthopaedic Center, University of Utah, 590 Wakara Way, Salt Lake City, UT 84108, USA

* Corresponding authors.

E-mail addresses: abarg@uhbs.ch; vvalderrabano@uhbs.ch

http://dx.doi.org/10.1016/j.fcl.2012.08.007

should not be used for evaluation of the inframalleolar alignment because in most cases the heel is hard to identify because of overlap of the midfoot, and the heel has a false lateral position (20° inner rotation of the foot and ankle). The Saltzman view is suggested for assessment of inframalleolar alignment.[15] In our experience, the physiologic inframalleolar alignment should be neutral or 1° to 2° of varus[7,8,16] and not 5° to 7° of valgus as reported in previous studies.[15,17–19]

Development of Osteoarthritis in Valgus Ankle

Valgus supramalleolar and/or inframalleolar deformities lead to an increase in pressure in the lateral part of the tibiotalar joint causing asymmetric lateral joint degeneration: distal tibial malunions, shortening fibula malunion, medial ankle ligament instability, hindfoot coalitios, posterior tibial tendon insufficiency, posttraumatic valgus sequelae of the hindfoot. Therefore, hindfoot malalignment has been identified as one of the most important risk factors of ankle osteoarthritis (OA) in numerous studies.[20–27] Steffensmeier and colleagues[28] analyzed the effects of medial and lateral displacement calcaneal osteotomies on tibiotalar joint contact stresses in cadavera. Lateral displacements unloaded the medial part of the tibiotalar joint whereas medial calcaneal displacements had the converse effect.[28] Recently, Knupp and colleagues[29] investigated changes in joint pressure and force transfer in cadaveric ankles with a supramalleolar deformity created by supramalleolar osteotomies. In specimens with an osteotomized fibula, valgus supramalleolar deformities led to a shift in force and peak pressure in the posterolateral direction.[29]

Valderrabano and colleagues[1] evaluated different causes leading to ankle OA and compared the important clinical and radiologic variables among the different groups. The mean radiologic alignment in the coronal plane was 88.0° (range 51–116°): 148 ankles (37%) had normal alignment, 225 ankles (55%) had varus alignment, and 33 ankles (8%) had valgus alignment. This distribution was similar in all 3 groups: patients with posttraumatic, secondary, and primary OA.[1] Similar results were observed by Chou and colleagues[30] with 13% of all patients with primary ankle OA presenting with planovalgus deformity.

Medial ligamental instability has been shown to be an important risk factor for pathogenesis of ankle OA.[31,32] Clarke and colleagues[33] developed a cadaveric ankle model and showed that sectioning of the deltoid ligament, regardless of fibular displacement, created up to 20° decrease in the contact area of the ankle joint. Harper[34] performed an anatomic study to evaluate the functions of the deltoid ligament, and showed that sectioning the superficial deltoid ligament did not result in increased anterior translation or lateral shift of the talus, whereas sectioning of the deep deltoid ligament did result in significant lateral shift and anterior translation of the talus.[34] Earll and colleagues[35] used 15 normal cadaveric lower extremities and observed the most significant changes in tibiotalar pressure after sectioning of the tibiocalcaneal fibers of the superficial deltoid ligament complex.[35] Michelson and colleagues[36] demonstrated that disruption of the deep deltoid ligament significantly increased the internal rotation of the foot.

Morthophological Type of Arthritic Valgus Ankle

Arthritic valgus ankles can be divided into 2 different morphologic types. The first type includes severe pes planovalgus deformity with insufficiency of the medial ligaments and advanced posterior tibial tendon insufficiency.[37–40] In the second type, osseous deformities are the primary factors. Osseous deformities and/or defects may result from malunion after fibular fractures or fractures of distal tibia (especially after intraarticular tibial plafond fractures).[6,37,41]

TREATMENT OPTIONS IN THE ARTHRITIC VALGUS ANKLE

Patients with an arthritic valgus ankle should be individually assessed and all concomitant pathologic conditions should be considered and addressed if necessary. Examples include: deltoid ligament insufficiency, dysfunction of the posterior tibial tendon, contracted heel cord, osseous deformities and/or defects of the distal tibia, shortening and/or deformity of the fibula, and inframalleolar deformities. Given the wide range of potential concomitant pathologic conditions, a generic approach in these patients may result in frequent clinical failure.[37]

Realignment Surgery for the Arthritic Valgus Ankle

In patients with arthritic valgus ankles, conservative treatment should be attempted first. Conservative treatment includes nonsteroidal antirheumatic therapy, shoe modifications with special insoles, physiotherapy, and semi-rigid orthoses.[42] The decision to plan realignment surgery should not be postponed too long because the development of degenerative changes is continuous and may proceed quickly.

The main indication for realignment surgery is lateral valgus ankle joint OA.[21,43] Cartilage of more than half of tibiotalar joint surface should be preserved. This may be assessed preoperatively by magnetic resonance imaging[44] and/or single photon emission-computed tomography (SPECT).[45,46] Furthermore, before realignment surgery, we recommend ankle arthroscopy or arthrotomy to assess the degree and localization of cartilage damage and ligamental instability.[21] We also recommend evaluation of cartilage degeneration according to the Outerbridge classification: grade 0, no cartilage damage; grade 1, cartilage softening; grade 2, cartilage damage with stripping of superficial cartilage layers; grade 3, deep cartilage ulceration without visible subchondral bone; grade 4, visible subchondral bone.[47]

Realignment surgery should not be performed in[21]

- patients in poor general health (especially patients who are unable to perform nonweight bearing exercises during the initial postoperative rehabilitation)
- patients with systemic joint disease
- patients with nonmanageable insufficiency of the deltoid ligament

The surgical realignment technique for arthritic valgus ankle has been described in detail previously.[21] The main surgery includes a medial-closing wedge osteotomy performed in the distal tibial metaphysis (**Fig. 1**). The aim of the surgery should be a final 2° to 5° varus orientation of the distal tibial joint.[21,48–50] In most cases, additional osseous and ligamental surgical procedures are necessary to achieve a well-balanced and stable hindfoot with restored physiologic biomechanics. Additional corrective surgeries should be performed depending on the stage and origin of the valgus deformity.[49] Patients with stage I deformity present with collapse of the lateral compartment of the tibial plafond and/or lateral malleolar gutter. In patients with stage I deformity with fibular malunion, a corrective lengthening osteotomy of the fibula should be performed. In patients with stage II deformity, lateral ankle joint degeneration is observed in combination with significant inframalleolar valgus alignment (heel valgus). In such cases, a medial sliding osteotomy[51,52] should be performed after correction of the tibiotalar joint deformity by supramalleolar osteotomy. In general, the heel-ground contact point should be shifted medially until a final position of 0 to 5 mm medial to the loading axis is achieved (Saltzman view). Stage III valgus deformity usually develops as a result of progressive flat foot deformity (eg, patients with stage III[53] or IV[38,54] dysfunction of the posterior tibial tendon). In these patients, inframalleolar deformity should be addressed by performing lateral calcaneal lengthening

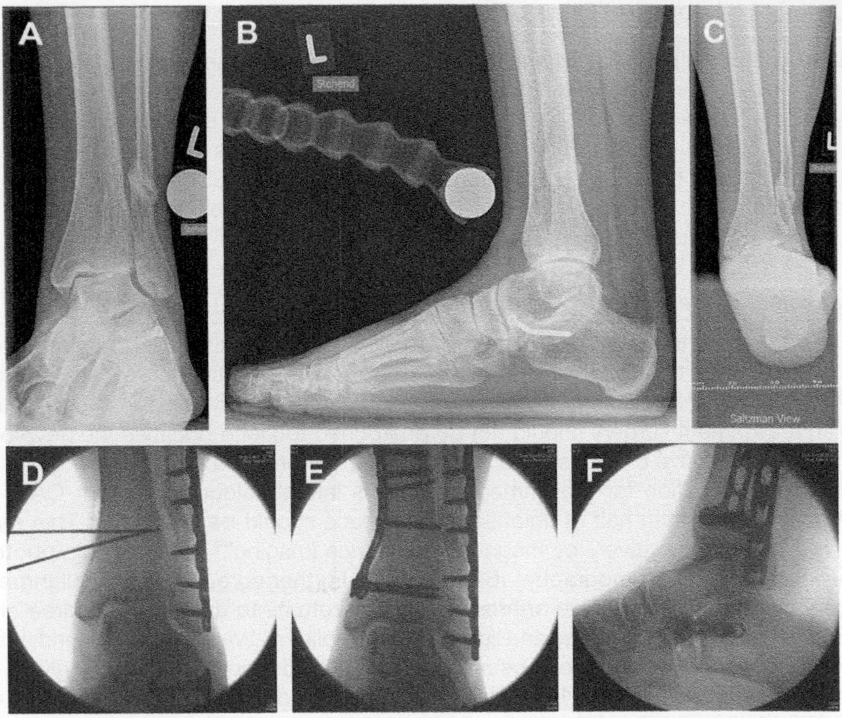

Fig. 1. A 58-year-old woman with progressive valgus malalignment of the hindfoot. (*A*) Anteroposterior radiograph shows the medial tilting of the talus with consecutive collapse of the lateral compartment of the tibiotalar joint. Significant shortening of the fibula is observed due to nonunion of a fibula stress fracture. (*B*) Lateral view shows nonunion of a previous attempt lengthening osteotomy of the calcaneus with a broken screw. (*C*) Saltzman view shows valgus malposition of the heel. (*D*) First, lengthening of the fibula has been performed with debridement of the nonunion area and stabilization with a plate. Also nonunion of the calcaneus osteotomy was debrided and refixed using a plate. Planning the supramalleolar medial-closing wedge osteotomy using 2 K-wires. (*E, F*) Physiologic alignment of the hindfoot with appropriate talus position within the mortise.

osteotomy to correct valgus abductus.[55] In some patients, additional forefoot correction surgery (eg, flexion osteotomy of the first metatarsal or medial cuneiform[56]) should be performed. Medial soft tissue procedures (posterior tibial tendon augmentation, reconstruction of medial ligaments) should be performed to achieve postoperative ligamental stability. In patients with fixed rigid pes planovalgus deformity, medial column procedures[57,58] or triple arthrodesis[59,60] should be performed to restore the physiologic medial arch of the foot.

Pitfalls of Realignment Surgery for Arthritic Valgus Ankle

In patients with undercorrected valgus deformity, the degenerative changes of the lateral part of the tibiotalar joint may progress. Therefore, realignment surgery should be repeated. Overcorrection after supramalleolar osteotomy is rare.[21] In patients with radiological delay or nonunion, immobilization in a stable walker or cast should be extended for 3 months postoperatively. We recommend computed tomography or SPECT scans to assess the status of the union 6 months after the primary surgery. In patients with symptomatic nonunion, internal fixation with grafting should be performed. The restricted range of motion of the realigned ankle should be treated first with intensive physiotherapy including stretching of triceps surae. In patients with chronic unmanageable triceps surae contracture, a percutaneous release may be performed. In patients with restriction of range of motion caused by osteophytes, open or arthroscopic debridement can be performed. In patients with progressive development of tibiotalar OA, joint-sacrificing procedures (ankle fusion or total ankle replacement [TAR]) should be discussed.

TAR in Patients with Valgus Deformity

Joint-sacrificing treatments include TAR (**Fig. 2**) and ankle fusion. They should be performed when joint-preserving procedures (eg, corrective osteotomies and/or ligament

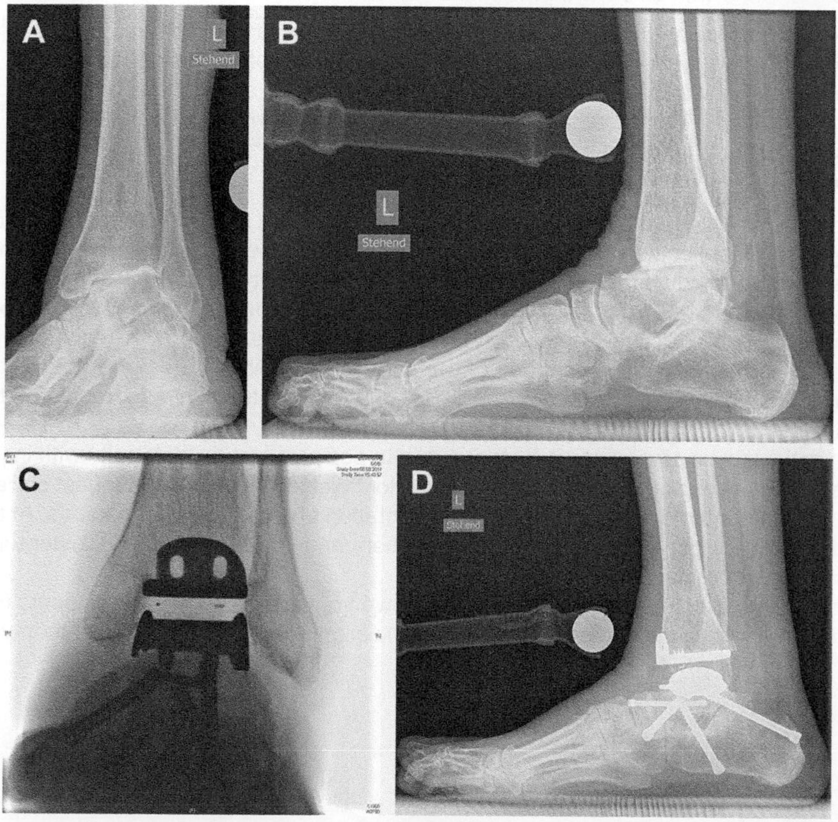

Fig. 2. An 82-year-old man with progressive valgus arthritic ankle and stage IV posterior tibial tendon dysfunction. The symptoms started 4 years previously and were progressive. The patient presented with significant impairment of mobility: maximal walking distance ca 100 m. (*A*) Anteroposterior radiograph shows a valgus arthritic ankle with subfibular impingement and lateralization of the heel. (*B*) Lateral view shows a collapsed tibiotalar joint line and degenerative changes of the subtalar and talonavicular joints. (*C, D*) Postoperative radiographs show appropriate alignment of prosthesis components. The hindfoot alignment was restored by modified triple arthrodesis (subtalar and talonavicular arthrodesis). (*Data from* De Wachter J, Knupp M, Hintermann B. Double-hindfoot arthrodesis through a single medial approach. Techniques in Foot & Ankle Surgery 2007;6:237–42; and Knupp M, Stufkens SA, Hintermann B. Triple arthrodesis. Foot Ankle Clin 2011;16:61–7.)

reconstruction) have failed. Ankle fusion may result in pain relief, at least in the short term,[61,62] however, mid-term and long-term problems include impaired mobility, difficulty walking on uneven surfaces, and difficulty running.[63–65] Increased load in the adjacent joints may lead to degenerative changes and painful OA.[61,64] Therefore, ankle fusion is no longer the gold standard therapy in patients with end-stage ankle OA.[66]

For TAR, we use the HINTEGRA prosthesis, a nonconstrained 3-component system.[67–70] A standardized surgical technique is used for implantation of the prosthesis components (see article by Barg and colleagues in this issue). In patients with valgus deformity of less than 10°, correction of the tibiotalar joint can be achieved by modification of bone cut. In patients with valgus deformity of more than 10°, additional surgeries should be performed depending on the localization and degree of the valgus deformity (**Fig. 3**):

- supramalleolar osteotomy (eg, medial-closing wedge osteotomy)[21,49,71,72]
- lengthening and (if necessary) rotational osteotomy of the distal fibula[73,74]
- corrective osteotomies of the calcaneus: medial displacement calcaneal osteotomy[51,52] or lateral column lengthening osteotomy of the calcaneus[49,75–77]
- reconstruction and repair of the medial ligaments[78,79]
- corrective subtalar fusion or triple arthrodesis[59,60]

In patients with severe hindfoot valgus malalignment due to significant valgus deformity and defects of the tibial plafond, we suggest the following chronologic sequence of surgical procedures. First, the supramalleolar deformity should be corrected by supramalleolar osteotomy followed by TAR. In patients with a remaining valgus position of the heel, calcaneal osteotomy or subtalar or triple arthrodesis (especially in patients with degenerative changes of the subtalar joint) should be performed. Ligamental instability should then be addressed by reconstruction and repair of the ligaments.

In patients with severe hindfoot valgus due to pes planovalgus deformity with insufficiency of the medial ligaments and/or posterior tibial tendon, we first suggest corrective subtalar or triple arthrodesis before implantation of prosthesis components. At the end of the surgery, ligamental reconstruction and fibula-lengthening osteotomy should be performed if necessary.

In patients with moderate hindfoot valgus, we implant prosthesis components first and then address the inframalleolar valgus malalignment by calcaneal osteotomy or

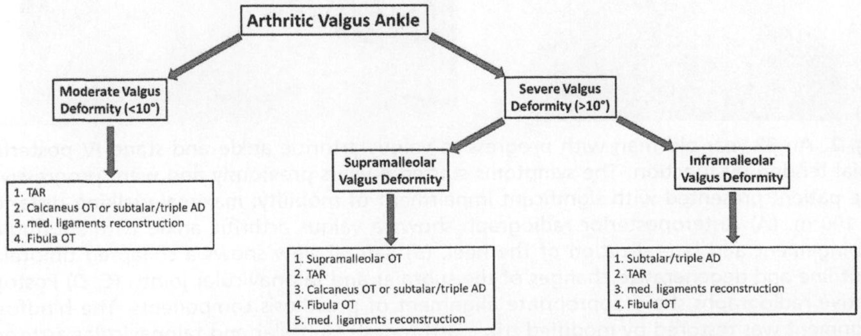

Fig. 3. Treatment strategy used for TAR in patients with preoperative valgus deformity of the hindfoot depends on the degree of the valgus deformity. AD, arthrodesis; med., medial; OT, osteotomy.

corrective subtalar or triple arthrodesis (patients with degenerative changes of the subtalar joint). In these patients, ligamental reconstruction and fibula-lengthening osteotomy should also be performed if necessary.

Pitfalls of TAR in Patients with Valgus Deformity

TAR is gaining acceptance among foot and ankle surgeons as an alternative treatment in patients with end-stage ankle OA. However, this procedure remains technically demanding and has a steep learning curve.[80–82] Correct positioning of the prosthesis components is one of the most demanding steps,[80,83] especially in patients with preoperative valgus or varus deformity. Malposition of the prosthesis components has biomechanical consequences, as shown in numerous cadaveric studies.[84–86] Recently, a clinical study showed that patients with neutrally aligned prosthesis components had the best clinical outcomes including range of motion and pain relief.[87] When the preoperative deformity was not sufficiently addressed, patients developed medial pain syndrome requiring revision surgery.[88] Furthermore, the patients who underwent TAR with a malaligned hindfoot were more likely to develop edge loading and are at higher risk for prosthesis failure.[14,89–92]

LITERATURE REVIEW: TAR EXPERIENCE IN PATIENTS WITH VALGUS DEFORMITY

The first clinical report addressing the feasibility and clinical outcomes of TAR recognized preoperative varus or valgus deformity as a possible source of prosthesis failure. Newton[93,94] performed 50 TAR procedures using the Newton Ankle Implant (a nonconstrained cemented prosthesis including high density polyethylene tibial and Vitallium talar components). Valgus or varus deformity of the talus greater than 20° was noted as an absolute contraindication for TAR.[93,94] In a later study,[95] Newton stated that although valgus or varus deformity of up to 15° could be corrected initially, the coronal deformity usually recurred. All ankles replaced with a talar tilt of more than 20° failed during the follow-up.[95] Kirkup[96] observed that severe valgus or varus deformity was common in many patients with rheumatoid OA. The author recognized that these deformities could not be corrected by cutting wedges, therefore, preoperative coronal deformity greater than 30° was a contraindication for TAR.[96] Stauffer and Segal[97] performed 102 TAR procedures using the Mayo Total Ankle, which is a highly congruent 2-component design including a polyethylene tibial component and cement fixation. The procedure was not performed in patients with preoperative coronal deformity (varus or valgus) of more than 20°.[97]

Pyevich and colleagues[98] analyzed the mid-term results of 100 consecutive Agility TAR procedures performed between 1984 and 1993 with a mean follow-up of 5 years. Preoperative valgus or varus malalignment was corrected using an external fixator. McIff and colleagues[99] and Vienne and Nothdurft[100] suggested the intraoperative correction of varus or valgus deformity using the external fixator with the Agility TAR. Pyevich and colleagues[98] observed that the position of the tibial component had a significant influence on the outcome. Patients with tibial components placed in more than 4° valgus had significantly more postoperative pain ($P<.05$) than the patients with neutrally aligned prosthesis components.

Saltzman[101] reviewed the state of the art in using TAR in 2000. He recognized that preoperative varus or valgus deformity, which was not sufficiently addressed during the TAR procedure, may lead to loading that accelerates the rate of polyethylene wear.[101]

Greisberg and Hansen[102,103] presented their strategies on how to address the associated deformities in patients with TAR. In patients with valgus foot due to medial collapse, the medial column should be restored, which may also regain the appropriate tension of the medial ligaments. The investigators suggest placing the tibial and talar components in a slightly lateral position. If the valgus malalignment of the hindfoot persists, a medial sliding osteotomy of the calcaneus should be performed. In patients with advanced flat foot deformity, a triple arthrodesis in addition to medial column stabilization may be performed to achieve proper alignment in the long term. The investigators stated that patients with persistent misalignment of the replaced ankle may have a higher risk of prosthesis failure.[102,103]

Conti and Wong[90,91] reviewed the possible complications of TAR. Varus or valgus malpositioning of the prosthesis components was a possible source of TAR failure. They stated that valgus positioning of the prosthesis component may be better tolerated that varus positioning. However, they recommended corrective osteotomy for supramalleolar deformity of more than 10° and cutting jig adjustment in ankles with any deformities of the distal tibial articular surface.[90,91]

Stamatis and Myerson[104] described how to avoid specific complications of TAR. They observed different pathologic conditions in valgus arthritic ankles including contracted lateral ligaments and insufficient medial ligaments, valgus heel, shortening and deformities of the fibula causing chronic impingement, and/or rupture of the spring ligament and posterior tibial tendon. The correction of the valgus deformity included several osseous and ligament procedures.[104]

Wood and Deakin[105] reviewed the results of 200 cementless, mobile-bearing Scandinavian TAR (STAR) procedures performed between 1993 and 2000. Preoperatively, 39 ankles had a significant coronal deformity of more than 15° (17 ankles with varus and 22 ankles with valgus deformity). Seven of these 39 ankles (18%) developed edge loading, whereas only 2 of the 161 ankles with neutral alignment (1%) had comparable problems. Of the 9 patients with edge loading 3 had additional surgery to improve realignment and stability of the hindfoot and 3 ankles ended up in conversion to ankle fusion. Therefore, the investigators stated that preoperative varus or valgus deformity of the talus of more than 10° was a relative contraindication for TAR.[105] Similar findings were observed in a later study including the same 200 STAR procedures.[106] Wood and colleagues[107] performed a review and addressed the outcomes of currently available TAR designs. The investigators found that the failure rate was lower in ankles that were well aligned than in ankles with more than 15° of valgus or varus preoperative deformity.[107]

Assal and colleagues[108] presented a case report describing fracture of the polyethylene component in a patient who underwent Agility TAR caused by varus malalignment of the talar component. The investigators stated that uncorrected foot and hindfoot deformities may induce significant valgus or varus forces resulting in pathologic polyethylene wear patterns. Therefore, especially in patients who undergo Agility TAR, normal alignment is important because the Agility TAR system has little intrinsic stability.[108]

Hintermann and Valderrabano[69] reviewed the use of TAR in 2003. In earlier clinical studies, patients with significant preoperative varus or valgus deformities were excluded from TAR, and ankle fusion was performed. The investigators stated that, as long the deformities could be corrected before or during the TAR procedure, they were not a contraindication for TAR.[69]

Takakura and colleagues[109] reviewed 160 TARs performed between 1975 and 2000 using a TNK ceramic prosthesis, which underwent 3 generations of development. The investigators suggested that TAR should not be used in patients with varus or valgus deformities of the tibial articular surface exceeding 15°, because of observed loosening and subsidence of the prosthesis in the early postoperative period.[109,110]

Greisberg and colleagues[111] addressed the importance of hindfoot alignment in patients undergoing TAR and described how to achieve a well-balanced hindfoot. Two different reasons for valgus malalignment in the ankle were described: posttraumatic arthritic ankle with loss of bone from the lateral plafond and advanced flatfoot with insufficient medial ligaments. The investigators recommended medial ligament reconstruction and, if necessary, restoration of the medial column. For valgus ankles, the bone cuts were not performed too close to the medial malleolus. After implantation of the final prosthesis components, the position of the hindfoot and the heel were checked and if the ankle remained in valgus, a medial sliding calcaneal osteotomy was performed.[111]

Haskell and Mann[92] presented short-term results of 86 patients who underwent STAR with a mean follow-up of 2 years. Thirty-five of 86 patients had a preoperative coronal plane deformity of more than 10° (25 patients with varus deformity and 10 patients with valgus deformity). All patients were divided into 4 groups: varus congruent, valgus congruent, varus incongruent, and valgus incongruent. In ankles with talar and tibial deformities, talar and tibial alignment improved toward a neutral weight-bearing axis postoperatively. The alignment remained constant during the subsequent 2 years. Eight of 34 patients developed progressive edge loading requiring 4 additional procedures. The patients with preoperative incongruent joints were 10 times more likely to develop postoperative edge loading.[92]

Kofoed[112] described a special sculpting technique on the talus that allows intraoperative correction of varus or valgus ankle deformity of more than 45°. This technique included cutting 1- to 2-mm slices off the talus facets and the talar dome, followed by rotation of the entire hindfoot inside the ankle mortise until normal hindfoot alignment was achieved. The investigators presented a case of a patient with preoperative valgus deformity of about 50°, with only a slight postoperative valgus alignment of the hindfoot.[112]

Doets and colleagues[113] performed a prospective single-center study including 19 low contact stress mobile-bearing TARs and 74 Buechel-Pappas TARs. The 8-year survivorship for both prostheses, with revision or conversion to an arthrodesis for any reason as the end point, was 85% (95% CI 73%–93%). However, the same survivorship in 17 ankles with a preoperative varus or valgus deformity of more than 10° was significantly lower ($P = .03$) at 48% (95% CI 6%–90%), whereas survivorship in ankles with a neutral preoperative alignment was 90% (95% CI 82%–98%). In 2 ankles with preexisting valgus deformity, a medial malleolar fracture occurred intraoperatively with nonunion in the further course. Both ankles also developed a stress fracture of the lateral malleolus resulting in nonmanageable valgus instability requiring ankle fusion. Therefore, the investigators defined preoperative valgus or varus deformity of more than 10° as an absolute contraindication for TAR. The investigators suggested that corrective surgery (eg, triple arthrodesis) should be performed before TAR to restore normal biomechanics and alignment of the hindfoot.[113]

Henricson and Ågren[114] performed 196 second-generation TARs in 186 patients with a mean follow-up of 4 years: 109 STAR, 62 Buechel-Pappas, and 22 AES (Ankle Evolutive System; Transystem, France) ankles. All ankles were divided into 3 groups: (1) normal hindfoot alignment (normal value was set to 5° valgus) n = 92; (2) varus alignment (mean 9.6°, range 5–30°) n = 55; (3) valgus alignment (mean 11°, range 5–30°) n = 46. The preoperative valgus malalignment was neutralized in 20 ankles, 1 overcorrected in slight varus, and 23 ankles stayed in a valgus position (mean 7.6°, range 5–15°). The overall revision rate was 21%. The revision rate was 31% in the preoperative varus group and 17% in the valgus and neutral groups, respectively. Therefore, the investigators stated that additional surgeries should be performed to achieve neutral alignment and TAR should be limited only to experienced foot and ankle surgeons.[114]

Coetzee[89] presented his strategies on how to perform TAR in patients with varus or valgus deformities. He identified that most valgus deformities are secondary to chronic posterior tibial tendon dysfunction. A lateral release could be done to get the talus in the correct position in the mortise. A primary deltoid repair can be performed; however, it is never strong enough. The following corrective procedures were suggested: posterior tibial tendon repair with augmentation of the flexor digitorum longus tendon, gastrocnemius slide, and stabilization of the medial ray. In patients with severe and rigid valgus deformities, a triple arthrodesis was performed to achieve long-term stability. The author suggested 15° of varus or valgus ligamentous instability as the arbitrary cut-off point and 10° as the hard cut-off point for performing ankle fusion.[89]

Bluman and Chiodo[37] described the anatomy and biomechanics of valgus arthritic ankles and presented different therapeutic strategies. In patients with preoperative coronal deformities of more than 15°, there was a higher risk of mechanical failure. However, in valgus arthritic ankles, all concomitant deformities (proximal and distal to the tibiotalar joint) should be sufficiently addressed.[37]

Wood and colleagues[14] performed a randomized, prospective, single-center study including 200 TARs to compare Buechel-Pappas and STAR implants with a minimum follow-up of 3 years. The 6-year survivorship was comparable ($P = .09$) in both groups: 79% (95% CI 63.4%–88.5%) and 95% (95% CI 87.2%–98.1%) in the Buechel-Pappas and STAR groups, respectively. However, the investigators observed a significantly higher ($P = .02$) incidence of prosthesis failure in ankles with preoperative varus or valgus deformity, especially when the deformity was greater than 15°, resulting in a predicted failure rate at 6 years exceeding 10% for the STAR prosthesis and 25% for the Buechel-Pappas prosthesis. When the preoperative deformity was 15° or less, the estimated 6-year survivorship was 86.7% for the Buechel-Pappas group and 95.5% for the STAR group.[14] Wood and colleagues[115] also shared their experience of TAR in patients with rheumatoid ankle OA. Nearly 50% of all patients with rheumatoid OA requiring either fusion or TAR presented with valgus deformity. In patients who underwent TAR, the heel should be well aligned under the tibia, which can be achieved by hindfoot fusion, as a 1-stage procedure, or 6 or 12 weeks before the ankle replacement.[115] In some patients, the valgus deformity had been corrected without ligamental release, but an alarming gap on the lateral side between the malleolus and prosthesis component was seen.[116]

Karantana and colleagues[117] retrospectively reviewed 45 patients with 52 TARs using the STAR prosthesis with a minimum follow-up of 5 years. Thirteen ankles (27%) had a preoperative coronal deformity of more than 10° (range 11–25°); most of them were in preoperative varus. The investigators believed that the preoperative hindfoot deformity was not an absolute contraindication for TAR, as long the deformity was manageable by additional realignment procedures including soft tissue releases, ligament reconstructions, calcaneal osteotomies, and corrective subtalar fusion.[117]

Wood and colleagues[118] reported short-term clinical and radiological results of a prospective case series including 100 Mobility TARs with a minimum follow-up of 3 years. There were 15 ankles with a preoperative coronal deformity between 16° and 20°. A varus or valgus deformity was observed in 33 (in 17 of these it was more than 10°) and in 29 (in 13 of these it was more than 10°) ankles, respectively. Postoperatively, there were 5 cases of edge loading of the mobile insert due to varus or valgus deformity. Of 5 ankles requiring revision surgery, 4 had significant preoperative coronal deformity: 3 patients with valgus deformity (11°, 12°, and 15°) and 1 patient with varus deformity (19°). Therefore, the investigators do not undertake TAR in patients with preoperative valgus or varus deformity of more than 20°. In these cases, the investigators recommend ankle fusion.[118]

Ellis and DeOrio[119] described the surgical technique using the INBONE prosthesis in detail. The investigators described how to correct slight varus or valgus deformity intraoperatively using a laminar spreader with teeth; the desired position of the talus should be 5° of valgus. However, the investigators stated that valgus deformity is more difficult to correct using this technique.[119,120]

Skyttä and colleagues[121] presented the survivorship analysis of the Finnish Arthroplasty Register included 515 TARs performed between 1982 and 2006. Nine different TAR prostheses were used. The most common TAR types were AES, STAR, ICLH, and HINTEGRA prostheses with 298, 217, 32, and 11 cases, respectively. The proportion of revisions done for instability in primary TAR was 39%. One of the reasons for prosthesis failure was preoperative valgus or varus deformity with insufficient ligaments.[121]

Morgan and colleagues[122] presented the outcomes in 38 consecutive patients who underwent TAR using the AES ankle with a minimum follow-up of 4 years. Twenty-eight patients had normal hindfoot alignment preoperatively, 10 patients had a valgus alignment ranging from 7° to 30°, and 7 patients had a varus alignment ranging from 4° to 23°. Postoperatively, 10 patients presented with edge loading; 5 and 2 of them had preoperative varus and valgus alignment, respectively.[122]

Kim and colleagues[123] reported the clinical and radiological outcomes of TAR in association with hindfoot fusion. Three ankles (5%) in the hindfoot fusion group and 10 ankles (3.5%) in the control group had preoperative coronal deformity of more than 15°. Significant valgus or varus deformity was not associated with a worse functional outcome or higher failure rate.[123]

Bonasia and colleagues[124] presented a review regarding indications for TAR and their surgical techniques. For small minimal distal tibial deformities less than 10°, realignment can be achieved by modification of the tibial cut. For more severe deformities, a dome or wedge osteotomy should be performed before TAR.[124]

Bonnin and colleagues[125] retrospectively reviewed 98 TARs performed in 97 ankles between 1997 and 2000 using the Salto prosthesis. The investigators did not consider substantial preoperative varus or valgus deformity as a contraindication for TAR. However, all hindfoot deformities were corrected as a first step with an associated procedure (eg, triple arthrodesis).[125] In some patients with preoperative valgus deformity, a special cemented lateral malleolar component was implanted to normalize load transfer in this patient cohort.[126]

Recently, Trincat and colleagues[127] presented their results of using TAR in patients with coronal plane deformities. Of a total of 131 TARs, 21 TARs (16 AES ankles, 4 Salto ankles, and 1 New-Jersey ankle) were performed in ankles with preoperative coronal deformities of more than 10°. There were 4 congruent and 2 incongruent valgus ankles. The following additional 1-stage surgeries were performed to achieve osseous and ligamental balancing: lateral malleolus lowering (2), Achilles tendon lengthening (4), reconstruction of medial ligaments (1), and triple arthrodesis (1). For congruent valgus ankles, surgery resulted in significant improvement in overall alignment from $14.7 \pm 2.5°$ to $0 \pm 2.5°$. There were no complications or failures in this subgroup. In preoperative incongruent valgus ankles, improvement in overall alignment from $19 \pm 5.5°$ to $2 \pm 4.2°$ was observed. Failure occurred in 1 patient who presented with a 23° deformity caused by a bimalleolar fracture with insufficiency of the medial ligaments and posterior tibial tendon dysfunction. In conclusion, the short-term results of TAR in patients with preoperative coronal deformities of more than 10° are comparable to those observed in patients with no deformities. However, several associated procedures were necessary to address the concomitant instabilities and deformities. Residual defects may compromise the longevity of prosthesis components and warrant further correction.[127]

SUMMARY

A clinically and radiologically well-aligned hindfoot and proper position of prosthesis components are the keys to long-term prosthesis stability and reliable functional outcomes in patients who undergo TAR. In patients with preoperative coronal deformities (valgus or varus), alignment and biomechanics should be restored. Our clinic typically strives to obtain a medial distal tibial angle of 90° and neutral inframalleolar alignment (as assessed using the Saltzman view). A moderate preoperative valgus deformity of less than 10° can be corrected intraoperatively by modification of bone cuts. In other patients, the deformity should be accurately corrected on the supramalleolar and/or inframalleolar levels before TAR. In patients with ligamental instability, reconstruction surgery should be performed to achieve a stable hindfoot.

REFERENCES

1. Valderrabano V, Horisberger M, Russell I, et al. Etiology of ankle osteoarthritis. Clin Orthop Relat Res 2009;467:1800–6.
2. Saltzman CL, Salamon ML, Blanchard GM, et al. Epidemiology of ankle arthritis: report of a consecutive series of 639 patients from a tertiary orthopaedic center. Iowa Orthop J 2005;25:44–6.
3. Knupp M, Valderrabano V, Hintermann B. Anatomical and biomechanical aspects of total ankle replacement. Orthopade 2006;35:489–94 [in German].
4. Kitaoka HB, Luo ZP, An KN. Three-dimensional analysis of normal ankle and foot mobility. Am J Sports Med 1997;25:238–42.
5. Glazebrook M, Daniels T, Younger A, et al. Comparison of health-related quality of life between patients with end-stage ankle and hip arthrosis. J Bone Joint Surg Am 2008;90:499–505.
6. Horisberger M, Valderrabano V, Hintermann B. Posttraumatic ankle osteoarthritis after ankle-related fractures. J Orthop Trauma 2009;23:60–7.
7. Frigg A, Nigg B, Davis E, et al. Does alignment in the hindfoot radiograph influence dynamic foot-floor pressures in ankle and tibiotalocalcaneal fusion? Clin Orthop Relat Res 2010;468:3362–70.
8. Frigg A, Nigg B, Hinz L, et al. Clinical relevance of hindfoot alignment view in total ankle replacement. Foot Ankle Int 2010;31:871–9.
9. Knupp M, Ledermann H, Magerkurth O, et al. The surgical tibiotalar angle: a radiologic study. Foot Ankle Int 2005;26:713–6.
10. Inman VT. The joints of the ankle. Baltimore (MD): Williams & Wilkins; 1976.
11. Stufkens SA, Barg A, Bolliger L, et al. Measurement of the medial distal tibial angle. Foot Ankle Int 2011;32:288–93.
12. Backer M, Kofoed H. Passive ankle mobility. Clinical measurement compared with radiography. J Bone Joint Surg Br 1989;71:696–8.
13. Buck P, Morrey BF, Chao EY. The optimum position of arthrodesis of the ankle. A gait study of the knee and ankle. J Bone Joint Surg Am 1987;69:1052–62.
14. Wood PL, Sutton C, Mishra V, et al. A randomised, controlled trial of two mobile-bearing total ankle replacements. J Bone Joint Surg Br 2009;91:69–74.
15. Saltzman CL, el Khoury GY. The hindfoot alignment view. Foot Ankle Int 1995;16:572–6.
16. Valderrabano V, Frigg A, Leumann A, et al. Total ankle arthroplasty in valgus ankle osteoarthritis. Orthopade 2011;40:971–7 [in German].

17. Brinker M. Review of orthopaedic trauma. Philadelphia: Saunders-Elsevier; 2001.
18. Johnson JE, Lamdan R, Granberry WF, et al. Hindfoot coronal alignment: a modified radiographic method. Foot Ankle Int 1999;20:818–25.
19. Miller M. Review of orthopaedics. Philadelphia: Saunders-Elsevier; 2004.
20. Thomas RH, Daniels TR. Ankle arthritis. J Bone Joint Surg Am 2003;85:923–36.
21. Pagenstert GI, Hintermann B, Barg A, et al. Realignment surgery as alternative treatment of varus and valgus ankle osteoarthritis. Clin Orthop Relat Res 2007;462:156–68.
22. Takakura Y, Takaoka T, Tanaka Y, et al. Results of opening-wedge osteotomy for the treatment of a post-traumatic varus deformity of the ankle. J Bone Joint Surg Am 1998;80:213–8.
23. Stamatis ED, Cooper PS, Myerson MS. Supramalleolar osteotomy for the treatment of distal tibial angular deformities and arthritis of the ankle joint. Foot Ankle Int 2003;24:754–64.
24. Buckwalter JA, Saltzman C, Brown T. The impact of osteoarthritis: implications for research. Clin Orthop Relat Res 2004;S6–15.
25. Buckwalter JA, Brown TD. Joint injury, repair, and remodeling: roles in post-traumatic osteoarthritis. Clin Orthop Relat Res 2004;7–16.
26. Felson DT. Risk factors for osteoarthritis: understanding joint vulnerability. Clin Orthop Relat Res 2004;S16–21.
27. McKinley TO, Rudert MJ, Koos DC, et al. Pathomechanic determinants of post-traumatic arthritis. Clin Orthop Relat Res 2004;S78–88.
28. Steffensmeier SJ, Saltzman CL, Berbaum KS, et al. Effects of medial and lateral displacement calcaneal osteotomies on tibiotalar joint contact stresses. J Orthop Res 1996;14:980–5.
29. Knupp M, Stufkens SA, van Bergen CJ, et al. Effect of supramalleolar varus and valgus deformities on the tibiotalar joint: a cadaveric study. Foot Ankle Int 2011;32:609–15.
30. Chou LB, Coughlin MT, Hansen S Jr, et al. Osteoarthritis of the ankle: the role of arthroplasty. J Am Acad Orthop Surg 2008;16:249–59.
31. Deland JT, de Asla RJ, Segal A. Reconstruction of the chronically failed deltoid ligament: a new technique. Foot Ankle Int 2004;25:795–9.
32. Valderrabano V, Hintermann B, Horisberger M, et al. Ligamentous posttraumatic ankle osteoarthritis. Am J Sports Med 2006;34:612–20.
33. Clarke HJ, Michelson JD, Cox QG, et al. Tibio-talar stability in bimalleolar ankle fractures: a dynamic in vitro contact area study. Foot Ankle 1991;11:222–7.
34. Harper MC. Deltoid ligament: an anatomical evaluation of function. Foot Ankle 1987;8:19–22.
35. Earll M, Wayne J, Brodrick C, et al. Contribution of the deltoid ligament to ankle joint contact characteristics: a cadaver study. Foot Ankle Int 1996;17:317–24.
36. Michelson JD, Hamel AJ, Buczek FL, et al. Kinematic behavior of the ankle following malleolar fracture repair in a high-fidelity cadaver model. J Bone Joint Surg Am 2002;84:2029–38.
37. Bluman EM, Chiodo CP. Valgus ankle deformity and arthritis. Foot Ankle Clin 2008;13:443–70, ix.
38. Bluman EM, Myerson MS. Stage IV posterior tibial tendon rupture. Foot Ankle Clin 2007;12:341–62, viii.
39. Bohay DR, Anderson JG. Stage IV posterior tibial tendon insufficiency: the tilted ankle. Foot Ankle Clin 2003;8:619–36.
40. Francisco R, Chiodo CP, Wilson MG. Management of the rigid adult acquired flatfoot deformity. Foot Ankle Clin 2007;12:317–27, vii.

41. Giannini S, Faldini C, Acri F, et al. Surgical treatment of post-traumatic malalignment of the ankle. Injury 2010;41:1208–11.
42. Noll KH. The use of orthotic devices in adult acquired flatfoot deformity. Foot Ankle Clin 2001;6:25–36.
43. Hintermann B, Knupp M, Barg A. Osteotomies of the distal tibia and hindfoot for ankle realignment. Orthopade 2008;37:212–3 [in German].
44. Hintermann B. What the orthopaedic foot and ankle surgeon wants to know from MR imaging. Semin Musculoskelet Radiol 2005;9:260–71.
45. Knupp M, Pagenstert GI, Barg A, et al. SPECT-CT compared with conventional imaging modalities for the assessment of the varus and valgus malaligned hindfoot. J Orthop Res 2009;27:1461–6.
46. Pagenstert GI, Barg A, Leumann AG, et al. SPECT-CT imaging in degenerative joint disease of the foot and ankle. J Bone Joint Surg Br 2009;91:1191–6.
47. Outerbridge RE. The etiology of chondromalacia patellae. J Bone Joint Surg Br 1961;43:752–7.
48. Cheng YM, Huang PJ, Hong SH, et al. Low tibial osteotomy for moderate ankle arthritis. Arch Orthop Trauma Surg 2001;121:355–8.
49. Pagenstert G, Knupp M, Valderrabano V, et al. Realignment surgery for valgus ankle osteoarthritis. Oper Orthop Traumatol 2009;21:77–87.
50. Takakura Y, Tanaka Y, Kumai T, et al. Low tibial osteotomy for osteoarthritis of the ankle. Results of a new operation in 18 patients. J Bone Joint Surg Br 1995;77:50–4.
51. Stufkens SA, Knupp M, Hintermann B. Medial displacement calcaneal osteotomy. Techniques in Foot & Ankle Surgery 2009;8:85–90.
52. Rodriguez RP. Medial displacement calcaneal tuberosity osteotomy in the treatment of posterior tibial insufficiency. Foot Ankle Clin 2001;6:545–67, viii.
53. Kelly IP, Easley ME. Treatment of stage 3 adult acquired flatfoot. Foot Ankle Clin 2001;6:153–66.
54. Kelly IP, Nunley JA. Treatment of stage 4 adult acquired flatfoot. Foot Ankle Clin 2001;6:167–78.
55. Hintermann B, Valderrabano V. Lateral column lengthening by calcaneal osteotomy. Techniques in Foot & Ankle Surgery 2003;2:84–90.
56. Tankson CJ. The Cotton osteotomy: indications and techniques. Foot Ankle Clin 2007;12:309–15, vii.
57. Barg A, Brunner S, Zwicky L, et al. Subtalar and naviculocuneiform fusion for extended breakdown of the medial arch. Foot Ankle Clin 2011;16:69–81.
58. Cohen BE, Ogden F. Medial column procedures in the acquired flatfoot deformity. Foot Ankle Clin 2007;12:287–99, vi.
59. De Wachter J, Knupp M, Hintermann B. Double-hindfoot arthrodesis through a single medial approach. Techniques in Foot & Ankle Surgery 2007;6:237–42.
60. Knupp M, Stufkens SA, Hintermann B. Triple arthrodesis. Foot Ankle Clin 2011;16:61–7.
61. Coester LM, Saltzman CL, Leupold J, et al. Long-term results following ankle arthrodesis for post-traumatic arthritis. J Bone Joint Surg Am 2001;83:219–28.
62. Nihal A, Gellman RE, Embil JM, et al. Ankle arthrodesis. Foot Ankle Surg 2008;14:1–10.
63. Boobbyer GN. The long-term results of ankle arthrodesis. Acta Orthop Scand 1981;52:107–10.
64. Fuchs S, Sandmann C, Skwara A, et al. Quality of life 20 years after arthrodesis of the ankle. A study of adjacent joints. J Bone Joint Surg Br 2003;85:994–8.
65. Mazur JM, Schwartz E, Simon SR. Ankle arthrodesis. Long-term follow-up with gait analysis. J Bone Joint Surg Am 1979;61:964–75.

66. Saltzman CL, Mann RA, Ahrens JE, et al. Prospective controlled trial of STAR total ankle replacement versus ankle fusion: initial results. Foot Ankle Int 2009; 30:579–96.
67. Hintermann B, Valderrabano V, Dereymaeker G, et al. The HINTEGRA ankle: rationale and short-term results of 122 consecutive ankles. Clin Orthop Relat Res 2004;424:57–68.
68. Hintermann B, Barg A. The HINTEGRA total ankle arthroplasty. In: Wiesel SW, editor. Operative techniques in orthopaedic surgery. 1st edition. Philadelphia: Lippincott Williams & Wilkins; 2010. p. 4022–31.
69. Hintermann B, Valderrabano V. Total ankle replacement. Foot Ankle Clin 2003;8: 375–405.
70. Hintermann B. Total ankle arthroplasty: historical overview, current concepts and future perspectives. Vienna: Springer; 2004.
71. Knupp M, Stufkens SA, Bolliger L, et al. Total ankle replacement and supramalleolar osteotomies for malaligned osteoarthritis ankle. Techniques in Foot & Ankle Surgery 2010;9:175–81.
72. Knupp M, Stufkens SA, Bolliger L, et al. Classification and treatment of supramalleolar deformities. Foot Ankle Int 2011;32:1023–31.
73. Hintermann B, Barg A, Knupp M. Corrective supramalleolar osteotomy for malunited pronation-external rotation fractures of the ankle. J Bone Joint Surg Br 2011;93:1367–72.
74. Brooke BT, Harris NJ, Morgan SS. Fibula lengthening osteotomy to correct valgus mal-alignment following total ankle arthroplasty. Foot Ankle Surg 2009; 18(2):144–7.
75. Bolt PM, Coy S, Toolan BC. A comparison of lateral column lengthening and medial translational osteotomy of the calcaneus for the reconstruction of adult acquired flatfoot. Foot Ankle Int 2007;28:1115–23.
76. Hintermann B, Valderrabano V, Kundert HP. Lengthening of the lateral column and reconstruction of the medial soft tissue for treatment of acquired flatfoot deformity associated with insufficiency of the posterior tibial tendon. Foot Ankle Int 1999;20:622–9.
77. Sands AK, Tansey JP. Lateral column lengthening. Foot Ankle Clin 2007;12: 301–8, vii.
78. Hintermann B. Medial ankle instability. Foot Ankle Clin 2003;8:723–38.
79. Valderrabano V, Wiewiorski M, Frigg A, et al. Chronic ankle instability. Unfallchirurg 2007;110:691–9 [in German].
80. Lee KT, Lee YK, Young KW, et al. Perioperative complications of the MOBILITY total ankle system: comparison with the HINTEGRA total ankle system. J Orthop Sci 2010;15:317–22.
81. Myerson MS, Mroczek K. Perioperative complications of total ankle arthroplasty. Foot Ankle Int 2003;24:17–21.
82. Saltzman CL, Amendola A, Anderson R, et al. Surgeon training and complications in total ankle arthroplasty. Foot Ankle Int 2003;24:514–8.
83. Schuberth JM, Patel S, Zarutsky E. Perioperative complications of the Agility total ankle replacement in 50 initial, consecutive cases. J Foot Ankle Surg 2006;45:139–46.
84. Espinosa N, Walti M, Favre P, et al. Misalignment of total ankle components can induce high joint contact pressures. J Bone Joint Surg Am 2010;92:1179–87.
85. Fukuda T, Haddad SL, Ren Y, et al. Impact of talar component rotation on contact pressure after total ankle arthroplasty: a cadaveric study. Foot Ankle Int 2010;31:404–11.

86. Tochigi Y, Rudert MJ, Brown TD, et al. The effect of accuracy of implantation on range of movement of the Scandinavian Total Ankle Replacement. J Bone Joint Surg Br 2005;87:736–40.
87. Barg A, Elsner A, Anderson AE, et al. The effect of three-component total ankle replacement misalignment on clinical outcome: pain relief and functional outcome in 317 consecutive patients. J Bone Joint Surg Am 2011;93(21): 1969–78.
88. Barg A, Suter T, Zwicky L, et al. Medial pain syndrome in patients with total ankle replacement. Orthopade 2011;40:991–9 [in German].
89. Coetzee JC. Management of varus or valgus ankle deformity with ankle replacement. Foot Ankle Clin 2008;13:509–20, x.
90. Conti SF, Wong YS. Complications of total ankle replacement. Clin Orthop Relat Res 2001;105–14.
91. Conti SF, Wong YS. Complications of total ankle replacement. Foot Ankle Clin 2002;7:791–807, vii.
92. Haskell A, Mann RA. Perioperative complication rate of total ankle replacement is reduced by surgeon experience. Foot Ankle Int 2004;25:283–9.
93. Newton SE. An artificial ankle joint. Clin Orthop Relat Res 1979;142:141–5.
94. Newton SE 3rd. An artificial ankle joint. Clin Orthop Relat Res 2004;424:3–5.
95. Newton SE 3rd. Total ankle arthroplasty. Clinical study of fifty cases. J Bone Joint Surg Am 1982;64:104–11.
96. Kirkup J. Richard Smith ankle arthroplasty. J R Soc Med 1985;78:301–4.
97. Stauffer RN, Segal NM. Total ankle arthroplasty: four years' experience. Clin Orthop Relat Res 1981;160:217–21.
98. Pyevich MT, Saltzman CL, Callaghan JJ, et al. Total ankle arthroplasty: a unique design. Two to twelve-year follow-up. J Bone Joint Surg Am 1998;80:1410–20.
99. McIff TE, Alvine FG, Saltzman CL, et al. Intraoperative measurement of distraction for ligament tensioning in total ankle arthroplasty. Clin Orthop Relat Res 2004;111–7.
100. Vienne P, Nothdurft P. OSG-Totalendoprothese Agility: Indikationen, Operationstechnik und Ergebnisse. FussSprungg 2004;2:17–28 [in German].
101. Saltzman CL. Perspective on total ankle replacement. Foot Ankle Clin 2000;5: 761–75.
102. Greisberg J, Hansen ST Jr. Ankle replacement: management of associated deformities. Foot Ankle Clin 2002;7:721–36, vi.
103. Greisberg J, Hansen ST Jr. Total ankle arthroplasty in the advanced flatfoot. Techniques in Foot & Ankle Surgery 2003;2:152–61.
104. Stamatis ED, Myerson MS. How to avoid specific complications of total ankle replacement. Foot Ankle Clin 2002;7:765–89.
105. Wood PL, Deakin S. Total ankle replacement. The results in 200 ankles. J Bone Joint Surg Br 2003;85:334–41.
106. Wood PL, Prem H, Sutton C. Total ankle replacement: medium-term results in 200 Scandinavian total ankle replacements. J Bone Joint Surg Br 2008;90:605–9.
107. Wood PL, Clough TM, Smith R. The present state of ankle arthroplasty. Foot Ankle Surg 2008;14:115–9.
108. Assal M, Al-Shaikh R, Reiber BH, et al. Fracture of the polyethylene component in an ankle arthroplasty: a case report. Foot Ankle Int 2003;24:901–3.
109. Takakura Y, Tanaka Y, Kumai T, et al. Ankle arthroplasty using three generations of metal and ceramic prostheses. Clin Orthop Relat Res 2004;424:130–6.
110. Tanaka Y, Takakura Y. The TNK ankle: short- and mid-term results. Orthopade 2006;35:546–51 [in German].

111. Greisberg J, Hansen ST, DiGiovanni C. Alignment and technique in total ankle arthroplasty. Oper Tech Orthop 2004;14:21–30.
112. Kofoed H. Scandinavian Total Ankle Replacement (STAR). Clin Orthop Relat Res 2004;424:73–9.
113. Doets HC, Brand R, Nelissen RG. Total ankle arthroplasty in inflammatory joint disease with use of two mobile-bearing designs. J Bone Joint Surg Am 2006; 88:1272–84.
114. Henricson A, Agren PH. Secondary surgery after total ankle replacement. The influence of preoperative hindfoot alignment. Foot Ankle Surg 2007;13:41–4.
115. Wood PL, Crawford LA, Suneja R, et al. Total ankle replacement for rheumatoid ankle arthritis. Foot Ankle Clin 2007;12:497–508.
116. Wood PL. Experience with the STAR ankle arthroplasty at Wrightington Hospital, UK. Foot Ankle Clin 2002;7:755–64.
117. Karantana A, Hobson S, Dhar S. The Scandinavian total ankle replacement: survivorship at 5 and 8 years comparable to other series. Clin Orthop Relat Res 2010;468:951–7.
118. Wood PL, Karski MT, Watmough P. Total ankle replacement: the results of 100 mobility total ankle replacements. J Bone Joint Surg Br 2010;92:958–62.
119. Ellis S, Deorio JK. The INBONE total ankle replacement. Oper Tech Orthop 2010;20:201–10.
120. Deorio JK, Easley ME. Total ankle arthroplasty. Instr Course Lect 2008;57: 383–413.
121. Skytta ET, Koivu H, Eskelinen A, et al. Total ankle replacement: a population-based study of 515 cases from the Finnish Arthroplasty Register. Acta Orthop 2010;81:114–8.
122. Morgan SS, Brooke B, Harris NJ. Total ankle replacement by the Ankle Evolution System: medium-term outcome. J Bone Joint Surg Br 2010;92:61–5.
123. Kim BS, Knupp M, Zwicky L, et al. Total ankle replacement in association with hindfoot fusion: outcome and complications. J Bone Joint Surg Br 2010;92: 1540–7.
124. Bonasia DE, Dettoni F, Femino JE, et al. Total ankle replacement: why, when and how? Iowa Orthop J 2010;30:119–30.
125. Bonnin M, Gaudot F, Laurent JR, et al. The Salto total ankle arthroplasty: survivorship and analysis of failures at 7 to 11 years. Clin Orthop Relat Res 2011;469: 225–36.
126. Bonnin M, Judet T, Colombier JA, et al. Midterm results of the Salto Total Ankle Prosthesis. Clin Orthop Relat Res 2004;424:6–18.
127. Trincat S, Kouyoumdjian P, Asencio G. Total ankle arthroplasty and coronal plane deformities. Orthop Traumatol Surg Res 2012;98:75–84.

Surgical Treatment of the Arthritic Varus Ankle

Mark E. Easley, MD

KEYWORDS

• Ankle • Arthritis • Varus • Osteotomy • Arthrodesis • Arthroplasty

KEY POINTS

- Surgical correction of the varus arthritic ankle is challenging; rarely does an isolated procedure provide satisfactory outcome.
- Many of the principles applied to joint-preserving realignment procedures may be applied to total ankle arthroplasty.
- Varus ankle arthritis exists on a continuum that prompts the treating surgeon to be familiar with a spectrum of surgical solutions, including joint-sparing realignment, arthroplasty, and arthrodesis.

INTRODUCTION

Within the past several years, the arthritic varus ankle has been addressed extensively in *Foot and Ankle Clinics*, with numerous excellent reviews by knowledgeable authors.[1–8] To support these outstanding contributions, this article provides a practical approach to this challenging constellation of foot and ankle abnormalities. Varus ankle arthritis exists on a continuum prompting the treating surgeon to be familiar with a spectrum of surgical solutions, including joint-sparing realignment, arthroplasty, and arthrodesis. Each of these treatment options is addressed with several expanded case examples, and the management approaches supported with the available pertinent literature.

EVALUATION

Apostle and Sangeorzan[9] and Thevendran and Younger[10] recently reviewed the anatomy and examination of the varus ankle, respectively. The reader is strongly urged to read these important interpretations of the salient features of the varus ankle; their insight provides a valuable foundation for this review. In addition, Easley and Vineyard[11] recently published a review article on varus ankle deformity. The following paragraphs borrow from this article to summarize what was deemed important in evaluating the varus ankle.

Department of Orthopaedic Surgery, Duke University Medical Center, 4709 Creekstone Drive, Box 2950, Durham, NC 27703, USA
E-mail address: mark.e.easley@duke.edu

Foot Ankle Clin N Am 17 (2012) 665–686
http://dx.doi.org/10.1016/j.fcl.2012.09.002
foot.theclinics.com

Clinical and Radiographic Evaluation of Limb Alignment and Ankle Stability

Varus alignment may not be isolated to the ankle, and the history and physical examination should include the entire affected extremity, from hip to foot. In cases of prior trauma or surgery proximal to the ankle and/or when the weight-bearing physical examination suggests potential proximal limb deformity, the author typically obtains weight-bearing full-length hip-to-ankle mechanical axis radiographs. Occasionally, deformity proximal to the ankle joint must be treated to effectively realign the ankle.

Varus alignment necessitates a comprehensive clinical and radiographic evaluation of the foot, because talar position depends on hindfoot position and the ankle and foot function in concert via the ankle–hindfoot ligamentous couple.[12] Weight-bearing examination of the foot may demonstrate heel varus, cavus, and/or first-ray plantarflexion (forefoot-driven hindfoot varus). The author recommends that the contribution of the first ray to varus hindfoot position and hindfoot flexibility be assessed using the Coleman Block test.[13] Routine anteroposterior and lateral foot radiographs generally define a cavus foot posture, particularly in the presence of talo-first metatarsal axis incongruence in both planes.

Despite varus ankle alignment, the hindfoot may be in a compensatory valgus position.[14,15] With ankle realignment from varus to a physiologic position, the ankle–hindfoot ligament couple may correct the hindfoot to its anatomic position. However, occasionally compensatory subtalar valgus position will not correct with ankle realignment, resulting in greater than physiologic heel valgus and potential subfibular impingement. The author recommends that preoperative hindfoot position be assessed on weight-bearing Saltzman hindfoot axis views.[16,17]

Varus alignment may be associated with lateral ankle ligament instability/peroneal tendon attenuation and medial ankle ligament/posterior tibial tendon contracture, particularly in an incongruent varus ankle deformity.[8,18] Some investigators emphasize that ankle malalignment should not be evaluated independent of lateral ankle ligament stability.[8,15] In patients with varus alignment, the author routinely performs anterior drawer testing and evaluate peroneal tendons/muscles with palpation and active eversion against resistance. Medial contractures are assessed through attempting passive correction of the ankle and hindfoot deformity. Moreover, during passive correction from varus to a neutral ankle and hindfoot position, peroneus longus contracture may be evidenced with increased first ray plantarflexion or rigidity; a peroneus longus-to-brevis tendon transfer should be considered in this situation. As suggested by several authors, varus alignment may be one component of multiplanar deformity, often associated with concomitant sagittal plane malposition on the lateral radiograph.[19–21] Congruent varus malalignment may be affiliated with recurvatum deformity; incongruent varus deformity may exist with anterior talar subluxation relative to the tibial plafond.[18,20–23]

MRI is rarely indicated in the workup of varus alignment, but clinical suspicion of peroneal tendon abnormality may be confirmed. CT is useful in defining the extent of ankle arthritis and identifying potential hindfoot arthritis; this may have some bearing on surgical management.

Evaluation of Ankle Arthritis

Joint-sparing procedures are rarely indicated for end-stage ankle arthritis; however, in select cases, realignment alone provided excellent relief despite advanced ankle arthritis (see **Fig. 4**). Except for in severe varus deformity and the rare associated ligament abnormality that cannot be rebalanced, the author favors ankle arthroplasty for end-stage ankle arthritis. Another exception is a young patient with mild-to-moderate varus deformity and end-stage ankle arthritis who plans to maintain high-demand activity on the ankle.

Knupp and colleagues[18] recently reinterpreted and modified the original classification of varus ankle arthritis presented by Takakura and colleagues,[20] providing a comprehensive treatment algorithm for joint-sparing procedures. Mann and colleagues,[24,25] in 2 separate investigations, noted that results of total ankle arthroplasty (TAA) for incongruent varus ankle arthritis are inferior to those for congruent deformity, suggesting that severe incongruent varus ankle arthritis is best treated with arthrodesis. In the author's experience, modern soft tissue rebalancing procedures have allowed the results of TAA in incongruent ankle arthritis to be comparable to those of TAA in congruent varus ankle arthritis.[26,27]

When extrapolating Mann and colleagues' experience to joint-sparing procedures, ankle realignment in incongruent ankle arthritis presents a challenge. Despite comprehensive supramalleolar realignment, soft tissue balancing, and foot correction, residual varus talar tilt is common, a finding confirmed by Knupp and colleagues.[18] Particularly challenging in joint-sparing procedures for varus ankle arthritis is Takakura stage III and Knupp type III deformity, in which the varus talus creates end-stage arthritis of the medial gutter (see **Fig. 3**A).[18,20] These classification schemes are valuable in determining optimal treatment. Although Mann and colleagues[28] recommend a joint-sparing intra-articular plafondplasty osteotomy to address the stage/type III deformity, the author favors either arthroplasty or arthrodesis for such complex deformity, with arthrodesis favored in severe deformity and patients who plan to maintain high-demand activity on their ankle.

CASE PRESENTATIONS

Joint-Sparing Procedures

Case I

A 38-year-old man presented with severe incongruent tibiotalar varus associated with cavus foot deformity. The patient failed to improve with bracing. A supramalleolar osteotomy was performed in combination with soft tissue rebalancing and realignment osteotomies of the foot, as recommended by Knupp and colleagues[18] The patient had a marked reduction in pain and no longer experienced symptomatic lateral foot overload (**Fig. 1**).

Case IA

A 63-year-old man presented with similar deformity to the patient in Case I (**Fig. 2**A, B). The deformity progressed to being unbraceable. He underwent similar surgical treatment to the patient in Case I: (1) medial opening wedge supramalleolar osteotomy, (2) deltoid ligament release, (3) posterior tibial tendon transfer to peroneal tendons, (4) lateral ankle ligament reconstruction, (5) peroneus longus-to-brevis tendon transfer, with longus tendon secured to base of fifth metatarsal, (6) lateralizing/lateral closing wedge calcaneal osteotomy, (7) plantar fascia release, and (8) dorsiflexion midfoot osteotomy. The patient had successful realignment to a plantigrade foot position and resolution of symptoms related to lateral foot overload (see **Fig. 2**C, D).

Case IB

A 50-year-old man presented with Knupp type III varus ankle arthritis (Takakura stage III) who desired a joint-sparing procedure despite concerns for the reported challenges in correcting type III/stage III deformity with a joint-sparing procedure (**Fig. 3**A).[18,20] Ideally, preoperative axial heel views should have been obtained to objectively evaluate the heel position, specifically if the patient had compensatory preoperative heel valgus.[16,17]

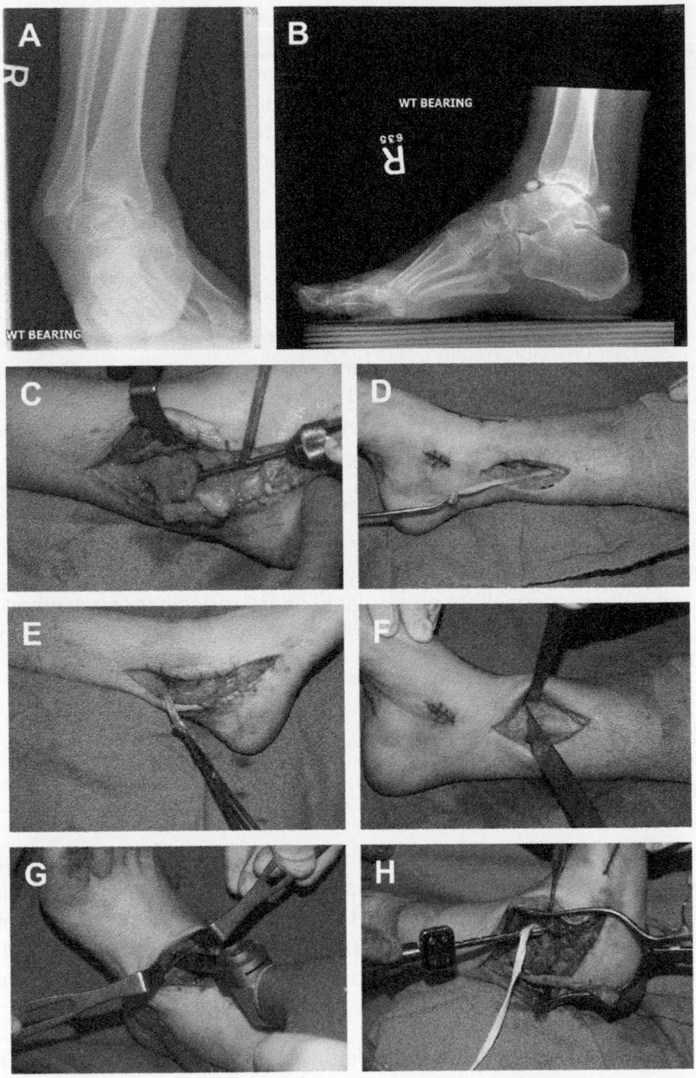

Fig. 1. (*A*) Anteroposterior (AP) ankle preoperative weight-bearing radiographs in a 38-year-old man. (*B*) Lateral foot of preoperative weight-bearing radiographs in same patient. (*C*) Drill holes for planned allograft lateral ankle ligament reconstruction. (*D, E*) Posterior tibialis tendon harvest and transfer to lateral foot. (*F*) Medial tibial opening wedge osteotomy. (*G*) Dorsiflexion midfoot osteotomy to correct global cavus deformity. (*H*) Lateral ankle ligament reconstruction using gracilis allograft. (*I, J*) Two-year follow-up weight-bearing radiographs: (*I*) ankle mortise, (*J*) lateral ankle and foot. (*Data from* Easley ME, Vineyard JC. Varus ankle and osteochondral lesions of the talus. Foot Ankle Clin 2012;17(1):21–38.)

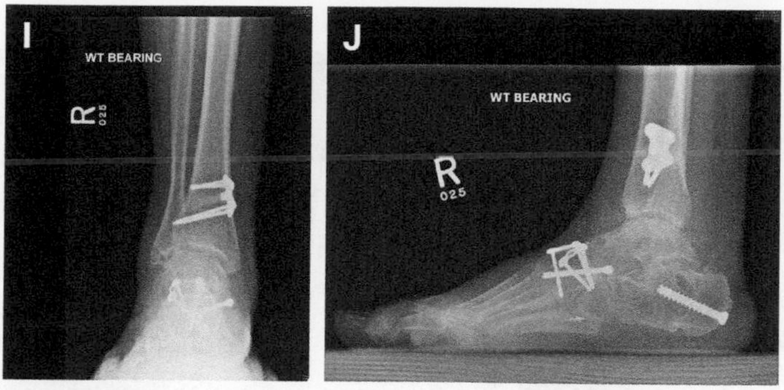

Fig. 1. (*continued*)

In addition to pain, he complained of lateral foot overload and lateral ankle instability; he failed multiple attempts at orthotic management and bracing.

In the author's opinion, the patient had a nonanatomic flare of the medial malleolus that could not be effectively managed with a traditional supramalleolar osteotomy. Mann and colleagues[28] suggested that the plafondplasty is indicated for intra-articular varus arthritis associated with lateral ankle instability, including ankles with the dysplasia from chronic pressure of the medially driven talus. Therefore, a plafondplasty was planned in combination with soft tissue rebalancing, lateral ankle allograft ligament reconstruction, and realignment osteotomy of the foot. Through a utilitarian lateral approach, the author performed a lateralizing/lateral closing wedge calcaneal osteotomy and debridement of peroneal tendinopathy, and prepared for a peroneus longus-to-brevis tendon transfer and a lateral ankle allograft ligament reconstruction.

With an adequate skin bridge, a traditional anterior approach to the ankle was taken, through which impinging anterolateral osteophytes and the lateral ankle gutter were debrided. In anticipation of the plafondplasty, a comprehensive medial soft tissue release was not performed; the author believes that simultaneous medial soft tissue release and medial malleolar osteotomy risks avascular necrosis of the medial malleolus. Passive hindfoot valgus stress after lateral gutter debridement and osteophyte removal confirmed the nonanatomic flare of the medial malleolus, prompting the author to proceed with plafondplasty. Plafondplasty differs from medial malleolar osteotomy described for TAA in that plafondplasty aims to correct angular medial malleolar deformity rather than simply translating the medial malleolus distally to effectively lessen deltoid ligament tension.

The author considered performing the plafondplasty through the anterior approach, but decided that access for structural bone grafting and hardware would be best via a separate medial incision. Although introducing greater risk to the soft tissues, the judiciously performed additional approach afforded an optimal working portal to complement the anterior approach that was used to monitor the medial malleolar reduction (see **Fig. 3**B). The osteotomy was straightforward, similar to a generous medial malleolar osteotomy for cartilage repair procedures. However, maintaining the medial malleolar fragment on an articular hinge was difficult (see **Fig. 3**C). Because this patient only had medial gutter wear and medial malleolar deformity and not medial tibial plafond impaction/varus deformity, the author believed that a more oblique and even more generous medial osteotomy, one that approached the tibial plafond subchondral bone but did not violate it, would have led to an intra-articular incongruency with the lateral tibial plafond; however, in retrospect, perhaps that would have made the medial malleolar fragment position easier to control. Nonetheless, the author was able to

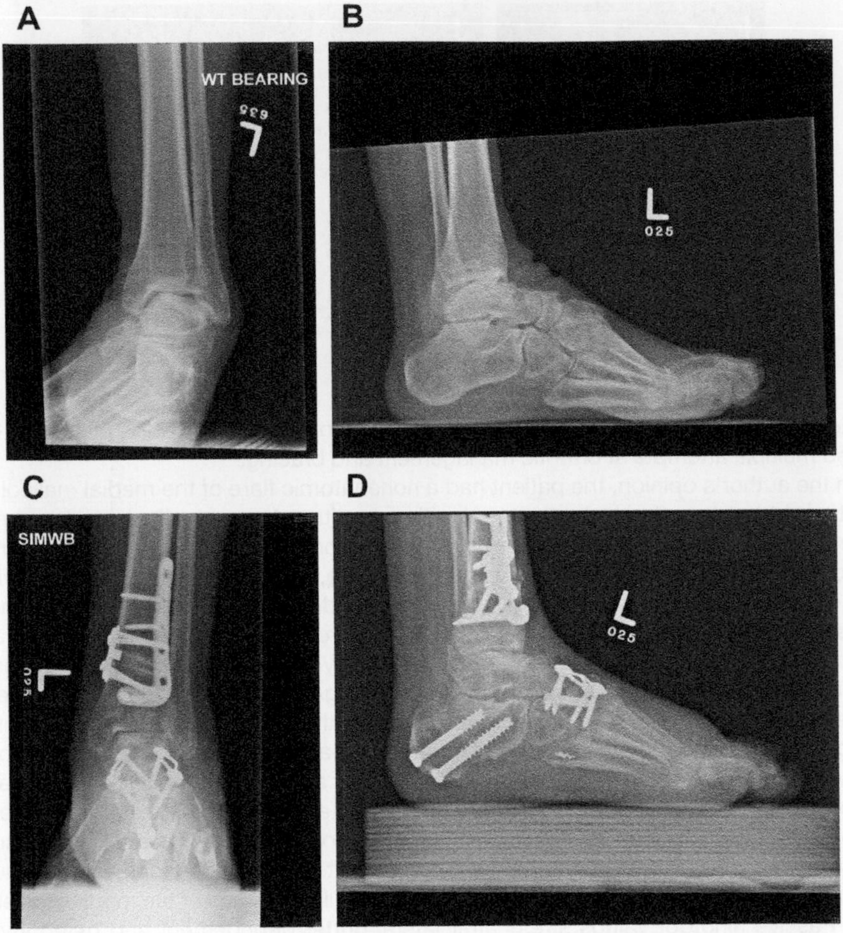

Fig. 2. Radiographs of a 63-year-old man with varus ankle arthritis and cavovarus foot managed with supramalleolar osteotomy, multiple foot realignment osteotomies, and soft tissue rebalancing. (*A*) Preoperative anteroposterior ankle radiograph. (*B*) Preoperative lateral ankle foot radiograph. (*C*) Postoperative anteroposterior ankle radiographs. (*D*) Postoperative lateral ankle and foot radiograph.

improve the mortise alignment with an interpositional structural graft and medial fixation. After the plafondplasty, the author completed the lateral ankle ligament and tendon reconstructions. Despite the 3 incisions, skin compromise was not an issue.

At 1-year follow-up, clinical alignment was optimal and symmetric to the contralateral side, and the patient showed improved ankle stability (see **Fig. 3**D). Continued pain, albeit less than experienced preoperatively, is attributable to residual varus talar tilt and high medial tibiotalar joint contact stresses noted radiographically. Although Knupp and colleagues[18] suggested that the plafondplasty may be best suited for the stage/type III deformities, Mann and colleagues,[28] in their review of the plafondplasty procedure, observed that the 4 failures in their study were type/stage III deformities. As the author discussed with patient preoperatively, TAA or ankle arthrodesis may eventually be warranted.

Case IC A 65-year-old woman presented with extra-articular distal tibial varus malunion and associated ankle arthritis (**Fig. 4**A). She had a distal tibia/fibula fracture

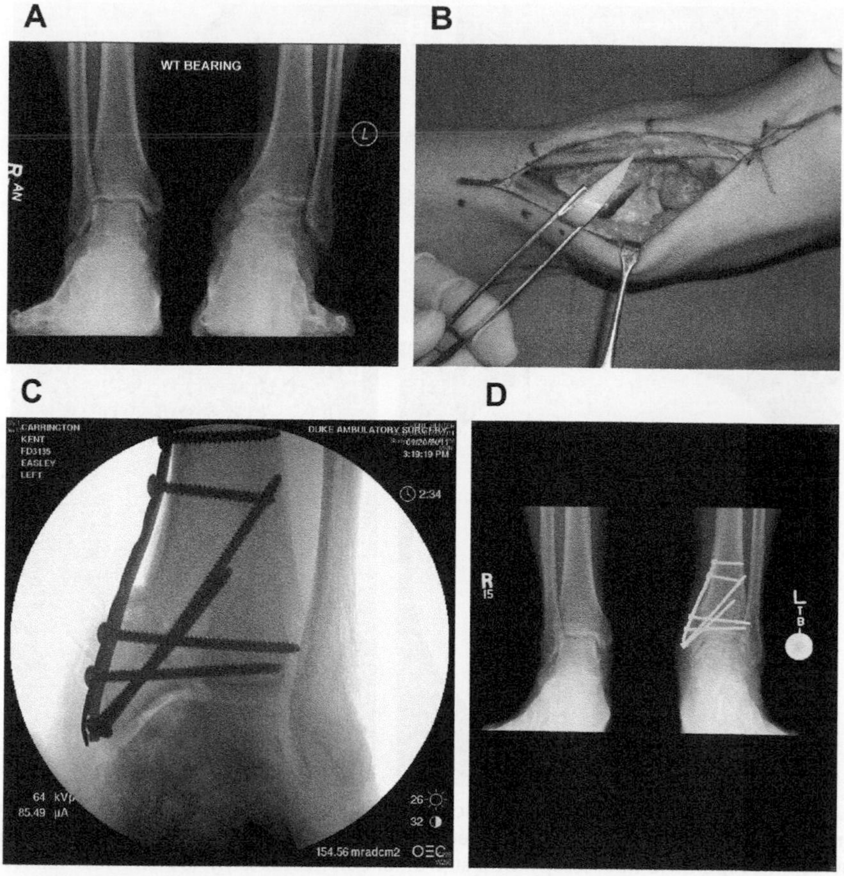

Fig. 3. Knupp type III varus ankle arthritis in a 50-year-old man. (*A*) Preoperative ankle radiograph. (*B*) Intra-articular medial malleolar osteotomy (ie, plafondplasty) with structural femoral head allograft. (*C*) Intraoperative anteroposterior ankle fluoroscopy after osteotomy fixation and realignment. (*D*) One-year follow-up anteroposterior ankle radiograph.

30 years earlier and reported progressively worsening symptoms that no longer responded to nonoperative treatment. The author consented her for distal tibial and fibular osteotomy and possible concomitant TAA, with the understanding that TAA would be considered in the same operation only if the osteotomy could be performed safely and efficiently with adequate residual tourniquet time. After removing the rod from the fibula, a utilitarian anterior approach was used to expose both the ankle and the distal tibia and fibula. The author removed the anterior osteophytes from the tibiotalar joint and proceeded with the realignment osteotomy. A dome osteotomy of both the distal tibia and fibula were performed through the anterior approach, while protecting the deep neurovascular bundle (see **Fig.** 4B). On completion of the osteotomy, the distal tibia was realigned through the dome osteotomy, reestablishing physiologic tibial alignment with anatomic valgus heel position (see **Fig.** 4C). After provisional fixation with pins, the osteotomy was stabilized with anterolateral and medial plates that were positioned so that they would not interfere with the TAA. Through a separate lateral incision with an adequate skin bridge from the anterior incision, a fibular plate was also placed to stabilize the fibular osteotomy. The author

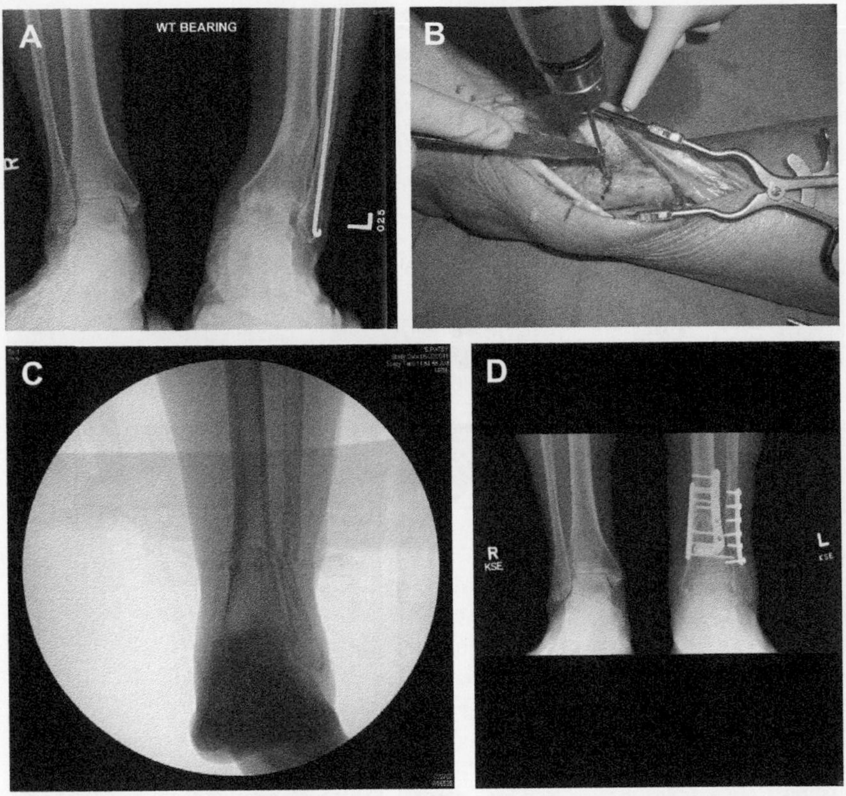

Fig. 4. Extra-articular varus tibial malunion and endstage ankle arthritis in a 65-year-old woman. (*A*) Preoperative anteroposterior ankle radiograph. (*B*) Supramalleolar dome osteotomy. (*C*) Intraoperative fluoroscopy after supramalleolar osteotomy. (*D*) One-year follow-up anteroposterior ankle radiograph.

deemed it safer to stage the TAA. At 1-year follow-up the author was planning to schedule the patient for a TAA, but she claimed that realignment alone (with osteophyte removal) markedly reduced her symptoms and she was functioning well, brace-free, with no intention to pursue TAA (see **Fig. 4**D). The author was admittedly surprised, particularly given her end-stage ankle arthritis, and although this represents anecdotal experience, this patient reinforced the significance of optimal alignment.[7,21,29–32]

TAA

Case II

A 72-year-old woman presented with incongruent varus ankle arthritis that failed to respond to nonoperative management (**Fig. 5**A). Several authors have cautioned that moderate-to-severe varus ankle malalignment, particularly incongruent varus malalignment, is a challenging problem in TAA.[24,27,33–40] The author, however, believes that techniques for soft tissue rebalancing for TAA have evolved to the point that even severe varus malalignment may be rebalanced. The author first performed a medial soft-tissue release.[27] The medial tibial periosteum was elevated, leaving the superficial deltoid fibers intact while the deep deltoid fibers were divided. This

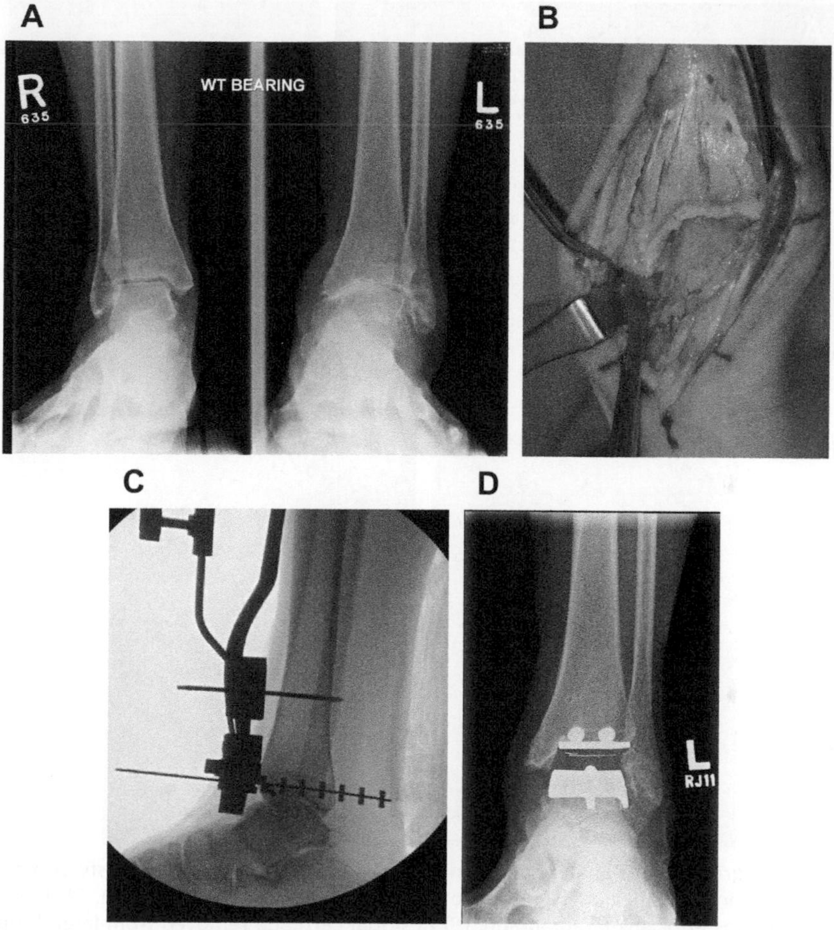

Fig. 5. Incongruent varus ankle arthritis managed with total ankle arthroplasty and medial (deltoid) release in a 72-year-old woman. (*A*) Preoperative anteroposterior ankle radiograph. (*B*) Medial soft tissue release. (*C*) Minimal bone resection from distal tibia. (*D*) One-year follow-up anteroposterior ankle radiograph.

maneuver allowed for the talus to congruently realign in the ankle mortise (see **Fig. 5**B). A mobile-bearing total ankle replacement was then performed, but with minimal bone resection because the contracted medial ligaments were being lengthened to balance the loose lateral ligaments (see **Fig. 5**C). Although the author was prepared to perform a lateral ankle ligament reconstruction, medial release alone sufficed to balance the lax lateral ligaments. At 1-year follow-up the ankle functioned well, remained well balanced (with the polyethylene and talar component well centered under the tibial component), and afforded excellent pain relief (see **Fig. 5**D).

Case IIA

A 54-year-old man presented with incongruent varus ankle arthritis that failed to respond to nonoperative management (**Fig. 6**A). Given the severe deformity, the author consented him for both TAA and ankle arthrodesis, with the plan to convert to ankle arthrodesis if the ankle could not be rebalanced. A medial release[27] was

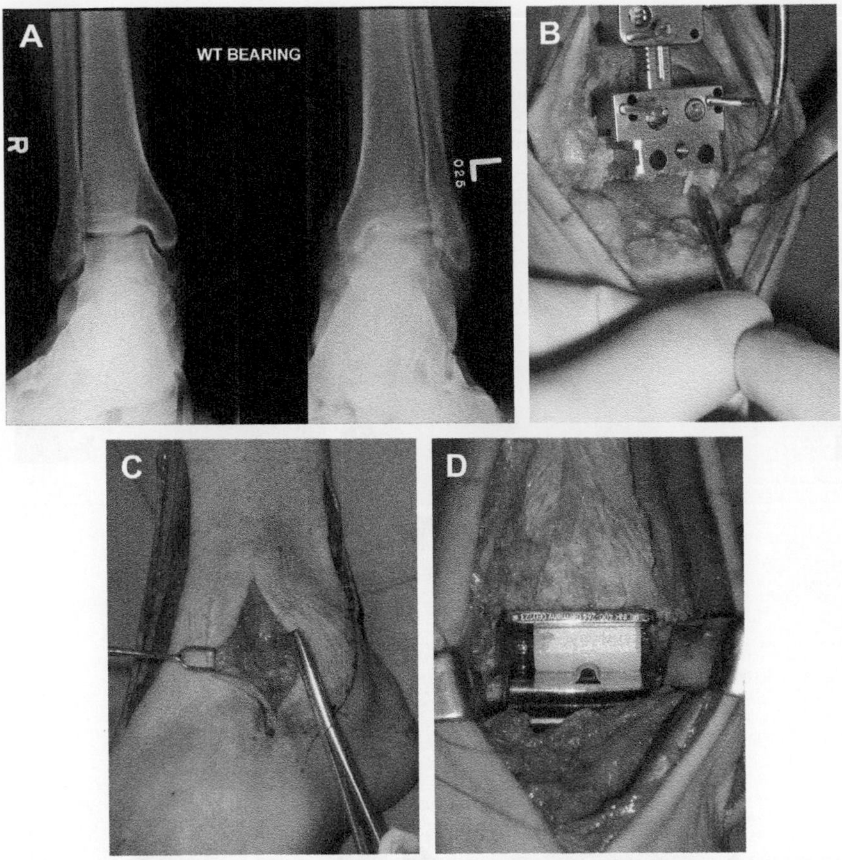

Fig. 6. Incongruent varus ankle arthritis managed with total ankle arthroplasty, soft tissue rebalancing, and dorsiflexion osteotomy of the first ray in a 54-year-old man. (*A*) Preoperative anteroposterior ankle radiograph. (*B*) Residual cartilage removed from lateral aspect of talar dome to avoid varus talar cut. (*C*) Modified Brostrom lateral ankle ligament repair. (*D*) Intraoperative photo of balanced mobile bearing total ankle arthroplasty.

performed as described for Case II, and the lateral ankle gutter was debrided to promote correct the talar tilt. Given the lax lateral ligaments and released medial ligaments, minimal bone resection from the distal tibia was performed. Even with minimal bone resection from the tibia, the ankle had a balanced but considerable ligament laxity. The cartilage wear for this varus ankle was on the medial talar dome, with well-preserved cartilage laterally. To avoid a varus talar cut and optimally rebalance the talus, the author removed the residual cartilage from the lateral talar dome (see **Fig. 6**B), thereby allowing the talar cutting guide to congruently seat on the talar dome. The author then completed the bony preparation of the talus and tibia, performed more lateral gutter debridement, and inserted the true talar component and trial tibial and polyethylene components to determine soft tissue balance. Because of residual varus instability even with a thick polyethylene component on balanced bone preparation, the author performed a peroneus-to-brevis tendon transfer, dorsiflexion osteotomy of the first metatarsal, lateral ankle ligament reconstruction (see **Fig. 6**C),[41] and fractional lengthening of the posterior tibial tendon (by accessing the posterior tibial tendon through the anterior incision used to perform ankle replacement). The soft tissues were put at risk by having 3 surgical approaches (anterior, anterolateral, and posterolateral), but fortunately no postoperative wound complications developed. For the lateral ankle ligament reconstruction, the trial polyethylene was removed, which allowed the use of a thinner final polyethylene than the trial polyethylene used before lateral ligament tightening. Final alignment, both clinically and fluoroscopically, was satisfactory and the ankle was balanced with stress in the coronal plane (see **Fig. 6**D). A lateralizing calcaneal osteotomy was not performed, because the patient had a preoperative compensatory valgus heel position. Ideally, the author would have obtained a heel alignment view to confirm the compensatory heel valgus in this patient with varus talar tilt, but the radiology unit at this site did not have this capability. At 1-year follow-up the patient had minimal pain and excellent function, and showed satisfactory alignment on weight-bearing radiographs.

Case IIB

A 50-year-old man presented with severe incongruent varus ankle arthritis that failed to respond to nonoperative management (**Fig. 7**A). The author consented him for TAA and possible ankle arthrodesis. A TAA was performed with medial malleolar osteotomy and lateral ankle ligament reconstruction, but with skepticism that TAA was feasible until the final components were implanted. The medial malleolar osteotomy was performed first (see **Fig. 7**B).[42] After lateral gutter debridement to remove any lateral obstruction to talar reduction, a modified Brostrom procedure was performed through a judiciously placed separate incision (see **Fig. 7**C). Then, a provisional pin was placed from the tibia to the talus to maintain the talus in anatomic position for bone preparation, position the cutting guide, and protect the lateral ankle ligament reconstruction (see **Fig. 7**D). The author implanted the metal components and trial polyethylene, allowing the medial malleolus to find its new resting tension, and then the medial malleolus was provisionally secured. With the ankle having acceptable alignment and balance, the author removed the trial polyethylene, inserted the true polyethylene, and performed open reduction and internal fixation for the medial malleolus. At 1 year follow-up, the patient is pleased enough with the procedure that he desires a similar procedure for a similar deformity on the contralateral ankle (see **Fig. 7**E).

Ankle Arthrodesis

Case III

A 60-year-old man presented with severe fixed varus ankle deformity, weak eversion function, and a tendency toward cavus with a plantarflexed first ray (**Fig. 8**A).

In addition, he had a prior infected total shoulder arthroplasty with limited use of his right upper extremity. The author had a detailed preoperative educational discussion with him and advised ankle arthrodesis.[43]

The arthrodesis was performed, reducing the talus anatomically within the ankle mortise; the ankle anatomy was preserved, leaving both malleoli intact. The arthrodesis was stabilized with dual anterior plates, compressing the lateral of the 2 plates to promote valgus.[44–47] The peroneus longus tendon was transferred to the brevis tendon to promote hindfoot eversion and relax the plantarflexed first ray. The plantar fascia was also released and a dorsiflexion osteotomy of the first ray performed. The author anticipates that his residual hindfoot motion, dorsiflexion osteotomy the first metatarsal, and soft tissue transfers/releases will lead to a plantigrade foot position. At 1-year follow-up he is pain-free and feels balanced on his foot despite the radiographs suggesting that he will still require a lateralizing calcaneal osteotomy (see **Fig. 8**B, C). Over the long term, he is at risk for developing hindfoot arthritis, but the author believes the benefits of ankle arthrodesis far outweigh the risk of adjacent joint arthritis in this patient.[48–51]

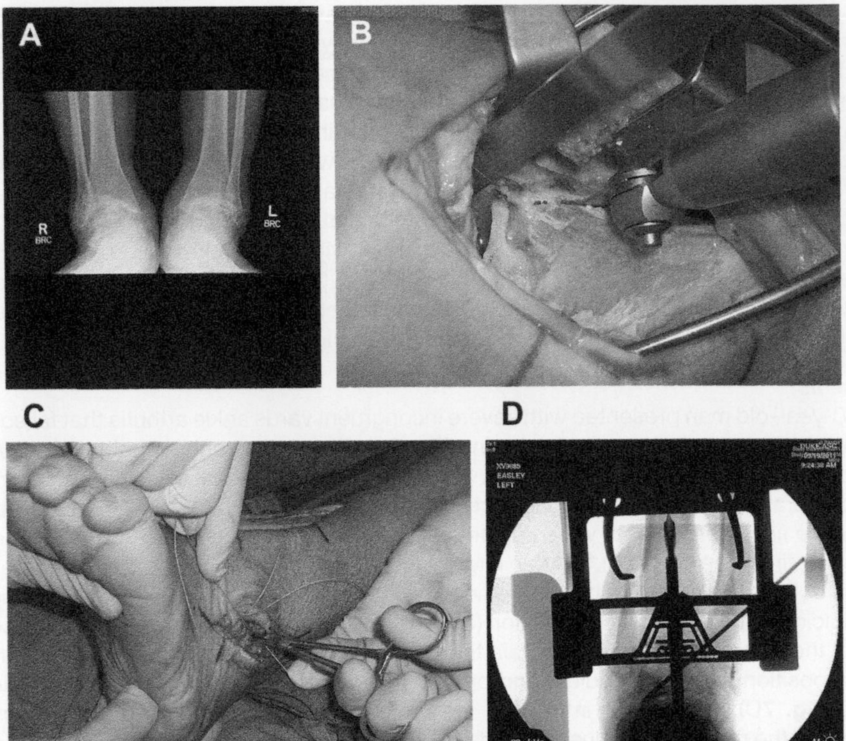

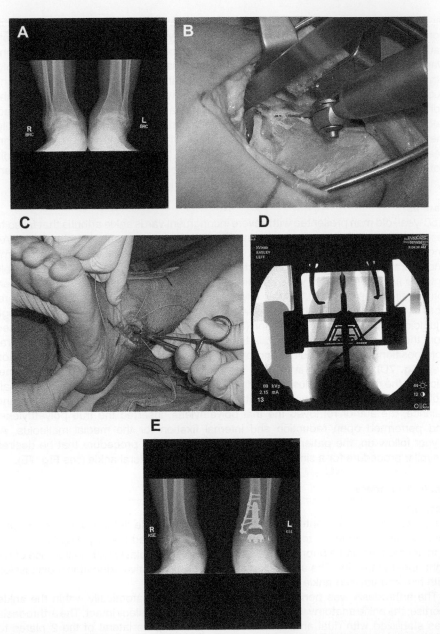

Fig. 7. Severe incongruent ankle arthritis in 50-year-old man. (*A*) Preoperative anteroposterior ankle radiograph. (*B*) Medial malleolar osteotomy (*C*) modified Brostrom lateral ankle ligament repair. (*D*) Cutting block aligned intramedullary reference guide (note talus provisionally pinned in anatomic position). (*E*) One-year follow-up anteroposterior ankle radiographs.

Case IIIA

A 43-year-old man with high-demand job presented with posttraumatic varus ankle arthritis (**Fig. 9**A). Given the demands he planned to place on the ankle, the author recommended ankle arthrodesis with realignment. After hardware removal, a routine

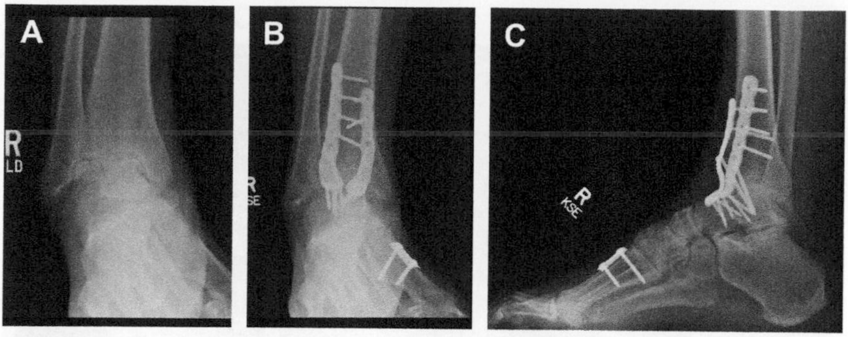

Fig. 8. Severe varus ankle arthritis, weak eversion function, and cavovarus foot position in a 60-year-old man. (*A*) Preoperative mortise ankle radiograph. (*B*) One-year follow-up mortise ankle radiograph. (*C*) Lateral ankle and foot follow-up radiograph.

ankle arthrodesis was performed through an anterior approach, using his prior anterior ankle approach. Subchondral bone was removed from the lateral tibial plafond in an effort to correct the varus deformity. The author effectively corrected varus at the joint with satisfactory bony apposition while preserving the medial and lateral malleoli. The arthrodesis was secured with 3 screws and an anterior plate. At 6 months' follow-up, symptoms at the ankle had resolved and radiographs suggested successful fusion. However, the patient reported overload of his lateral foot despite efforts to correct varus with eccentric joint preparation to promote physiologic valgus. Clinically, he had residual varus ("peek-a-boo" heel sign when viewed from the front), and hindfoot varus was suggested on inspection of posterior hindfoot (see **Fig. 9**B). Careful inspection of the radiographs did not suggest varus ankle malunion at the tibiotalar joint, but given the preoperative varus deformity of the distal tibia, residual varus was apparent for the ankle and hindfoot (see **Fig. 9**C).

Although the patient, with well-preserved hindfoot motion, noted improvement with a valgus-producing orthotic, the lateral foot symptoms could not be effectively managed nonoperatively. Therefore, the hardware was removed through the previous anterior approach and an opening wedge medial tibial osteotomy was performed first with an oscillating saw (see **Fig. 9**D) followed by osteotomes. Through carefully stacking 3 osteotomes in succession, the osteotomy could be opened medially while maintaining the lateral hinge. To promote greater hindfoot valgus, the author performed a concomitant lateralizing/lateral closing wedge calcaneal osteotomy (see **Fig. 9**E). The stable oblique distal tibial osteotomy was secured, in which a lateral hinge was able to be preserved as a pivot for correction, with a dedicated distal medial wedge plate. The author considered fibular shortening osteotomy, but did not deem it necessary at the time. The tibial osteotomy was bone grafted with the wedge of bone that was removed from the lateral calcaneus.

Perhaps because of the insufficient hardware and stiff adjacent ankle, the patient progressed to tibial nonunion above his malunited ankle arthrodesis (see **Fig. 9**F).

The author performed a revision supramalleolar osteotomy with a structural allograft (see **Fig. 9**G). The osteotomy was secured with a stout medial locking plate, using a combination of locking and nonlocking screws (see **Fig. 9**H). In retrospect, it may have been best to use a strictly nonlocking plate to allow the graft to experience compression that may promote healing. However, the author believes the graft was already being compressed, even before fixation, simply by being placed in the opening wedge osteotomy site, suggesting that a locking construct would not be detrimental to graft incorporation. A dorsiflexion osteotomy of the first metatarsal was also added to

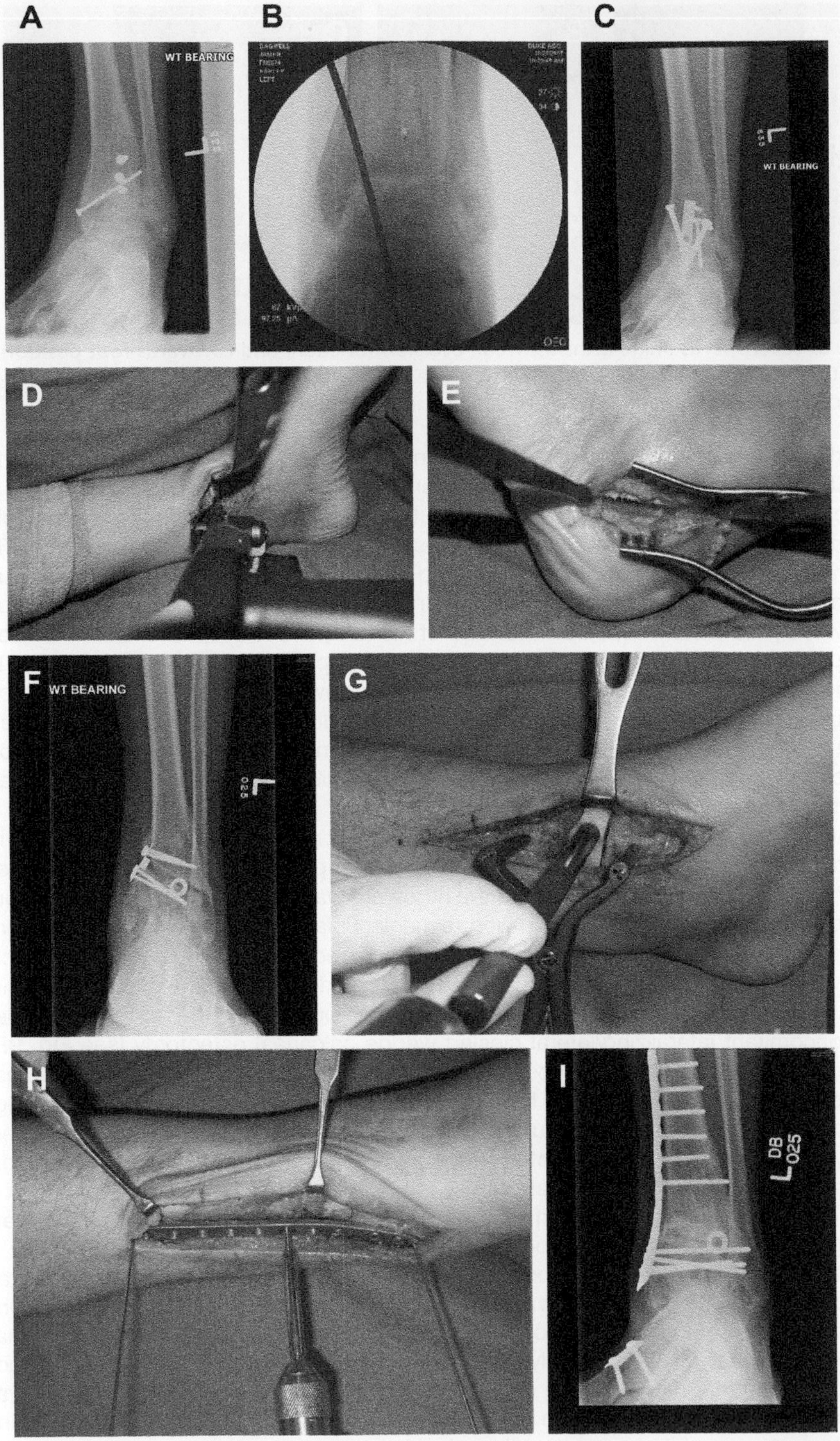
A
WT BEARING
B
C
WT BEARING
D
E
F
WT BEARING
L
025
G
H
I
L
DB
025

optimize foot position. A fibular osteotomy perhaps should have been considered; however, the patient's malleoli remain intact in the event that he could be considered for conversion to TAA, develops adjacent hindfoot arthritis, or transitions to a lower-demand job. After patiently waiting through 3 lengthy postoperative periods, the osteotomy successfully healed and the foot alignment was physiologic (see **Fig. 9**I).

DISCUSSION

Joint-Sparing Procedures

Knupp and colleagues[18] recently reported on 94 supramalleolar osteotomies (92 patients) for ankle arthritis, with 33 supramalleolar osteotomies being performed for varus ankle arthritis. Additional procedures in the varus group included fibular osteotomy (n = 6), calcaneal osteotomy (n = 6), midfoot osteotomy/arthrodesis (n = 5), lateral ligament repair (n = 18), and medial ligament repair (n = 3). The investigators corrected varus deformity with a medial opening wedge osteotomy for varus deformity less than 10° and a lateral closing wedge osteotomy for varus deformity greater than 10°. For the varus group, the mean Visual Analog Scale (VAS) score improved from 4.3 to 2.7 ($P = .001$) and the mean American Orthopaedic Foot and Ankle (AOFAS) Hindfoot-Ankle Score improved from 55.2 to 70.6 points (P = .002). Radiographic parameters also improved, with the mean Saltzman hindfoot assessment improving significantly from 17.2° to 8.7° at follow-up. However, for all patients, including those with varus and valgus talar tilt, only 25 of 60 patients experienced correction of talar tilt within the ankle mortise. The overall Takakura ankle arthritis score did not improve significantly, except for patients with stage III arthritis, albeit with better improvement in the valgus group compared with the varus group. Five supramalleolar osteotomies performed for patients with varus deformity failed to improve and were converted to either ankle arthrodesis or total ankle replacement.

From their investigation, Knupp and colleagues[18] introduced a modification of Takakura's classification of varus ankle arthritis that may be applied in joint-sparing procedures for ankle arthritis. As suggested by Takakura and colleagues,[22] stage III or type III varus ankle arthritis (varus malalignment with medial arthritis at the articulation of the medial talus and medial malleolus) may be at highest risk for failure with correction via supramalleolar osteotomy. For these type III deformities, the authors suggest that a plafondplasty may be indicated. Mann and colleagues[28] recently reported on a case series of intra-articular opening medial tibial wedge osteotomies (plafondplasty) performed for varus ankle osteoarthritis with an average follow-up of nearly 60 months (range, 14–98 months). Nineteen patients underwent a plafondplasty, with 18 having concomitant lateral ligament reconstruction. Although the average correction of talar tilt was significant, average talar tilt only improved from 18° to 10°. Fifteen of the patients were satisfied at the most recent follow-up, with 2 patients undergoing TAA and 2 ankle arthrodesis.

Fig. 9. Posttraumatic varus ankle arthritis in a 43-year-old man. (*A*) Preoperative mortise ankle radiograph. (*B*) Follow-up hindfoot alignment after ankle arthrodesis suggesting residual varus alignment. (*C*) Follow-up mortise ankle radiograph after ankle arthrodesis and suggesting residual varus alignment. (*D, E*) Revision surgery with supramalleolar opening wedge and lateral calcaneal closing wedge osteotomies. (*F*) Follow-up anteroposterior ankle radiograph showing nonunion of medial tibial supramalleolar osteotomy. (*G*) Re-revision surgery with structural femoral head allograft to re-prepared medial tibial opening wedge supramalleolar osteotomy. (*H*) Fixation with a long, stout, dedicated medial tibial plate. (*I*) Final follow-up anteroposterior ankle radiograph (note dorsiflexion osteotomy of first metatarsal).

Other investigators have reported results of supramalleolar osteotomy for varus ankle arthritis. Lee and colleagues[15] evaluated 16 supramalleolar osteotomies (16 patients) for moderate varus ankle osteoarthritis. All procedures included a concomitant fibular osteotomy. At a mean follow-up of 2.3 years, the authors noted significant improvements in the mean AOFAS score and mean radiographic parameters. In contrast to Knupp and colleagues,[18] the authors also observed a significant improvement in the Takakura ankle arthritis stage when comparing preoperative and follow-up radiographs. Despite the small patient cohort, the authors observed that a high preoperative talar tilt correlated with a high postoperative talar tilt and noted higher mean AOFAS scores and lower radiographic arthritis stages in patients with lower talar tilt. They suggested that the threshold for predicting postoperative talar tilt was a preoperative talar tilt of 7.3° or greater. They also cautioned that patients with varus ankle arthritis and preoperative compensatory heel valgus may develop symptomatic subfibular impingement after corrective supramalleolar osteotomy.

TAA

The current literature suggests that the outcome of TAA in ankle arthritis with neutral alignment is more favorable than that associated with varus malalignment, in fact suggesting that the greater the deformity, the worse the outcome.[24,25,40,52–55] In the past decade, several authors have offered absolute numbers for coronal plane deformity above which total ankle replacement is, in their experience, contraindicated. In a 2003 study, Wood and Deakin[52] suggested that coronal plane deformity exceeding 15° leads to worrisome edge-loading and potential component failure. Coronal plane deformity of 15° as a contraindication is also supported by Takakura and colleagues,[54] based on their series of TAAs in which concerning early postoperative loosening and subsidence were observed for this subset of patients. In 2009, Wood and colleagues[40] supported this concern with 6-year failure rate data for 2 mobile-bearing implants. In their comparative study, 10% of Scandanavian Total Ankle Replacement (STAR; Small Bone Innovations, Inc.) prostheses and 25% of Buechel-Pappas (Endotec) prostheses implanted for ankles with 15° or more of preoperative coronal plane malalignment failed at 6-year follow-up. In 2010, Wood and colleagues[56] reported on the outcome of 100 Mobility (DePuy) prostheses, suggesting that TAA for coronal plane deformity greater than 20° is contraindicated, and cautioned that TAA for deformity greater than 10° is manageable but challenging. Doets and colleagues[53] also suggested that TAA for coronal plane deformity exceeding 10° is perhaps contraindicated; in their series, 8-year survivorship was 90% and 48% for neutral and greater than 10° coronal plane deformity, respectively. However, review of these reported methods revealed that little mention is made of associated procedures to correct coronal plane malalignment.

Surgical techniques are evolving to improve outcomes of TAA in varus ankle arthritis. Proposed procedures include talar sculpting, lateral ligament reconstruction, medial (deltoid ligament) release, realignment osteotomies, hindfoot arthrodesis, tendon transfers, and any combination of these procedures, with perhaps the greatest development being the medial release.[2,27,36,41,57–60] This evolution is particularly evident in reports of TAA by the same investigators. In their long-term follow-up of a series of mobile-bearing TAAs performed between 2000 and 2003, Mann and colleagues[37] found that only 75% of the 36 ankles with preoperative coronal plane malalignment greater than 10° maintained physiologic alignment at an average follow-up of 9.1 years. All but one of these malaligned ankles lost neutral alignment by 2-year follow-up.[24] Subsequently, in a more recent series of 45 TAAs performed by the same senior investigator, with mean preoperative coronal plane deformity of 18° (range, 10–30°) and average follow-up of 38 months, physiologic correction was maintained in 82% of patients.[25] The original series included 7 lateral ligament reconstructions and only one deltoid release; in contrast, the more recent series included 12 deltoid ligament release and only a single lateral ligament repair. Bonnin and colleagues[27] also concluded that with an adequate medial release, lateral ("convex side") ligament reconstruction was rarely necessary. Whereas Bonnin and colleagues[27] describe the medial release as being performed first from the medial tibia and if necessary from the talus, Reddy and colleagues[25] suggest that it is transected midsubstance, in a graduated manner, from anterior to posterior. Coetzee[41] suggests that the medial release should be performed from the talus; Ryssman and Myerson[59,60] caution that this may compromise the vascular supply to the medial talar dome. An alternative to medial deltoid ligament release is a medial malleolar osteotomy.[42,59,60] The series by Cornelis Doets and colleagues[42] of 15 TAAs in 13 patients with varus ankle arthritis suggests that varus malalignment can be effectively corrected with medial malleolar osteotomy. In their series, only 2 of the 15 osteotomies were secured with internal fixation and 13 united. Medial malleolar osteotomy appears to be an attractive alternative to medial deltoid release; to avoid vascular compromise to the medial malleolus, medial release and medial malleolar osteotomy are mutually exclusive.

In 3 different reports, Mann and colleagues[24,25,37] have suggested that incongruent varus deformity is more difficult to correct than congruent varus malalignment. At a mean follow-up of 41 months in a recent study of 43 TAAs performed in patients with coronal plane deformity, 10 congruent varus osteoarthritic ankles showed no recurrence, whereas 4 of 13 incongruent varus ankles showed recurrent deformity.[25] The investigators concluded that irrespective of type of varus deformity, a medial release is necessary when varus exceeds 18° and, in their hands, TAA is contraindicated when varus exceeds 25°, even with soft tissue rebalancing.

Most surgeons agree that the tibial preparation for tibial component positioning in the coronal plane should be perpendicular to the tibial shaft axis[2,36,41]; this often necessitates an eccentric resection of the eroded distal tibia, with more bone being removed from the lateral than medial tibial plafond.[36] However, some flexibility for slight divergence from this perpendicular position may be possible. Although Mann and colleagues[37] and Wood and Deakin[52] observed that slight varus malposition (3°–5°) of the tibial component did not have an adverse effect on clinical outcomes, Saltzman and colleagues[61] cautioned that even minor component malpositioning may lead to atypical length change in the periankle ligaments, putting the implants at risk for eccentric loading. Barg and colleagues,[33] in a series of 317 mobile-bearing total ankles, emphasized the importance of proper talar component position and optimal sagittal plane relationship between the tibial and talar components, noting that tibio-talar component malpositioning or offset leads to decreased function and increased pain compared with TAAs in their series with optimal talar component position.

In 2 recent surgical technique articles, Ryssman and Myerson[59,60] provide a stepwise approach to performing TAA for the arthritic varus ankle. Although these articles are not supported by these authors' clinical data, their systematic approach represents a practical recipe for varus correction, with techniques of ligament balancing, tendon lengthening and transfer, and realignment osteotomies. Hobson and colleagues[62] compared mobile-bearing TAA in 91 ankles with coronal plane deformity less than or equal to 10° to 32 ankles with coronal plane deformity between 11° and 30°. Most of the ankles had varus deformity. The authors report that most correction was achieved through bone preparation with infrequent ligament rebalancing. A few patients had staged procedures, most of which were performed postoperatively, to improve alignment and stability. At mean follow-up of 4 years, no significant differences were noted in implant survivorship, range of motion, or complications, and the group with greater deformity had a significantly greater mean AOFAS hindfoot-ankle score. Although these authors suggest that TAA may be successfully performed in ankle arthritis with coronal plane deformity up to 30°, they acknowledge that in their experience, 27% of TAAs performed for ankle arthritis associated with coronal plane deformity between 11° and 30° failed because of gross instability. Kim and colleagues[36] also provide clinical outcomes in their comparative study of 23 TAAs performed in moderate-to-severe varus ankle arthritis (range, 10°–28° of varus malalignment) and 22 TAAs performed in ankle arthritis with neutral alignment. Their stepwise approach to correcting the varus deformity is detailed in their investigation and includes (1) medial release, (2) lateral ligament stabilization, (3) neutralizing tibial preparation, (4) calcaneal osteotomy, and (5) dorsiflexion first metatarsal osteotomy. Applying their stepwise approach, at mean follow-up of 27 months these authors observed satisfactory outcomes in both groups without a significant difference. One failure with need for conversion of TAA to ankle arthrodesis occurred in each group.

Ankle Arthrodesis

Ankle arthrodesis in the management of the varus arthritic ankle was thoroughly reviewed by Hennessy and colleagues[3] in the September 2008 *Foot and Ankle Clinics* volume. The literature on ankle arthrodesis for varus ankle arthritis does not seem to have dramatically changed. Smith and Wood[43] reported on 25 ankle arthrodesis for coronal plane deformity exceeding 20°, with 20 of the procedures performed for varus malalignment. The investigators performed the arthrodesis through an anterior approach with screw fixation and added a distal fibular resection in 13 cases. Eighteen of the 25 procedures were corrected to within 5° of neutral, and the mean AOFAS hindfoot-ankle score improved for function and pain from 25.5 to 43.7 points and from 10.5 to 35.2 points, respectively. In a smaller case series of open ankle arthrodeses performed for ankle arthritis associated with cavovarus foot alignment, Fortin and colleagues[63] reported that dorsiflexion first metatarsal osteotomies were necessary to achieve a plantigrade foot position, as shown in Case III.

Although most authors agree that arthroscopic ankle arthrodesis should be reserved for patients with minimal coronal plane deformity,[64–66] 2 investigations in particular suggest that, with experience, even greater deformity may be corrected using an arthroscopic technique. Gougoulias and colleagues[67] retrospectively evaluated 78 arthroscopic ankle arthrodesis, comparing 30 ankles with preoperative coronal plane deformity with a mean coronal plane deformity of 24.7° versus 48 ankles with mean coronal plane deformity of 5.6°. The technique for the ankles with greater deformity included an eccentric distal tibia preparation and debridement to realign the ankle and hindfoot. Four ankles required extension of the arthrodesis to the subtalar joint. The investigators did not observe any significant differences between the groups, with hindfoot alignment being 0.4° and 0.7° for the ankles with less and more preoperative coronal plane deformity, respectively. Each group had a single nonunion. Winson and colleagues[68] also suggested that ankle arthrodesis may be performed with large coronal plane deformity. In their series of 105 arthroscopic ankle arthrodeses, with preoperative coronal plane malalignment ranging from 28° of varus to 22° of valgus, the investigators identified 83 patients with good-to-excellent results and a union rate of 92.4%. In 4 patients, concomitant calcaneal osteotomies were required to achieve a satisfactory hindfoot alignment.

SUMMARY

Surgical correction of the varus arthritic ankle is challenging and rarely does an isolated procedure provide satisfactory outcome. Many principles applied to joint-preserving realignment procedures may be applied to TAA. Comprehensive ankle and foot realignment may relieve symptoms in most patients with varus ankle arthritis, but intra-articular distortion often does not allow for physiologic correction in joint-sparing surgery. Although considerable correction may be achieved with isolated TAA, optimal balance and load distribution is rarely possible without the realignment principles applied to joint-sparing surgery for varus ankle arthritis. Likewise, ankle arthrodesis may require concomitant procedures to achieve a plantigrade foot position. More investigation with longer follow-up is needed to determine optimal treatment of this complex deformity.

REFERENCES

1. Ahmad J, Raikin SM. Ankle arthrodesis: the simple and the complex. Foot Ankle Clin 2008;13(3):381–400, viii.
2. Coetzee JC. Management of varus or valgus ankle deformity with ankle replacement. Foot Ankle Clin 2008;13(3):509–20, x.
3. Hennessy MS, Molloy AP, Wood EV. Management of the varus arthritic ankle. Foot Ankle Clin 2008;13(3):417–42, viii.
4. Knupp M, Bolliger L, Hintermann B. Treatment of posttraumatic varus ankle deformity with supramalleolar osteotomy. Foot Ankle Clin 2012;17(1):95–102.
5. LaClair SM. Reconstruction of the varus ankle from soft-tissue procedures with osteotomy through arthrodesis. Foot Ankle Clin 2007;12(1):153–76, x.
6. Mayich DJ, Daniels TR. Total ankle replacement in ankle arthritis with varus talar deformity: pathophysiology, evaluation, and management principles. Foot Ankle Clin 2012;17(1):127–39.
7. Stamatis ED, Myerson MS. Supramalleolar osteotomy: indications and technique. Foot Ankle Clin 2003;8(2):317–33.
8. Klammer G, Benninger E, Espinosa N. The varus ankle and instability. Foot Ankle Clin 2012;17(1):57–82.
9. Apostle KL, Sangeorzan BJ. Anatomy of the varus foot and ankle. Foot Ankle Clin 2012;17(1):1–11.
10. Thevendran G, Younger AS. Examination of the varus ankle, foot, and tibia. Foot Ankle Clin 2012;17(1):13–20.
11. Easley ME, Vineyard JC. Varus ankle and osteochondral lesions of the talus. Foot Ankle Clin 2012;17(1):21–38.
12. Leardini A, Stagni R, O'Connor JJ. Mobility of the subtalar joint in the intact ankle complex. J Biomech 2001;34(6):805–9.
13. Coleman SS, Chesnut WJ. A simple test for hindfoot flexibility in the cavovarus foot. Clin Orthop Relat Res 1977;123:60–2.
14. Hayashi K, Tanaka Y, Kumai T, et al. Correlation of compensatory alignment of the subtalar joint to the progression of primary osteoarthritis of the ankle. Foot Ankle Int 2008;29(4):400–6.
15. Lee WC, Moon JS, Lee K, et al. Indications for supramalleolar osteotomy in patients with ankle osteoarthritis and varus deformity. J Bone Joint Surg Am 2011;93(13):1243–8.
16. Frigg A, Nigg B, Davis E, et al. Does alignment in the hindfoot radiograph influence dynamic foot-floor pressures in ankle and tibiotalocalcaneal fusion? Clin Orthop Relat Res 2010;468(12):3362–70.

17. Saltzman CL, el-Khoury GY. The hindfoot alignment view. Foot Ankle Int 1995; 16(9):572–6.
18. Knupp M, Stufkens SA, Bolliger L, et al. Classification and treatment of supramalleolar deformities. Foot Ankle Int 2011;32(11):1023–31.
19. Stufkens SA, van Bergen CJ, Blankevoort L, et al. The role of the fibula in varus and valgus deformity of the tibia: a biomechanical study. J Bone Joint Surg Br 2011;93(9):1232–9.
20. Takakura Y, Tanaka Y, Kumai T, et al. Low tibial osteotomy for osteoarthritis of the ankle. Results of a new operation in 18 patients. J Bone Joint Surg Br 1995;77(1): 50–4.
21. Horn DM, Fragomen AT, Rozbruch SR. Supramalleolar osteotomy using circular external fixation with six-axis deformity correction of the distal tibia. Foot Ankle Int 2011;32(10):986–93.
22. Takakura Y, Takaoka T, Tanaka Y, et al. Results of opening-wedge osteotomy for the treatment of a post-traumatic varus deformity of the ankle. J Bone Joint Surg Am 1998;80(2):213–8.
23. Tanaka Y, Takakura Y, Hayashi K, et al. Low tibial osteotomy for varus-type osteoarthritis of the ankle. J Bone Joint Surg Br 2006;88(7):909–13.
24. Haskell A, Mann RA. Ankle arthroplasty with preoperative coronal plane deformity: short-term results. Clin Orthop Relat Res 2004;(424):98–103.
25. Reddy SC, Mann JA, Mann RA, et al. Correction of moderate to severe coronal plane deformity with the STAR ankle prosthesis. Foot Ankle Int 2011;32(7):659–64.
26. Merian M, Glisson RR, Nunley JA. J. Leonard Goldner Award 2010. Ligament balancing for total ankle arthroplasty: an in vitro evaluation of the elongation of the hind- and midfoot ligaments. Foot Ankle Int 2011;32(5):S457–472.
27. Bonnin M, Judet T, Colombier JA, et al. Midterm results of the Salto Total Ankle Prosthesis. Clin Orthop Relat Res 2004;(424):6–18.
28. Mann HA, Filippi J, Myerson MS. Intra-articular opening medial tibial wedge osteotomy (plafond-plasty) for the treatment of intra-articular varus ankle arthritis and instability. Foot Ankle Int 2012;33(4):255–61.
29. Hintermann B, Barg A, Knupp M. Corrective supramalleolar osteotomy for malunited pronation-external rotation fractures of the ankle. J Bone Joint Surg Br 2011;93(10):1367–72.
30. Knupp M, Stufkens SA, van Bergen CJ, et al. Effect of supramalleolar varus and valgus deformities on the tibiotalar joint: a cadaveric study. Foot Ankle Int 2011; 32(6):609–15.
31. Stamatis ED, Cooper PS, Myerson MS. Supramalleolar osteotomy for the treatment of distal tibial angular deformities and arthritis of the ankle joint. Foot Ankle Int 2003;24(10):754–64.
32. Kupcha PC. RE: supramalleolar osteotomy for the treatment of distal tibial angular deformities and arthritis of the ankle joint stamatis, ED, et al. Foot Ankle Int 2003 24(10):754–63. Foot Ankle Int 2004;25(7):516.
33. Barg A, Elsner A, Anderson AE, et al. The effect of three-component total ankle replacement malalignment on clinical outcome: pain relief and functional outcome in 317 consecutive patients. J Bone Joint Surg Am 2011;93(21):1969–78.
34. Bonnin M, Gaudot F, Laurent JR, et al. The Salto total ankle arthroplasty: survivorship and analysis of failures at 7 to 11 years. Clin Orthop Relat Res 2011;469(1): 225–36.
35. Gougoulias N, Khanna A, Maffulli N. How successful are current ankle replacements?: a systematic review of the literature. Clin Orthop Relat Res 2010; 468(1):199–208.

36. Kim BS, Choi WJ, Kim YS, et al. Total ankle replacement in moderate to severe varus deformity of the ankle. J Bone Joint Surg Br 2009;91(9):1183–90.
37. Mann JA, Mann RA, Horton E. STAR ankle: long-term results. Foot Ankle Int 2011; 32(5):S473–484.
38. Saltzman CL, Mann RA, Ahrens JE, et al. Prospective controlled trial of STAR total ankle replacement versus ankle fusion: initial results. Foot Ankle Int 2009;30(7): 579–96.
39. Wood PL, Prem H, Sutton C. Total ankle replacement: medium-term results in 200 Scandinavian total ankle replacements. J Bone Joint Surg Br 2008;90(5):605–9.
40. Wood PL, Sutton C, Mishra V, et al. A randomised, controlled trial of two mobile-bearing total ankle replacements. J Bone Joint Surg Br 2009;91(1):69–74.
41. Coetzee JC. Surgical strategies: lateral ligament reconstruction as part of the management of varus ankle deformity with ankle replacement. Foot Ankle Int 2010;31(3):267–74.
42. Cornelis Doets H, van der Plaat LW, Klein JP. Medial malleolar osteotomy for the correction of varus deformity during total ankle arthroplasty: results in 15 ankles. Foot Ankle Int 2008;29(2):171–7.
43. Smith R, Wood PL. Arthrodesis of the ankle in the presence of a large deformity in the coronal plane. J Bone Joint Surg Br 2007;89(5):615–9.
44. Mohamedean A, Said HG, El-Sharkawi M, et al. Technique and short-term results of ankle arthrodesis using anterior plating. Int Orthop 2010;34(6):833–7.
45. Plaass C, Knupp M, Barg A, et al. Anterior double plating for rigid fixation of isolated tibiotalar arthrodesis. Foot Ankle Int 2009;30(7):631–9.
46. Tarkin IS, Mormino MA, Clare MP, et al. Anterior plate supplementation increases ankle arthrodesis construct rigidity. Foot Ankle Int 2007;28(2):219–23.
47. Yasui Y, Takao M, Miyamoto W, et al. Technique tip: open ankle arthrodesis using locking compression plate combined with anterior sliding bone graft. Foot Ankle Int 2010;31(12):1125–8.
48. Coester LM, Saltzman CL, Leupold J, et al. Long-term results following ankle arthrodesis for post-traumatic arthritis. J Bone Joint Surg Am 2001;83(2): 219–28.
49. Fuchs S, Sandmann C, Skwara A, et al. Quality of life 20 years after arthrodesis of the ankle. A study of adjacent joints. J Bone Joint Surg Br 2003;85(7):994–8.
50. Hendrickx RP, Stufkens SA, de Bruijn EE, et al. Medium- to long-term outcome of ankle arthrodesis. Foot Ankle Int 2011;32(10):940–7.
51. Ahmad J, Pour AE, Raikin SM. The modified use of a proximal humeral locking plate for tibiotalocalcaneal arthrodesis. Foot Ankle Int 2007;28(9):977–83.
52. Wood PL, Deakin S. Total ankle replacement. The results in 200 ankles. J Bone Joint Surg Br 2003;85(3):334–41.
53. Doets HC, Brand R, Nelissen RG. Total ankle arthroplasty in inflammatory joint disease with use of two mobile-bearing designs. J Bone Joint Surg Am 2006; 88(6):1272–84.
54. Takakura Y, Tanaka Y, Kumai T, et al. Ankle arthroplasty using three generations of metal and ceramic prostheses. Clin Orthop Relat Res 2004;(424):130–6.
55. Espinosa N, Walti M, Favre P, et al. Misalignment of total ankle components can induce high joint contact pressures. J Bone Joint Surg Am 2010;92(5):1179–87.
56. Wood PL, Karski MT, Watmough P. Total ankle replacement: the results of 100 mobility total ankle replacements. J Bone Joint Surg Br 2010;92(7):958–62.
57. Hintermann B, Valderrabano V, Dereymaeker G, et al. The HINTEGRA ankle: rationale and short-term results of 122 consecutive ankles. Clin Orthop Relat Res 2004;(424):57–68.

58. Rippstein PF, Huber M, Coetzee JC, et al. Total ankle replacement with use of a new three-component implant. J Bone Joint Surg Am 2011;93(15):1426–35.
59. Ryssman D, Myerson MS. Surgical strategies: the management of varus ankle deformity with joint replacement. Foot Ankle Int 2011;32(2):217–24.
60. Ryssman DM, Myerson MS. Total ankle arthroplasty: management of varus deformity at the ankle. Foot Ankle Int 2012;33(4):347–54.
61. Saltzman CL, Tochigi Y, Rudert MJ, et al. The effect of agility ankle prosthesis misalignment on the peri-ankle ligaments. Clin Orthop Relat Res 2004;(424): 137–42.
62. Hobson SA, Karantana A, Dhar S. Total ankle replacement in patients with significant pre-operative deformity of the hindfoot. J Bone Joint Surg Br 2009;91(4): 481–6.
63. Fortin PT, Guettler J, Manoli A. Idopathic cavovarus and lateral ankle instability: recognition and treatment implications relating to ankle arthritis. Foot Ankle Int 2002;23(11):1031–7.
64. Ferkel RD, Hewitt M. Long-term results of arthroscopic ankle arthrodesis. Foot Ankle Int 2005;26(4):275–80.
65. Glick JM, Morgan CD, Myerson MS, et al. Ankle arthrodesis using an arthroscopic method: long-term follow-up of 34 cases. Arthroscopy 1996;12(4):428–34.
66. Myerson MS, Quill G. Ankle arthrodesis. A comparison of an arthroscopic and an open method of treatment. Clin Orthop Relat Res 1991;(268):84–95.
67. Gougoulias NE, Agathangelidis FG, Parsons SW. Arthroscopic ankle arthrodesis. Foot Ankle Int 2007;28(6):695–706.
68. Winson IG, Robinson DE, Allen PE. Arthroscopic ankle arthrodesis. J Bone Joint Surg Br 2005;87(3):343–7.

Revision Total Ankle Replacement

Jacques Heinrich Jonck, MB, ChB, FC ORTH[a],
Mark S. Myerson, MD[b,*]

KEYWORDS

- Revision total ankle arthroplasty • Revision ankle replacement
- Ballooning osteolysis • Component subsidence • Ankle arthritis

KEY POINTS

- Several factors, including patient selection, implant characteristics, surgical technique, or a combination of these, can lead to failure of a total ankle replacement (TAR).
- Pain following TAR may be a symptom of implant failure, but other causes for pain, especially in the absence of radiographic abnormalities, should be considered and may include infection, periarticular inflammation caused by soft-tissue strain, and gutter impingement.
- Limited range of motion in a TAR is an unfortunate complication. Several factors may play a role, including the level of preoperative stiffness, technical error (overstuffing of the joint or inadequate release of soft tissue), prolonged postoperative immobilization, component subsidence, gutter impingement, heterotopic ossification, or arthrofibrosis.
- Ballooning osteolysis can be a silent process, progressively growing in size and eventually leading to implant loosening and failure. Computed tomography is superior to standard radiography in both detecting cysts and accurately determining their size. A sensible approach to this problem would be to actively look for cyst formation in the early postoperative period and monitor for signs of progression over time. Signs of cyst progression on imaging should prompt a surgical intervention. Surgical options are curettage and bone graft of cysts, with or without polyethylene liner exchange, or metal component revision with bone graft.
- The tibial component can be revised to another standard component if good medial and lateral bone support and a good-quality bleeding cancellous bone base of more than 50% is available after bone cuts and debridement. If structural stability in the distal tibia is severely compromised because of massive cyst formation or osteolysis, revision with a custom made tibial component should be considered.
- It is important to fill all bone defects under the weight-bearing surface of the tibial base plate with impaction bone grafting. This action should be taken before insertion of the revision tibial component. The tibial base plate should cover all bone graft to prevent it from falling into the joint and becoming loose bodies.

Continued

Disclosure.

[a] Department of Orthopaedics, Windhoek Central Hospital, Namibia, PO Box 9819, Windhoek, 9000 Namibia; [b] Institute for Foot and Ankle Reconstruction at Mercy, 301 Saint Paul Place, Baltimore, MD 21202, USA
* Corresponding author.
E-mail address: mark4feet@aol.com

Foot Ankle Clin N Am 17 (2012) 687–706
http://dx.doi.org/10.1016/j.fcl.2012.08.008
foot.theclinics.com

Continued

- If a failed talar component is to be revised, 3 surgical options exist: revision with a standard component of the same design, revision with a standard component of a different design, or revision with a custom-made stemmed prosthesis. When deciding on which implant to use, the factors that should be considered are patient factors (obesity, osteopenia, level of activity), level of subsidence, osteolysis or cyst formation, and symptomatic subtalar joint arthritis.
- When faced with severe prosthesis failure, loosening, and subsidence, the options are really limited to either a patient-customized device, a large structural bone graft arthrodesis, or an amputation. The structural bone graft arthrodesis does not have a predictable outcome, and a poor rate of arthrodesis at best. Fortunately patient-customized devices for the ankle can still be used, although because of recent restrictions imposed on the industry, currently the only manufacturer of these implants in the United States is Tornier (Edina, MN), these being based on the Salto Talaris 2-part component system.

INTRODUCTION

Since the first total ankle replacement (TAR) in 1970, orthopedic surgeons have struggled with the sequelae of implant failure. The first-generation prostheses mostly consisted of cemented tibial and talar implants that did not adequately reproduce the complex natural anatomy of the ankle joint. Unacceptably poor patient satisfaction outcomes and high failure rates of these older-generation implants brought prosthetic replacement of the ankle joint into disrepute, and arthrodesis of the ankle joint remained the gold standard for surgical treatment of end-stage arthritis of the ankle.

The mid-1980s saw newer generations of TAR prosthesis designs with uncemented implant bone interfaces, less constrained kinematics, and a meniscus-type polyethylene insert together with improved surgical techniques. Improved patient satisfaction levels and lower failure rates led to new enthusiasm among foot and ankle surgeons for this technique as the surgical procedure of choice for end-stage ankle arthritis in selected patients.[1,2]

Despite current best efforts regarding implant design, surgical technique, and patient selection, the intermediate and long-term survival of TAR is still unpredictable and remains inferior to that of hip and knee replacement. Labek and colleagues[3] reviewed revision rates for hip, knee, ankle, shoulder, and elbow replacement as reported in the different National Joint Registries. The results were indicated as "revisions per 100 observed component years" as originally introduced by the Australian Arthroplasty Register. The mean revision rate of 1.29 per 100 observed component years for total hip replacement (THR) was comparable with the mean of 1.28 revisions per 100 observed component years for total knee replacement (TKR). Revisions after TAR were only reported in 3 of the 6 countries, namely New Zealand, Norway, and Sweden. The mean revision rate of 3.29 per 100 observed component years was significantly higher than that for hips and knees. This finding therefore has to be taken into consideration by surgeons who are performing primary TAR, who should have the knowledge, technical skill, and know-how to revise the inevitable failed implants during their careers.

TAR is often associated with secondary surgery that may follow the index procedure. The literature is confusing in this regard, as these procedures are labeled as "revisions," "reoperations," or "additional procedures" without consensus about the definition of each. Henricson and colleagues[4] proposed definitions for these 3 terms after reviewing the literature. The proposed definition for "revision" was "the removal or exchange of one or more of the prosthetic components with the exception of incidental exchange of the polyethylene insert." Incidental polyethylene exchange can occur during secondary surgery involving the joint, but not specifically the prosthetic components. Indications for this type of surgery could be early deep infection, bone overgrowth, or joint impingement. The reason for exchanging the polyethylene insert in these cases would be to create space to adequately debride the joint and not primarily for failure of the insert; therefore, it is believed that these surgeries should not be counted as revisions. The proposed definition for "reoperation" was "nonrevisional secondary surgery involving the joint." Examples of these procedures are joint debridements, joint washouts, and incidental polyethylene exchange. The term "additional procedure" was proposed to be defined as "nonrevisional secondary surgery not involving the joint." Examples of this include ligament reconstruction, soft-tissue release, Achilles lengthening, and calcaneal osteotomy. This article discusses revision TAR as defined by Henricson and colleagues.[4]

FAILURE OF TOTAL ANKLE REPLACEMENTS

Several factors, including patient selection, implant characteristics, surgical technique, or a combination of these can lead to failure of a TAR.[2] Patient factors that can negatively affect the outcome are physiologic (medical comorbidities, drugs, obesity), psychological, lifestyle, and habits (smoking, occupation, and recreation). Several studies have highlighted the negative predictive value of obesity on hip and knee replacements, but the only study (level 4) evaluating the effect of obesity on survivorship of TAR showed comparable results between obese and nonobese patients. In this study by Barg and colleagues,[5] 118 patients (123 ankles) with a minimum body mass index (BMI) of 30 kg/m^2 were reviewed retrospectively. An overall implant survivorship of 93% at 6 years was comparable with other reported results of nonobese patients. However, it should be noted that 98 patients (83.1%) were of the group Obesity grade I (BMI 30.0–34.9 kg/m^2) and only 1 patient (0.8%) was classified as Obesity grade III (BMI >40.0 kg/m^2).

The implant features that can potentially jeopardize longevity of the prosthesis are: the implant-bone interface; whether cemented or uncemented; and in the uncemented whether the undersurface is hydroxyapatite coated, grit blasted or trabecular metal, the level of constrained motion, the footprint size of the individual components, and the amount of bone that needs resection for implantation of these components.[1,2,5] To date there is scant evidence to suggest superiority of any of the newer-generation implants over another. Henricson and colleagues[6] found statistically improved outcomes in the double-coated Scandinavian Total Ankle Replacement (STAR; Waldemar Link, Hamburg, Germany) prosthesis versus the single-coated STAR prosthesis in their review of the Swedish Ankle Registry. Wood and colleagues[7] published their results from a prospective randomized trial comparing 2 third-generation mobile-bearing prostheses, the STAR and Buechel-Pappas (Endotech, South Orange, NJ, USA and Wright Cremascoli, Toulon, France), and although their medium-term results were better with the STAR prosthesis, they were not statistically significant. Gougoulias and colleagues[8] reviewed the literature regarding 1105 TARs with currently used prostheses (Agility [DePuy Orthopedics, Inc, Warsaw, IN, USA], STAR, Buechel-Pappas, HINTEGRA [New Deal, Lyon, France], Salto [Tornier, Saint Ismier, France], TNK [Kyocera, Kyoto, Japan], Mobility [Depuy International, Leeds, UK]), and found no superiority of one implant over another.

Surgical technique plays a critical role in the long-term survival of TARs, and improvement in outcome over time that is due to the so-called learning curve is well described.[6,9,10] Careful handling of the tenuous soft-tissue envelope, choosing the correct size of implant, correctly placing it in 3 planes, addressing ankle instability adequately, and correcting preexisting malalignment in the ankle, as well as proximal and distal to it, should positively influence the short-term, medium-term, and long term outcomes.

Glazebrook and colleagues[11] reviewed the literature for complications associated with TAR and the relative risk of failure attributable to each complication. This study reviewed 20 series with a total of 2386 ankles, and found 9 main complications reported, namely:

- Intraoperative fracture
- Postoperative fracture
- Wound-healing problems
- Deep infection
- Aseptic loosening
- Nonunion
- Implant failure
- Subsidence
- Technical error

Although deep infection was the least commonly reported complication, the investigators found that, as is the case with aseptic loosening and implant failure, it resulted in failure of the TAR in more than 50% of cases, and therefore these 3 complications were classified as high grade. Technical error, subsidence, and postoperative bone fracture each resulted in failure of the TAR less than 50% of the time in cases where it was reported, and therefore these 3 complications were classified as intermediate grade. Intraoperative bone fracture and wound-healing problems never resulted in TAR failure, and were therefore classified as low-grade complications.

Coronal plane deformity and ankle instability must be addressed during TAR. Even trivial malalignment or instability will increase edge loading on the polyethylene liner with increased wear, and a higher incidence of loosening and failure. It is also important to simultaneously correct abnormal foot architecture for the same reason (**Fig. 1**).[12,13]

Vaupel and colleagues[14] examined 10 failed Agility implants for macroscopic and microscopic wear patterns. Six surface damage modes were investigated, namely burnishing, embedding, grooving/scratching, pitting, dishing, and abrasion. All 6 of these patterns were observed on the retrieved polyethylene liners. A visible area of material removal on the polyethylene liner was a constant finding. This "talar footprint" correlates with the surface area on the polyethylene liner where the talar component primarily articulated. The areas of maximum surface damage to the polyethylene liners correlated with the edges of the contact area between the talar component and the liner. Titanium particles were also found embedded in the polyethylene liner in the area of the talar footprint. This third-body particle-wear process can intensify the damage done to the polyethylene liner. Intentional mismatching of the talar component size with the total contact area of the polyethylene liner to potentially increase freedom of mobility in the implant created a smaller ratio of footprint area versus total liner contact area; this invariably leads to higher contact stresses and in some cases may exceed the yield stress for polyethylene. Pitting and abrasion are 2 wear patterns associated with high contact stresses, often seen in TKR. These 2 wear patterns produce the most wear particles.[15] Six of the 8 retrieved liners showed evidence of abrasion, and all of them had evidence of pitting. Kobayashi and colleagues[16] found polyethylene wear particle concentrations in synovial fluid to be similar in TAR and

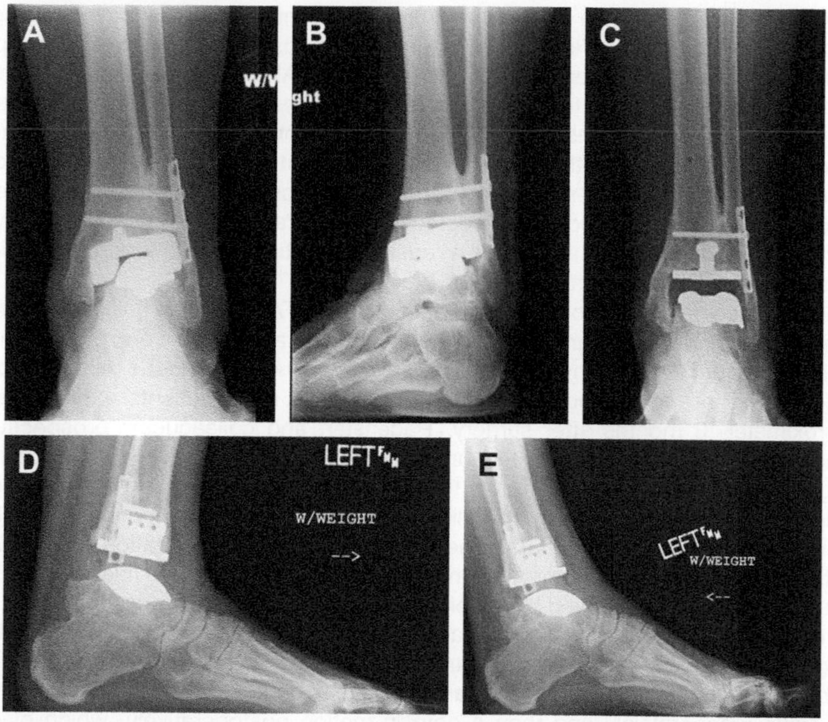

Fig. 1. This patient had an ankle arthrodesis taken down and converted to an Agility (DePuy, Warsaw, IN) TAR in 2005 for persistent ankle and hindfoot pain. In 2006 a subtalar arthrodesis was added for painful subtalar arthritis. In 2010 the patient developed lateral-sided ankle pain, and a CT scan confirmed tibial component loosening and medial gutter impingement. She was revised to a Salto Talaris (Tornier, Edina, MN) prosthesis and at last follow-up was doing well. On the preoperative radiographs (*A, B*) note the valgus malalignment of the tibial component and intra-articular varus failure that was perfectly corrected with the revision implant (*C, D, E*).

posterior stabilized TKR. Progressive peri-implant osteolysis and eventual implant loosening is therefore related in many cases to the production and accumulation of polyethylene wear particles. Several of the TAR systems currently in use have a stemmed tibial component that needs a large anterior distal tibia bone window for insertion. Although these bone windows are bone grafted after insertion, increased initial micromotion was noted with these implants. This initial instability may lead to fibrous tissue ingrowth and subsequent failure of fixation.[17]

CLINICAL DILEMMAS

Pain with Normal Radiographs

Ongoing, substantial pain following total ankle replacement that is not adequately responding to pain management measures is one of the most common reasons for revision surgery to the ankle.[18] The primary symptom indicating early failure following TAR is pain. This pain is often described as start-up pain or mechanical pain associated with increase in activity. Radiographic features including ballooning osteolysis, linear loosening lines, component subsidence, or liner failure will confirm the diagnosis of implant failure. Such presentations of failure can be either septic or aseptic. It is imperative to confirm or rule out the diagnosis of deep infection, because the management for each is vastly different.[19] The surgical options for management of aseptic failure are generally narrowed down to either revision TAR or hindfoot and ankle (ankle or tibiotalocalcaneal [TTC]) fusion. Septic failure requires 2-stage revision with antibiotic cement spacer to either revision TAR or hindfoot fusion, retention of cement spacer, or amputation. In their recent review of 9 patients with retained antibiotic impregnated cement spacers following hardware removal and debridement of deep infection after ankle arthrodesis or replacement, Ferrao and colleagues[20] showed that long-term use of these spacers is a reasonable option in the low-demand patient with medical or surgical comorbidities (**Fig. 2**).

However, some patients present with pain following TAR and no significant features of failure on standard radiographs. These patients pose a diagnostic and management challenge for the treating physician. An interesting phenomenon is the relapse in pain and swelling in and around the replaced ankle that most patients experience at approximately 3 months after surgery. Pagenstert and colleagues[21] prospectively observed 28 patients with isolated unilateral posttraumatic ankle arthritis treated surgically with TAR (HINTEGRA) over the first year following surgery. None of these patients had any postoperative complications. Scores measuring pain and swelling showed marked improvement at 6 weeks, with significant deterioration at 3 months and then constant, gradual improvement at 6, 9, and 12 months. This relapse in symptoms is most probably caused by a typical local inflammatory response related to the increased strain placed on the periarticular soft tissues when the rehabilitation program progresses out of the constraints of a surgical boot after 6 weeks. The authors have noted this too, particularly in patients who had limited movement of the ankle preoperatively and then a gain in motion postoperatively, which places a strain on the Achilles tendon in particular.

Intermittent episodes of pain and swelling with localized inflammation are often seen during periods of increased patient activity. Scarred and shortened periarticular soft tissues, associated with long-standing stiffness of the arthritic ankle joint, are subjected to increased strain owing to the improved mobility in the ankle joint following TAR, which can cause microtrauma and inflammation. Most TAR implant designs in clinical use today are semiconstrained or unconstrained (mobile bearing), in contrast to the relatively constrained, highly congruent natural ankle. This lack of constraint

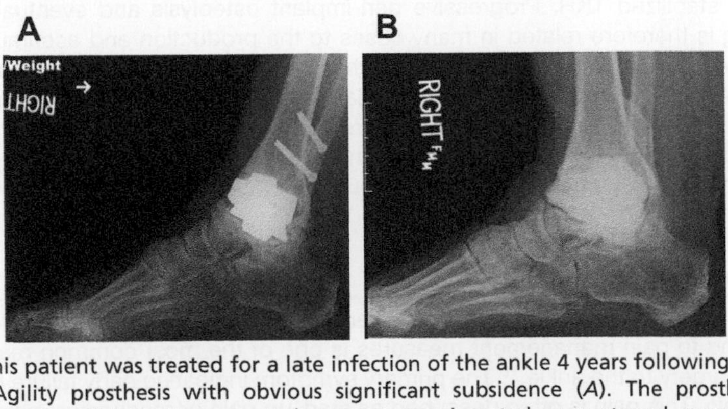

Fig. 2. This patient was treated for a late infection of the ankle 4 years following insertion of this Agility prosthesis with obvious significant subsidence (*A*). The prosthesis was removed and antibiotic impregnated cement was inserted as a staged procedure for management of the infection (*B*). However, following this procedure and with control of the infection, the patient noted that she was asymptomatic and the cement was left in place. This radiograph was taken 2 years following insertion of the cement.

may lead to shear forces being directed to the periarticular soft tissues, adding to the development of inflammation during increased activity.[21] Simple measures such as oral anti-inflammatories and rest, with or without the application of an ankle brace or boot, is usually enough to resolve these symptoms.

Uncomplicated local inflammation as a cause of pain should be a diagnosis by exclusion. Low-grade infection of a TAR must always be part of the differential diagnosis in a patient presenting with nonspecific pain and normal radiographs. This diagnosis can be very difficult to make, because the classic symptoms and signs of infection, such as fevers or chills, soft-tissue fluctuation, open wounds, or draining sinuses may be absent. A high index of suspicion is necessary and a standard blood workup including a full blood count, erythrocyte sedimentation rate, and C-reactive protein level should routinely be used. If the blood results are inconclusive, a percutaneous image-guided biopsy should be performed to rule out or confirm the diagnosis of infection.[19] The management of the infected TAR falls outside the scope of this article and is therefore not discussed here.

Another cause for postoperative pain in the presence of a normal-appearing implant on standard radiographs is gutter impingement. Bony impingement in the medial or lateral gutter can be associated with subsidence or loosening of the implant (most often the talar component), and can usually be appreciated on standard radiographs.[2,22] Some patients, however, may present with persistent gutter pain (commonly on the medial side), with no clear evidence of bony impingement on radiographs. These patients may have true soft-tissue impingement.[23] A cortisone injection mixed with a local anesthetic agent given under aseptic conditions in the affected gutter will serve a dual purpose by confirming the anatomic site of the pain as well as treating underlying synovitis, which may cause the pain. Kurup and Taylor[23] performed posterior tibial tendon (PTT) decompressions on 2 patients with persistent medial gutter impingement symptoms due to soft-tissue impingement, and found good symptomatic improvement in both. If patients seem to have localized medial or lateral joint pain that seems to be arising from gutter impingement, it is helpful to obtain a computed tomography (CT) scan to confirm what is going on in the gutter. Sometimes osteophytes that were not adequately removed during the primary procedure are present, and at times the prosthesis has been inserted too far medially or laterally. These medial or lateral joint impingements can be very difficult to appreciate on radiographs, and can be quite subtle. If there is clearly an osteophyte in the gutter that is not associated with incorrect positioning of the prosthesis, and if there is no loosening or subsidence of the talar component, then debridement, either arthroscopic or open, can be considered.

The authors have found that CT is far more reliable than radiography for persistent pain caused by a loose implant with no evidence of loosening on standard radiographs. CT was proved to be superior to standard radiographs in detecting peri-implant lucencies that were smaller in volume. Osteolytic lesions are also, on average, 3 times larger on CT scans than on radiographs.[24]

Postoperative Stiffness

The aim of surgical treatment for end-stage ankle arthritis is primarily to relieve pain. In general, the 2 options available are arthrodesis and TAR. However, mobility of the ankle joint following TAR does improve gait and may also serve to protect adjacent joints from early degeneration, as seen with ankle arthrodesis.[25,26] With data suggesting that intermediate- and long-term outcomes following TAR and ankle arthrodesis are comparable[27] and that similar improvement in pain relief and function can be expected at intermediate-term follow-up,[22] it is often the maintenance or improvement in ankle range of motion (ROM) that swings the pendulum toward TAR during the decision-making process. It is therefore unfortunate when a patient presents with significant stiffness of the ankle following TAR. It is important to try and find the underlying cause for the decreased ROM to successfully address this problem. Several factors may play a role, including the level of preoperative stiffness, technical error (overstuffing of the joint or inadequate soft-tissue release), prolonged postoperative immobilization, component subsidence, gutter impingement, heterotopic ossification, or arthrofibrosis. The best way of treating postoperative stiffness is to avoid it in the first place. Although preoperative stiffness is not a contraindication to primary TAR, Valderrabano and colleagues[28] found that 21 of the 22 ankles in their series that needed revision had posttraumatic osteoarthritis as their indication for primary TAR. These investigators suggested that preoperative scar tissue, stiffness, and altered mechanics of the ankle may all have a negative effect on the restoration of normal function with TAR.

Intraoperative ROM with trial components or the definitive implant will be the maximum that can be expected postoperatively. Because limited dorsiflexion in particular is poorly tolerated, at least 10° of dorsiflexion should be possible at the end of surgery.[29] ROM can be increased intraoperatively by using a thinner polyethylene liner, taking off more bone from the distal tibia, correcting excessive anterior translation of the talar component, or percutaneous Achilles lengthening/gastrocnemius recession. In general, the authors try to avoid lengthening of the Achilles or even the gastrocnemius recession if possible, and try to find another cause for the limited ROM intraoperatively, in particular, overstuffing of the joint, in which case a thinner polyethylene or more of a tibial cut is preferable.

No uniform postoperative rehabilitation protocol following TAR is evident from the current literature. Different implant designs, a high incidence of associated bony and soft-tissue procedures, and surgeon preference may be to blame. Pagenstert and colleagues[21] suggest that early motion during rehabilitation may decrease the formation of adhesions and improve function. Unfortunately the surgical incision in the poor soft-tissue envelope of the ankle does not tolerate early aggressive movement well, and the development of wound dehiscence and possible deep infection may have catastrophic consequences. Early ROM rehabilitation may also apply excessive shear forces to newly implanted cementless prostheses with subsequent failure of bony ingrowth. Early compressive forces, on the other hand, enhance bone ingrowth.[21] The authors' current early postoperative regime for uncomplicated primary TAR with a Salto Talaris uncemented prosthesis involves immobilization in a bulky posterior and mediolateral plaster-of-paris splint with the ankle in maximum dorsiflexion, and strictly no weight bearing for 2 weeks. At 2 weeks the surgical incision is evaluated and sutures are removed if applicable. A standard series of weight-bearing radiographs are also taken (anteroposterior [AP], mortise, lateral). At this visit the patient is placed in a surgical boot. Weight bearing in the boot as tolerated is encouraged. The patient is also instructed to remove the boot 5 times during the day and start controlled, in-line dorsiflexion and plantarflexion exercises at home. Walking in a swimming pool and swimming with a flipper on the affected foot is advised from approximately 3 weeks or after the surgical wound has sealed completely. At 6 weeks the patient starts to wean out of the surgical boot and a standard physical therapy program including stretching, strengthening, proprioception, and local modalities for pain and swelling is followed.

Patients with early postoperative ankle stiffness may benefit from forceful manipulation of the joint under general anesthesia. Fluoroscopic views of the ankle in maximum plantarflexion and dorsiflexion before and after the manipulation are useful to assess the amount of improvement obtained. This maneuver is most effective within the first 4 weeks following surgery, with very limited success thereafter. The authors do not believe that a lengthening of the Achilles following surgery is of much benefit to gain ROM in the ankle. No true increase in the ankle ROM occurs, and the increase is at the expense of strength of push off, which should not be compromised. If the stiffness is really disabling, then one may have to consider a revision of the prosthesis, starting again intraoperatively to ensure that maximum movement is present.

The most common causes for late presentation of postoperative ankle stiffness are bone impingement, heterotopic ossification or arthrofibrosis, and, in particular, subsidence of the talar component causing the bone to build up around the joint. Of course, this is not heterotopic ossification, which in fact rarely occurs around the ankle but is the development of osteophytes around the joint as the prosthesis subsides.

Valderrabano and colleagues[28] found periarticular ossification, mostly situated in the posteromedial aspect of the joint, in 43 of 68 ankles that were treated with the STAR prosthesis, despite postoperative use of indomethacin or other nonsteroidal anti-inflammatory drugs (NSAIDs). This high incidence may be related to excessive strain on the medial ligament complex caused by the nonanatomic cylindrical shape of the talar component. Twenty-three ankles had either revision surgery or other secondary surgery performed at a later stage, of which 11 was for progressive stiffening of the joint. No mention is made as to whether stiffness in these ankles were associated with periarticular ossification, how many underwent revision TAR versus other secondary surgery, or what type of secondary surgery was performed. Stiffness caused by intra-articular bone buildup is almost always associated with subsidence of either the talar or tibial component. During subsidence, the supportive rim of cortical bone that was suppose to keep the implant stable becomes the source of impingement as the implant is driven progressively deeper into the talar body or metaphysis of the distal tibia.[2] Radical debridement of protruding bone, either arthroscopically or as an open arthrotomy, and with or without polyethylene exchange, has been reported to improve ROM,[2,30] but the authors cannot agree with the use of this approach. However, the compromised base of bone is vulnerable for further subsidence and even fracture of the remaining talar body. Stiffness caused by subsidence is best treated surgically with revision TAR. Revision can be done with standard primary tibial and talar implants if adequate medial and lateral bone support is available after bone cuts were made and more than 50% of healthy bleeding bone is in contact with the undersurface of the implants to allow bony ingrowth. If not, custom-made stemmed prosthesis should be used to ensure adequate initial stability to allow bone ingrowth. Another reason why custom stemmed prostheses are an attractive option in this scenario is the fact that the same loads will be applied to the same (or weaker) quality bone with the same (or higher) risk of subsidence in ankles that were revised with standard components. Custom stemmed implants have a much better force distribution compared with healthy bone, and in theory should decrease the risk of recurrent subsidence. A larger polyethylene liner is often necessary because the bony defects and larger bone cuts usually prevent anatomic positioning of the metal components. The scarred and shortened capsule, ligaments, and tendons associated with subsidence are difficult to completely release, which prevents normal mobility of the joint during revision and often causes a nonanatomic center of rotation of the revised implant with a decreased effective ROM. Still, it is very important to try and remove all periarticular scar tissue, particularly posteriorly. The flexor hallucis longus and posterior neurovascular bundle are often trapped in the posterior capsular scar, therefore this maneuver must be done very carefully and under direct vision to avoid iatrogenic injuries to these structures.

Postoperative stiffness owing to true arthrofibrosis is the most difficult symptom to treat. Barg and colleagues[5] treated 7 patients with chronic pain and stiffness caused by arthrofibrosis following TAR with the HINTEGRA prosthesis with open arthrolysis and percutaneous Achilles lengthening, with good pain relief and increased ROM. Cui and colleagues[31] treated 5 patients with posttraumatic adhesive capsulitis, confirmed with an arthrogram and magnetic resonance imaging. Arthrofibrosis may be a similar pathologic process to adhesive capsulitis, which does not meet the strict inclusion criteria as outlined by Goldman because of incomplete involvement of the anterior or posterior ankle recess as seen on the arthrogram. All 5 ankles were treated with NSAIDs, physical therapy, and corticosteroid injections. Three ankles, which had no or only temporary relief with this treatment regime, had subsequent arthroscopic synovectomy and joint arthrolysis. Diagnostic arthroscopy found inflamed, thickened synovium with generalized synovial proliferation and fibrosis. Two of the 3 ankles treated with physical therapy, corticosteroid injection, and arthroscopy had improved pain and function, and 1 was unchanged. One of the 2 ankles that only had physical therapy and injection improved and the other remained unchanged. The investigators consider that neither arthroscopy nor revision arthroplasty provides predictable improvement of ROM in stiff ankles caused by arthrofibrosis.

MANAGING THE ASYMPTOMATIC CYST

Ballooning osteolysis can be a silent process, progressively growing in size and eventually leading to implant loosening and failure.[32] The radiography can be remarkably benign, and the authors have found that CT is superior to standard radiography both in detecting cysts as well as accurately determining its size. Revision surgery in some of these cases, whether revision to another implant or arthrodesis of the tibiotalar or TTC joints, may be exceedingly difficult because of the large structural defects left in the distal tibia and talar body. Very little is known of the etiology, pathophysiology, natural history, and optimal treatment of these cysts in the setting of TAR. Periprosthetic lucency and lysis has been defined on standard radiographs and CT imaging. On standard AP, mortise, and lateral radiographs lucency is defined as a lucent line at the prosthesis bone interface not exceeding 2 mm in width. Ballooning lysis is defined as lucency exceeding 2 mm.[24,33] Periprosthetic lucent lesions are defined as well-demarcated lucent lesions between the bone and prosthesis without osseous trabeculae using helical CT imaging with a metal artifact–minimizing protocol and 1.25-mm thick cuts.[24] The size of these lesions is measured on standard radiographs by measuring the longest axis in millimeters, and the length of the axis perpendicular to the long axis can be multiplied with the long axis to obtain a surface area in square millimeters. The same measurements can be used on coronal CT images.[24]

The development of these lytic lesions is probably multifactorial.[32] Small nonprogressive cysts may be mechanical in nature and may be related to stress shielding and early bone remodeling after insertion of the biologically active implant surface. Pyevich and colleagues[33] found that lucent lines associated with the Agility prosthesis almost always occurred before 2 years and that it was mostly nonprogressive in nature. Ballooning osteolysis was almost always found on the lateral side of the prosthesis and was mostly associated with nonunion of the tibiofibular syndesmosis. Their hypothesis was that these lesions occurred in areas of high interfacial stresses between the implant and the loose lateral malleolus. Large cysts are most likely a chemical phenomenon related to the accumulation of wear particles in the periarticular tissues and the host's osteoclastic reaction to it. Polyethylene microparticles are thought to be the predominant source of wear particles, but titanium and hydroxyapatite can also contribute.[29] Rodriguez and colleagues[32] used CT analysis and found a 100% incidence of osteolysis in 18 ankles replaced with the Ankle Evolutive System (AES; Biomet, Valence, France) ankle prosthesis at a mean follow-up of 39.4 months. At that stage only 1 patient had surgery for moderate ankle pain associated with 3 large osteolytic lesions. The cysts were curettaged and packed with lyophilized allograft, with good pain relief and osseous integration on standard radiographs at 6 months' follow-up. No need for implant exchange was necessary at that stage. Of importance, the histology of the biopsy taken during cyst curettage revealed a hystiocytic foreign body reaction, and morphology on polarized light was compatible with polyethylene wear. Bonnin and colleagues[29] analyzed 85 patients (87 ankles) with a Salto TAR at a mean follow-up of 8.9 years, and found 19 ankles with tibial or talar cysts larger than 5 mm on CT. Eight of these ankles were treated with cyst curettage and packing with iliac crest cancellous autograft as well as routine polyethylene exchange. Biopsy again confirmed the presence of wear particles, with macrophage inflammatory reaction in all cases. Half of these cases showed complete osseous integration at last follow-up and the other 4 showed residual cysts, all smaller than 5 mm. Of the 19 ankles, 8 more remained asymptomatic and 3 ankles had implant removal with subsequent arthrodesis. Of the 8 ankles with cysts larger than 5 mm that remained asymptomatic, 4 showed spontaneous regression without activity modification and none were associated with implant subsidence or loosening.

The unpredictable natural history of asymptomatic peri-implant cysts makes it extremely difficult to formulate a treatment plan that is acceptable for both the surgeon and the patient. From a surgeon's perspective it is important to intervene early on and avoid the surgical difficulties associated with massive bone loss due to enlarging cysts. The patient, however, is asymptomatic and may be reluctant to undergo major surgery for a potential problem that is to them at that stage clinically irrelevant. A sensible approach to this problem would be to actively look for cyst formation in the early postoperative period and monitor for signs of progression over time. Such monitoring can be done either with standard radiographs at routine follow-up visits (despite the known limitations regarding underdiagnosing smaller cysts as well as underestimating cyst size) or by doing a CT scan on all patients at a predetermined postoperative interval (eg, 1 year). All patients with signs of cyst formation on standard radiographs must undergo a CT scan to accurately assess the number, position, and size of the cysts. Follow-up imaging should be 6-monthly and preferably by CT scan. However, the cost implications and excessive exposure to radiation makes CT follow-up over an extended period of time impractical.

Signs of cyst progression on imaging should prompt a surgical intervention. A preoperative CT scan is imperative for surgical planning. Surgical options are curettage and bone graft of cysts, with or without polyethylene liner exchange, or metal component revision with bone graft (**Fig. 3**). It is the authors' opinion that all polyethylene liners should be exchanged during surgery. Signs of excessive polyethylene wear during the early postoperative period (first 3 years) may indicate abnormal ankle biomechanics caused by ankle instability, loose or subsided implants, periarticular malalignment, or technical error during the index procedure. Care should be taken to completely correct these abnormalities in conjunction with the polyethylene exchange and bone graft procedure. The diagnosis of associated implant loosening or subsidence should be made preoperatively using standard radiographic parameters (change in implant position of more than 5° or 5 mm on serial radiographs).[33] This diagnosis enables the surgeon to plan the implant revision, because a custom stemmed prosthesis may be necessary in certain cases where large cysts are present. The talar and tibial components should, however, be probed for loosening

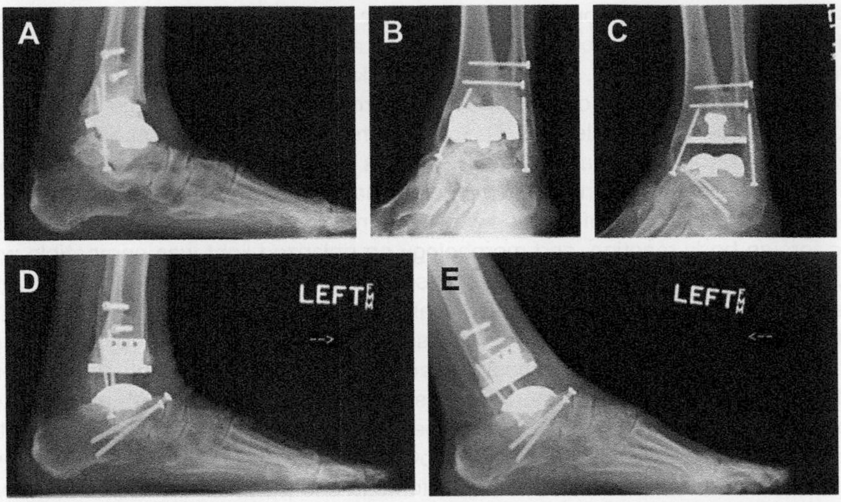

Fig. 3. This patient underwent the Agility replacement 5 years ago. Note significant cyst formation in the tibia, associated with subsidence and loosening of the tibial component (*A, B*). The patient was revised to a Salto Talaris prosthesis with cancellous bone graft (*C, D, E*). The range of motion at 2 years following revision was adequate but not excellent, owing to significant stiffness of the ankle at the time of the revision procedure.

intraoperatively despite a stable radiographic appearance and, if found to be loose, should be revised. Therefore, a full set of implants including a wide array of different polyethylene sizes should always be available in the operating room during this procedure.

The cysts should be curettaged onto healthy bleeding bone and the contents of the cyst must be transported to the laboratory in 2 containers, 1 containing normal saline for cell count, microbial culture, and sensitivity, and 1 containing formalin for histology. Impaction grafting of the cyst can be done with either cancellous autograft taken from the iliac crest or proximal tibial metaphysis, lyophilized cancellous allograft, or a mixture of cancellous allograft mixed with demineralized bone matrix (DBM). Curettage of the cysts, impaction bone grafting, and exchange of the polyethylene liner is usually all that is needed in these ankles. Cysts that present or start to show progression at a later stage (more than 3 years) are most probably due to normal polyethylene wear. It is useful to carefully evaluate the polyethylene during the revision and check if there is any abnormal wear pattern. If this is present, a revision of the polyethylene will not be enough to manage the cyst, because ankle instability or mechanical malalignment will be present. It should be noted that isolated polyethylene exchange is not so easy with the semiconstrained implants such as the Agility or the Salto, compared with the mobile-bearing 3-component implants. The earlier Agility tibial components had a bottom-loading mechanism of insertion of the polyethylene, which made isolated polyethylene exchange impossible without revision of the tibial and/or the talar component.

MANAGING THE DISTAL TIBIA

The biggest concern when revising the distal tibia is the amount and quality of the remaining bone stock. Reasons for bone loss are overresection during the primary procedure, loosening and subsidence of the tibial component, osteolysis and cyst formation, bone loss during implant removal, or previous infection. Revision of the infected tibial implant falls outside the scope of this article and is not discussed here. If good medial and lateral bone support and a good-quality bleeding cancellous bone base of more than 50% is available after bone cuts and debridement, standard tibial components can be used.[2] If bone loss is minimal, reimplantation with a component from the same design can be used. A thicker polyethylene insert must be used to compensate for the loss of tibial height. In cases that still fulfill the criteria for standard component revision, but with more extensive bone loss, a standard component with a larger bone implant surface area is applicable. The Agility tibial component uses both the medial and lateral malleoli for its press-fit implantation. Stable fixation of the distal tibiofibular joint with bony arthrodesis is necessary for implant stability. If structural stability in the distal tibia is severely compromised because of massive cyst formation or osteolysis, revision with a custom-made tibial component should be considered. One of the advantages of the custom prosthesis is that the base plate can be built up to compensate for irregular distal tibial bone loss. A peg or keel of varying shape, size, and length can be designed to fit snugly in the healthy distal diaphysis/metaphysis and can thereby increase initial stability to allow for bony ingrowth. Multiple holes for locking screws can be added to the design, which may also improve initial stability. The main disadvantage with the custom tibia remains the cost implication associated with custom implants. Other concerns are the intraoperative lack of modularity, the large anterior tibial bone window that has to be made for implantation of certain designs, and the surgical skill associated with implantation using nonstandard instrumentation.

A possible alternative for the custom prosthesis may be the standard INBONE prosthesis from Wright Medical (Arlington, TN).[34] This prosthesis has been available for clinical use in the United States since 2005, and is the only system that uses intramedullary referencing and intramedullary fixation with a long modular tibial stem. The authors have no personal experience with this implant; however, the sturdy intramedullary stem may provide stable fixation of the tibial component while bone graft of distal tibial defects incorporate. The most important apparent benefit is that the tibial stem is inserted through the base of the distal tibia without the need for an anterior tibial bone window. DeVries and colleagues[35] reviewed 5 patients with failed Agility TAR who were treated with revision surgery using the INBONE system. All 5 patients showed signs of implant migration during early follow-up. At last follow-up (range 7–25 months) 3 patients had signs of bony ingrowth with no signs of cyst formation or progression. Two patients had failure of revision due to deep infection. One had a transtibial amputation and the other a TTC fusion. No real conclusions can be made from this small group of patients with relative short follow-up. However, this is an interesting alternative to custom implant replacement, and further research should be encouraged (**Fig. 4**).

How does one fill the defect? If there is gross cystic change in the talus it can be filled, even if it includes the subtalar joint, because the graft is contained. However, this is not so with the tibia, because many of these cysts communicate with the joint surface, and graft will fall into the joint and may not support the load of the prosthesis. Can one use cement, large structural grafts, or even cages, or should one stick to well-tried procedures such as impaction cancellous bone grafting?

It is important to fill all bone defects under the weight-bearing surface of the tibial base plate with impaction bone grafting; this is necessary for bony ingrowth to be able to take place over the entire surface area of the implant-bone interface. Over time, as the graft consolidates, it will also provide structural support. For smaller defects the authors prefer cancellous autograft that can be taken either from the iliac

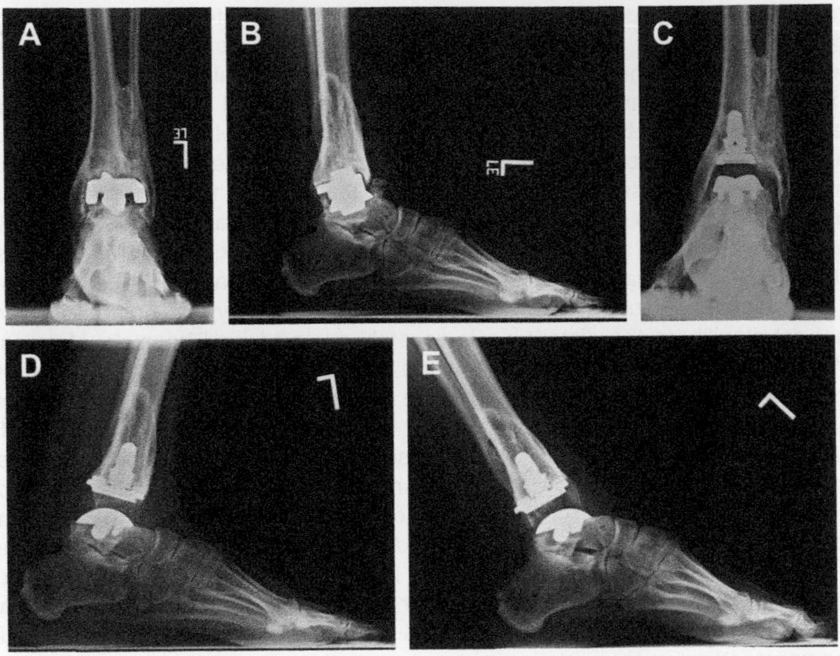

Fig. 4. Failure of Agility replacement (*A, B*). Revision to INBONE prosthesis with good postoperative range of motion (*C, D, E*). (*Courtesy of* Dr Steven Haddad.)

crest or from the proximal tibial metaphysis. Large defects can be filled with a combination of cancellous allograft and DBM.[2] Contained defects and irregularities of the distal tibia should be impacted with bone graft before insertion of the tibial component, which will create a smooth sturdy surface to accommodate the tibial component. Moreover, it is impossible to reach deep cysts and properly impact the graft once the tibial component is inserted. The authors do this using a standard anterior ankle approach after all other joint preparation has been completed. A very wide osteotome, corresponding with the width of the distal tibia, is inserted from anterior to posterior, resting on the posterior capsule. Bone graft, either cancellous autograft or cancellous allograft mixed with DBM, is inserted into the distal tibia from the distal surface. Combining the allograft with DBM makes it malleable and sticky, which helps prevent it from falling into the joint and becoming loose bodies. The osteotome is now hinged upwards around a point of rotation posterior to the distal tibia to impact the graft into the distal tibia. This process is repeated until a firm, flat surface is created on the distal tibia. It would be prudent to follow this step with insertion of the distal tibial component, but unfortunately most systems currently in use have the talar component inserted first with the tibial component subsequent to it. Care should be taken not to disturb the impaction graft during talar component insertion. The metal base plate of the tibial component must cover the entire area of impaction grafting to prevent the graft from entering the joint and becoming loose bodies. Remaining gaps between the implant and the bone as well as the anterior slot accommodating the insertion of a keel or peg should now be sealed and filled with the remainder of the graft. This action should prevent wear particles from accumulating along the implant-bone interface and should reduce cyst formation.[29]

Large defects involving the distal cortical rim could potentially be grafted with well-contoured structural fresh frozen allograft. The use of structural fresh frozen allograft in the foot and ankle has been well described, with good results.[36] However, no literature regarding the use of this type of graft for TAR augmentation could be found.

The spectacular failure of the earlier cemented TAR implants[37] is a stark reminder of the limited use of cement in modern TAR. The successful use of cement to fill small cystic lesions (less than 5 mm) in revision TKR has been well described.[38] However, taking into consideration the small surface area of the distal tibia and the fact that cement prevents bone ingrowth and remodeling, the use of cement in the distal tibia should be discouraged. The only vague indication during revision might be the use of cement around the peg, fin, or stem of the tibial implant in a very low-demand patient with poor-quality bone that needs to be able to weight bear early on (eg, rheumatoid arthritis).[2] Paucity of the literature on the use of cement in revision TAR is noted.

Highly porous tantalum metal has been used to fill tibial and femoral metaphyseal bone defects as an alternative to structural allograft in revision TKR, with good success, although follow-up is still short. Tantalum has a low stiffness (similar to that of bone), is biocompatible and corrosion resistant, and its high porosity enhances bone ingrowth. It does not lose structural integrity over time. The coarse surface enhances initial stability with a press fit. Tantalum can be manufactured in a wide array of shapes and sizes, which make it very modular.[38] Henricson and Rydholm[39] described ankle arthrodesis with a trabecular metal cone (TM Cone; Zimmer, Warsaw, IN), locked intramedullary fixation, and allograft or autograft in 13 patients with failed TAR. At mean follow-up of 1.4 years no nonunion was noted on radiographs and complete or good pain relief was achieved in 12 patients. These implants may have a role to play in revision TAR with bone loss, but to the authors' knowledge this has not been described.

MANAGING THE TALUS

If a failed talar component is to be revised, 3 surgical options exist: revision with a standard component of the same design, revision with a standard component of a different design, or revision with a custom-made stemmed prosthesis. When deciding on which implant to use, the factors that should be considered are patient factors (obesity, osteopenia, level of activity), level of subsidence, osteolysis or cyst formation, and symptomatic subtalar joint arthritis.

Standard weight-bearing radiographs can be used to assess radiographic signs of loosening (5° or 5 mm change), the level of subsidence, and arthritic changes in the subtalar joint. Ellington and Myerson[40] developed a radiographic grading system for subsidence that guides treatment and correlates with outcome following revision TAR. Grade 1 is no subsidence, grade 2 is subsidence but not to the level of the subtalar joint, and grade 3 is subsidence to the level of the subtalar joint or below. These investigators found that ankles with grade 1 subsidence could be revised using standard talar components and a standard technique, but ankles of grades 2 and 3 needed a long stem implant with fixation across the subtalar joint. The outcome after revision for grade-1 ankles was significantly better than for grades 2 or 3. A preoperative helical CT scan with metal artifact–limiting protocol and narrow cuts is necessary to evaluate lysis and cyst formation in the talus that may be obscured by the talar implant. It is also useful to assess the subtalar joint for signs of arthritis.

Patients with failure of a talar component who are overweight, more active, or have poor bone quality have a very high risk of recurrent failure with revision using standard implants. A custom talar component with a long stem is indicated for revision in these patients. Patients with limited ROM and pain in the subtalar joint and radiographic evidence of subtalar joint arthritis will need a subtalar arthrodesis in conjunction with the revision procedure. Joint preparation can be done through a separate sinus tarsi incision with standard screw fixation and a standard talar component revision. However, if doubt exists regarding the quality of the remaining talar bone for implant fixation, the presence of subtalar joint arthritis will tilt the scale toward a custom stemmed prosthesis. The long stem into the body of the calcaneus also gives added stability in cases where associated calcaneal osteotomies or triple arthrodesis are performed.

Revision with a standard component of the same design is preferable in cases where the tibial component is well incorporated and in a good position. Some systems (Salto, Agility) allow for mismatching of the talar and tibial component sizes, which makes it possible to put in a larger talar component to compensate for bone loss and ensure the biggest distribution of weight on the remaining talus as possible, without having to adjust the tibial component. However, this can only be done in grade 1 and early grade 2 subsidence if the talar component from the system in use will be able to achieve a cortical rim fit, and perfect apposition of the undersurface of the component on the remaining talus can be obtained. Decreased talar height caused by bone loss can be compensated for with a thicker polyethylene insert after proper coronal balancing.[40] Small cysts should be curettaged onto healthy bleeding bone and filled with cancellous bone graft before placement of the talar component.

Revision with a standard talar component from a different design is mainly indicated in 2 scenarios: where subsidence or osteolysis have weakened the structural integrity of the talus to the extent that stable fixation with an implant from the system in use would not be possible, or where the tibial component has to be revised to another system because of bone loss. A case report by Kharwadkar and Harris[41] of 2 STAR prostheses whereby only the subsided tibial components were revised to revision AES implants shows that some interchangeability between certain 3-component mobile-bearing systems does exist. Hintermann and colleagues[42] found components with a flat undersurface to work better in revision surgery. The HINTEGRA system provides a revision talar component with a flat undersurface.[17] The Agility talar component also has a flat undersurface with a short peg and a medial and lateral wing to maximize load distribution to the talar body.[43] The Agility was the standard implant of choice in Ellington and Myerson's[40] series on TAR revisions. The talar component of the INBONE system has a porous coated flat undersurface with a wide talar base and a short (10 mm) or long (14 mm) stem.[34,35] Despite these features, DeVries and colleagues[35] found implant subsidence in all 3 surviving implants.

An alternative option for failure of a talar component associated with subsidence or significant lysis is an ankle or TTC fusion, often using a structural bone graft.[44,45] However, this is a salvage procedure and the associated hindfoot stiffness causes obvious functional limitations for the patient.[40] The bone loss attributable to the original bone cuts, osteolysis, subsidence, or implant extraction may create enormous defects that are challenging to adequately fill with structural bone graft. Fixation is mostly done with retrograde intramedullary nailing, but ankle or TTC arthrodesis following failed TAR has a less predictable union rate when compared with primary arthrodesis, especially in patients with rheumatoid arthritis.[44,45]

The development of a talar component with a long stem for stable fixation in healthy calcaneal bone together with metal augmentation at the base to compensate for talar bone loss created a surgical alternative for the failed TAR with a structurally insufficient talus. The unique anatomy of the talus (absence of a shaft) makes intramedullary fixation impossible. If the structural integrity of the strong cortical bone has been breached by subsidence or lysis, the only way to obtain initial stable fixation for bony ingrowth that can withstand the forces of human ambulation may be to cross the subtalar joint with a press-fit long stem. This procedure is always done in conjunction with a formal subtalar joint arthrodesis. In patients with a normal subtalar joint, some hindfoot motion will be lost to benefit superior fixation of the talar component and improved ankle joint function. When patients reach the stage where revision of a failed TAR is being considered, the subtalar joint is often no longer normal, perhaps resulting from abnormal ankle and hindfoot biomechanics before the index TAR or during the phase of TAR failure. If the subtalar joint is painful, the arthrodesis will address the pain and if it is stiff, no worsening in function should be noted. Ankles with grade-3 subsidence cannot be treated surgically without incorporating the subtalar joint.

The custom prosthesis has some unique features. The implant dimensions and stem angles are precisely determined for each patient using radiographs and CT with standardized radiographic template markers in the AP and lateral views. Implant templates are than sent back to the surgeon for verification before the go-ahead is given for production of the final implant. Custom instrumentation is also produced, for example, a cannulated custom talar dome for correct placement of the guide pin in the calcaneus, custom cannulated reamers, and a custom stemmed trial talar component. Different sizes of polyethylene should be available intraoperatively to allow for some adjustments to the soft-tissue tension because the custom metal implants have predetermined sizes. Because of the variable amount of bone loss, it is often difficult to accurately reconstruct the anatomic joint level, which may decrease the effective ROM. The custom prosthesis is inserted through a standard anterior ankle approach, most often through the previous scar. Patients should be counseled regarding possible sensory deficits in the superficial and deep peroneal nerve distributions, because these nerves are commonly trapped in the old scar tissue. For revision with a custom long stem talus, a formal subtalar arthrodesis must be performed through a separate 2-cm sinus tarsi approach, using sharp osteotomes to denude the remaining cartilage and a 2-mm drill to perforate the subchondral bone of the inferior talus and superior calcaneus. A single 4.0-mm cannulated screw is placed from the dorsum of the talus, anterior to the position of the talar implant, in a plantar posterior direction into the calcaneus, for good compression. The rest of the subtalar joint stability is obtained from the talar stem. If the primary tibial component is from the same design and well fixed, only the polyethylene liner needs revision. If it is from a different design but no excessive bone loss is evident, it can be replaced with a standard tibial component from the designers of the custom talus. If it fulfills the criteria for a custom prosthesis, both the talus and tibia are replaced with custom prostheses. The standard principles regarding bone graft augmentation, as discussed earlier, applies (**Fig. 5**).

Ellington and Myerson[40] reviewed 53 patients with revision TAR and a minimum follow-up of 2 years. All were revised to another implant, either standard Agility or custom prosthesis from Agility, by the principal author (Myerson). Of the 34 patients who met the inclusion criteria, 17 had a custom talar component inserted. The most common reason for revision in all patients was talar subsidence. Despite poor improvement in postoperative radiographic position of the implants, good improvement in pain and function was noted. Seventy-four percent had good or excellent outcome with 79% back at previous employment duties at final follow-up; 85% would have agreed to have the surgery again. It was concluded that revision is a viable alternative for arthrodesis following failure of a TAR.

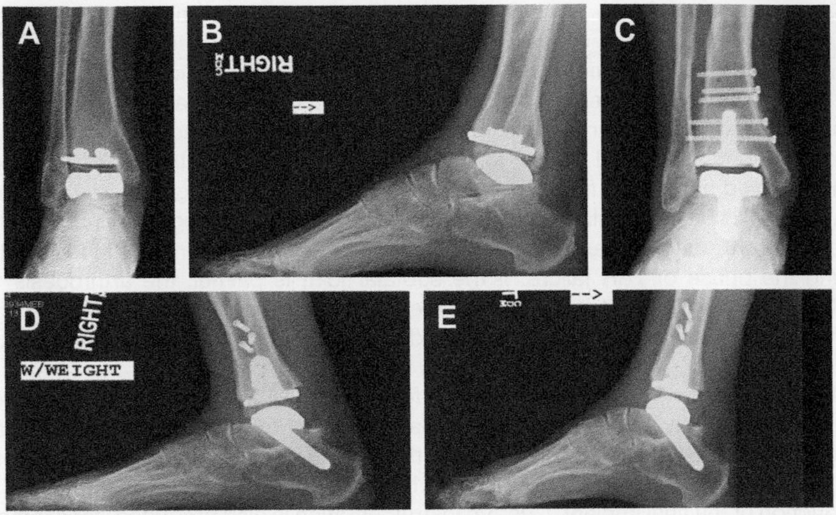

Fig. 5. Preoperatively the patient presented with findings and symptoms of a loose prosthesis, subsidence, and very limited range of motion of the ankle (*A*, *B*). The patient was revised to a long-stem patient-customized Salto prosthesis. (*C*, *D*, *E*) Anteroposterior view, and lateral flexion and extension views 6 months following revision. Note the screws in the distal tibia, inserted to stabilize a crack in the tibia that occurred during insertion of the tibial component.

SUMMARY

When faced with severe prosthesis failure, loosening, and subsidence, the options are limited to a patient-customized device, a large structural bone graft arthrodesis, or an amputation. The structural bone graft arthrodesis does not have a predictable outcome, and a poor rate of arthrodesis at best. Fortunately patient-customized devices can still be used for the ankle, although owing to recent restrictions imposed on industry, currently the only manufacturer of these implants in the United States is Tornier, these being based on the Salto Talaris 2-part component system.

REFERENCES

1. Gougoulias NE, Khanna A, Maffulli N. History and evolution in total ankle arthroplasty. Br Med Bull 2009;89:111–51.
2. Myerson MS, Won HY. Primary and revision total ankle replacement using custom-designed prostheses. Foot Ankle Clin 2008;13(3):521–38.
3. Labek G, Thaler M, Janda W, et al. Revision rates after total joint replacement: cumulative results from worldwide joint register datasets. J Bone Joint Surg Br 2011;93(3):293–7.
4. Henricson A, Carlsson A, Rydholm U. What is a revision of total ankle replacement? Foot Ankle Surg 2011;17(3):99–102.
5. Barg A, Knupp M, Anderson AE, et al. Total ankle replacement in obese patients: component stability, weight change, and functional outcome in 118 consecutive patients. Foot Ankle Int 2011;32(10):925–32.
6. Henricson A, Nilsson JÅ, Carlsson A. 10-year survival of total ankle arthroplasties: a report on 780 cases from the Swedish Ankle Register. Acta Orthop 2011;82(6):655–9.

7. Wood PL, Sutton C, Mishra V, et al. A randomised, controlled trial of two mobile-bearing total ankle replacements. J Bone Joint Surg Br 2009;91(1):69–74.
8. Gougoulias N, Khanna A, Maffulli N. How successful are current ankle replacements?: a systematic review of the literature. Clin Orthop Relat Res 2010; 468(1):199–208.
9. Anderson T, Montgomery F, Carlsson A. Uncemented STAR total ankle prostheses. J Bone Joint Surg Am 2004;86(Suppl Pt 2):103–11.
10. Henricson A, Ågren PH. Secondary surgery after total ankle replacement. Foot Ankle Surg 2007;13(1):41–4.
11. Glazebrook M, Arsenault K, Dunbar M. Evidence-based classification of complications in total ankle arthroplasty. Foot Ankle Int 2009;30(10):945–9.
12. Kim BS, Lee JW. Total ankle replacement for the varus unstable osteoarthritic ankle. Tech Foot Ankle Surg 2010;9(4):157–64.
13. Trincat S, Kouyoumdjian P, Asencio G. Total ankle arthroplasty and coronal plane deformities. Orthop Traumatol Surg Res 2012;98(1):75–84.
14. Vaupel Z, Baker E, Baker KC, et al. Analysis of retrieved agility total ankle arthroplasty systems. Foot Ankle Int 2009;30(9):815–23.
15. Bartel DL, Bicknell MS, Wright TM. The effect of conformity, total thickness, weight material on for stresses in ultra-high molecular components replacement. J Bone Joint Surg 1986;68(7):1041–51.
16. Kobayashi A, Minoda Y, Kadoya Y, et al. Ankle arthroplasties generate wear particles similar to knee arthroplasties. Clin Orthop Relat Res 2004;424(424):69–72.
17. Younger A, Penner M, Wing K. Mobile-bearing total ankle arthroplasty. Foot Ankle Clin 2008;13(3):495–508.
18. Spirt A, Assal M, Hansen ST. Complications and failure after total ankle arthroplasty. J Bone Joint Surg Am 2004;86(6):1172–8.
19. Kotnis R, Pasapula C, Anwar F, et al. The management of failed ankle replacement. J Bone Joint Surg 2006;88(8):1039–47.
20. Ferrao P, Myerson MS, Schuberth JM, et al. Cement spacer as definitive management for postoperative ankle infection. Foot Ankle Int 2012;33(3):173–8.
21. Pagenstert G, Horisberger M, Leumann AG, et al. Distinctive pain course during first year after total ankle arthroplasty: a prospective, observational study. Foot Ankle Int 2011;32(2):113–9.
22. Krause FG, Windolf M, Bora B, et al. Impact of complications in total ankle replacement and ankle arthrodesis analyzed with a validated outcome measurement. J Bone Joint Surg Am 2011;93(9):830–9.
23. Kurup HV, Taylor GR. Medial impingement after ankle replacement. Int Orthop 2008;32(2):243–6.
24. Hanna RS, Haddad SL, Lazarus ML. Evaluation of periprosthetic lucency after total ankle arthroplasty: helical CT versus conventional radiography. Foot Ankle Int 2007;28(8):921–6.
25. Brodsky JW, Polo FE, Coleman SC, et al. Changes in gait following the Scandinavian total ankle replacement. J Bone Joint Surg Am 2011;93(20):1890–6.
26. Sealey RJ, Myerson MS, Molloy A, et al. Sagittal plane motion of the hindfoot following ankle arthrodesis: a prospective analysis. Foot Ankle Int 2009;30(3): 187–96.
27. Haddad SL, Coetzee JC, Estok R, et al. Intermediate and long-term outcomes of total ankle arthroplasty and ankle arthrodesis. A systematic review of the literature. J Bone Joint Surg Am 2007;89(9):1899–905.
28. Valderrabano V, Hintermann B, Dick W. Scandinavian total ankle replacement. Clin Orthop Relat Res 2004;424:47–56.

29. Bonnin M, Gaudot F, Laurent J-R, et al. The Salto total ankle arthroplasty: survivorship and analysis of failures at 7 to 11 years. Clin Orthop Relat Res 2011;469(1):225–36.
30. Nunley JA, Caputo AM, Easley ME, et al. Intermediate to long-term outcomes of the STAR total ankle replacement: the patient perspective. J Bone Joint Surg Am 2012;94(1):43–8.
31. Cui Q, Milbrandt T, Millington S, et al. Treatment of posttraumatic adhesive capsulitis of the ankle: a case series. Foot Ankle Int 2005;26(8):602–6.
32. Rodriguez D, Bevernage BD, Maldague P, et al. Medium term follow-up of the AES ankle prosthesis: high rate of asymptomatic osteolysis. Foot Ankle Surg 2010;16(2):54–60.
33. Pyevich MT, Saltzman CL, Callaghan JJ, et al. Total ankle arthroplasty: a unique design. J Bone Joint Surg 1998;80(10):1410–20.
34. Unknown author. INBONE® total ankle replacement by Wright Medical Technology, Inc. Available at: http://www.inbone.com/DesignRationale.aspx. Accessed April 5, 2012.
35. DeVries JG, Berlet GC, Lee TH, et al. Revision total ankle replacement: an early look at agility to INBONE. Foot Ankle Spec 2011;4(4):235–44.
36. Myerson MS, Neufeld SK, Uribe J. Fresh-frozen structural allografts in the foot and ankle. J Bone Joint Surg Am 2005;87(1):113–20.
37. Bonasia DE, Dettoni F, Femino JE, et al. Total ankle replacement: why, when and how? Iowa Orthop J 2010;30:119–30.
38. Poultsides LA, Sculco TP. Bone loss management in revision total knee replacement. Tech Orthop 2011;26(2):84–93.
39. Henricson A, Rydholm U. Use of a trabecular metal implant in ankle arthrodesis after failed total ankle replacement. Acta Orthop 2010;81(6):745–7.
40. Ellington K, Myerson MS. Outcomes of revision TAR. J Bone Joint Surg Am, in press.
41. Kharwadkar N, Harris NJ. Revision of STAR total ankle replacement to hybrid AES-STAR total ankle replacement—a report of two cases. Foot Ankle Surg 2009;15(2):101–5.
42. Hintermann B, Barg A, Knupp M. Revision arthroplasty of the ankle joint. Der Orthopäde 2011;40(11):1000–7 [in German].
43. Cerrato R, Myerson MS. Total ankle replacement: the agility LP prosthesis. Foot Ankle Clin 2008;13(3):485–94.
44. Hopgood P, Kumar R, Wood PL. Ankle arthrodesis for failed total ankle replacement. J Bone Joint Surg Br 2006;88(8):1032–8.
45. Culpan P, Le Strat V, Piriou P, et al. Arthrodesis after failed total ankle replacement. J Bone Joint Surg Br 2007;89(9):1178–83.

Management of Specific Complications Related to Total Ankle Arthroplasty

Pascal F. Rippstein, MD*, Martin Huber, MD, Florian D. Naal, MD

KEYWORDS

• Total ankle arthroplasty • Total ankle replacement • Complications • Prosthesis

KEY POINTS

- Total ankle arthroplasty (TAA) has evolved over time, and modern 3-component implants offer good and reliable clinical results.
- When discussing complications after TAA, one should always remember that for most cases ankle fusion is a valuable alternative to TAA revision.
- The incidence of intraoperative complications is significantly associated with the experience of the treating surgeon, and beginning with TAA includes an obvious learning curve.[1–4]

INTRODUCTION

Total ankle arthroplasty (TAA) has been introduced in the 1970s as an alternative to ankle fusion for the treatment of end-stage ankle osteoarthritis (OA).[5] Although very high failure rates using first-generation prostheses have been observed, modern 3-component implants have demonstrated favorable clinical results and improved survivorship as reported in different case series.[1,6–14] Despite these improvements, TAA is still associated with a higher rate of revisions and complications when compared with total hip or knee arthroplasty.[15] One reason might be that ankle arthritis is by far less frequent than hip or knee OA; hence, the global number of TAAs implanted is comparatively low, resulting in limited experience of treating surgeons.[16] Hence, results reported by specialized centers should be analyzed carefully considering that these results are in general better than those based on registry data.[17] Furthermore, ankle fusion is still an excellent alternative to TAA that is not associated with the well-known limitations in function and activities of daily living after a hip or knee arthrodesis. Some complications seen in the clinical practice are specific to

Department of Foot and Ankle Surgery, Schulthess Klinik, Lengghalde 2, Zurich 8008, Switzerland
* Corresponding author.
E-mail address: pascal.rippstein@kws.ch

Foot Ankle Clin N Am 17 (2012) 707–717
http://dx.doi.org/10.1016/j.fcl.2012.08.010
1083-7515/12/$ – see front matter

the type of implant used, but most complications are common to all TAA designs currently available. The number of different designs available today highlights that a universal, ideal TAA does not yet exist and that considerable improvements still need to be achieved. It is not the intention of this contribution to point out specific design-related problems but to discuss the management of classic general complications that might occur with any implant used.

PRINCIPLES

When discussing complications after TAA, one should always remember that for most cases ankle fusion is a valuable alternative to TAA revision. On the one hand, multiple revision surgeries may make a final ankle fusion technically more difficult; on the other hand, patients might subjectively develop chronic pain, even if the last revision is considered successful from an objective point of view. Therefore, some considerations should be carefully made if the intention is to perform a revision preserving the TAA.

First, the complication must be correctly identified and well understood. A clear treatment solution should then exist that has a reasonable chance of success and that is as minimally invasive as possible at the same time. If the chance of success is considered only low or fair and/or if the revision will be more invasive than an ankle fusion, then one should have really good reasons to decide preserving the TAA. One such argument might be the presence of severe concomitant arthritis of other hind foot joints. Second, a TAA that has to be revised must still have a reasonable range of motion. A TAA without motion does not fulfill its primary function and is, therefore, not worthwhile to be preserved. In such cases, fusion might be the better option. Finally, patients must be well informed about ankle fusion as an alternative treatment option.

Specific Complications and Their Management

Intraoperative complications

The incidence of intraoperative complications is significantly associated with the experience of the treating surgeon, and beginning with TAA includes an obvious learning curve.[1–4] An incidence of up to 60% within the first cases has been reported.[2] Intraoperative complications are usually obvious and can be solved during the same surgery. The most classic intraoperative complications are the accidental cut of the lateral malleolus and the fracture of the medial malleolus.[1,4,18] Both need anatomic internal fixation allowing adhering to the routine postoperative protocol with early ankle mobilization. The lateral malleolus can be best fixed through a separate incision (plate and screws), whereas the medial malleolus can be easily fixed through the anterior approach used for the TAA (screws).

If situations such as unstable components on osteoporotic bone, insufficient bone stock for correct implant fixation, instable/nonanatomic fixation of fractured malleoli, ankle instability that cannot be corrected, or any other severe complication that cannot be addressed adequately are encountered during TAA surgery, TAA must be abandoned and an ankle fusion should be performed. At this stage, ankle fusion can be performed relatively easily because the bone stock is still available. An ankle fusion will always give a better result than a poorly implanted TAA. It is important to be prepared for such a change in the surgical plan and this must be, therefore, always preoperatively discussed with patients.

Soft tissue complications are rather rare.[1] The tibial nerve can be injured during the tibial resection, either directly by the saw blade or indirectly by the heat produced during the cut. This complication is typically noticed 1 to 2 days postoperatively. A proper electrophysiological examination is mandatory to determine if the nerve has been transected or if surgical repair is required. Flexor tendons can also be directly injured by the saw blade. Direct repair should be performed, using a separate posteromedial approach for this purpose.

Postoperative Complications

Delayed wound healing

Most TAAs are implanted through an anterior longitudinal approach. The ankle is a small joint and because of relatively big components, soft tissues are considerably stretched during surgery. Furthermore, mobilization of the ankle is usually initiated before soft tissue healing is completed, resulting in additional stress on the wound. To prevent wound dehiscence or skin necrosis, stress on the soft tissues should be reduced to a minimum during surgery. The authors recommend using a long incision, avoiding Hohmann retractors, releasing the tension on the soft tissues when not required, a careful hemostasis avoiding hematomas, and meticulously suturing the skin. A small wound dehiscence occurring during the early rehabilitation should be addressed by a secondary suture and previous debridement, if required. If larger skin areas become necrotic or dehiscent, or if tendons are exposed (tibialis anterior), covering by a musculo-cutaneus flap should be considered.

Postoperative loss of motion

A good intraoperative ankle motion can be lost during the first weeks following surgery.[1] To prevent this complication, the authors routinely apply a circular cast immediately at the end of the surgery before opening the tourniquet. This cast prevents postoperative swelling and the early equinus at the ankle that is difficult to correct during the first postoperative days because of pain and hematoma. After 7 to 10 days postoperatively, when swelling and pain are significantly decreased, the cast is removed and an aggressive early mobilization program is initiated. Best ankle motion can be achieved if such a rehabilitation program is performed intensively during the first 2 months following surgery. After 2 months, ankle motion cannot be significantly increased anymore, not by intensive physiotherapy or by open mobilization (adhesiolysis), which has always been disappointing in the authors' hands.

Stress fracture of the medial malleolus

Soft tissue tension is usually higher at the medial side if no extensive deltoid release has been performed during TAA. Ankle malalignment, particularly a residual varus deformity, might contribute to this tension imbalance. High medial tension can typically provoke a stress fracture of the medial malleolus (**Fig. 1**) that has been more or less weakened by the distal tibial cut required for implantation of the tibial component. Postoperative malleolar stress fractures may occur in 4% to 5%.[1] These stress fractures are usually only minimally displaced and can heal spontaneously. A fracture occurring more than 2 months postoperatively is best treated conservatively. If a fracture occurs within the first 2 months after TAA, it is best treated surgically. Without internal fixation, pain is produced during ankle mobilization and the intensity of the rehabilitation program needs to be reduced. As indicated before, this might result in poor final ankle motion. For this reason, the authors recommend percutaneous screw fixation for malleolar stress fractures when they occur during the early rehabilitation period.

Chronic anteromedial pain syndrome

Anteromedial ankle pain is a common finding after TAA. This pain is located in the anteromedial soft tissues, outside of the ankle joint itself, and can irradiate proximally

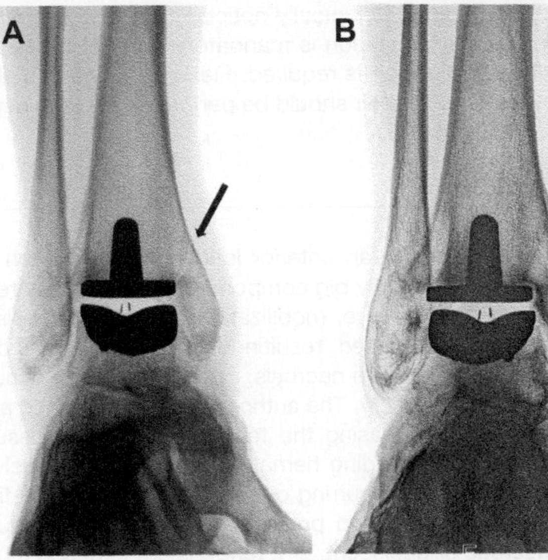

Fig. 1. (*A*) Stress fracture of the malleolus medialis (*arrow*) in a 63-year-old female patient 4 months after TAA. (*B*) Six months later, the stress fracture has spontaneously healed, leaving a small callus.

into the medial malleolus. Periosteal thickening can be sometimes observed radiographically. Clinically, the pain can constantly be provoked by direct palpation of the anteromedial soft tissues. Selective injections of local anesthesia into these soft tissues immediately relieve the pain, confirming its extra-articular location. This pain is also probably related to an increased medial soft tissue tension. The risk of such an anteromedial pain syndrome can be reduced by performing an extensive deltoid release during TAA. The authors now routinely perform such a release in all TAA cases and observe a decreased incidence of this source of pain. If patients present with an anteromedial pain syndrome after TAA, conservative treatment with steroid injections into the soft tissues should first be initiated. These infiltrations usually need to be repeated monthly 3 to 6 times to achieve definitive, long-lasting pain relief. Surgical release of the deltoid ligament is indicated when conservative treatment is not successful. The authors perform a deltoid release under ankle block anesthesia with a supramalleolar tourniquet. Through an anteromedial approach, the deep deltoid fibers are completely transected and the periost of the medial malleolus is detached from its tip proximally over a distance of 2 to 3 cm. Any scar tissue has to be removed. The release is sufficient when the ankle opens up symmetrically on the lateral and medial sides under axial distraction. If required, superficial deltoid fibers also have to be released. The authors have not observed any iatrogenic medial ankle instability, even when performing a very aggressive release.

Pain in the malleolar gutter

Arthritic changes are commonly observed in the malleolar joints, which are those parts of the ankle between the malleoli and the talus. Interestingly, malleolar joint OA is rarely painful. Load reduction and distraction of this part of the ankle after restoration of the joint line by TAA might explain this observation. For this reason, the malleolar joints do not need to be primarily debrided during TAA. Debridement of the malleolar gutter creates bleeding bony surfaces, potentially leading to painful new bone formation. In the authors' experience, painful malleolar joints are observed in less than 5% of all implanted TAAs. Patients report pain that is typically focal and subjectively located underneath the involved malleolus. In contrast to the anteromedial pain syndrome, this pain cannot be provoked by direct palpation. Treatment is always surgical. Under ankle block anesthesia and supramalleolar tourniquet, the malleolar gutters must be widely debrided, leaving a space of at least 5 mm between the malleolus and the talus (**Fig. 2**). The debrided bony surfaces should be sealed with bone wax to prevent new bone formation, which might lead to recurrent pain. The debridement sometimes has to be repeated after several years because bone can proliferate again within the gutter over time.

Painful osteophytes and ectopic bone

Osteophytes around an arthritic ankle are a very common observation preoperatively. When using the classic anterior approach, anterior osteophytes are automatically removed during TAA. Osteophytes at the tip of the malleoli (**Fig. 3**A) might be easily overseen and can lead to postoperative pain.[1] This pain is clearly localized, usually quite sharp, and can be temporarily eliminated with the injection of local anesthetics. Treatment is always surgical. The osteophytes can be removed through a small incision under ankle block anesthesia and a supramalleolar tourniquet (see **Fig. 3**B). Complete pain relief is achieved in most cases. Ectopic bone can also develop after TAA and lead to painful impingement with one or both TAA components, at the same time restricting more or less significantly ankle motion.[1,19,20] The diagnosis is made radiographically (plain radiographs or computed tomography [CT] scans), and the treatment is surgical. All ectopic bone has to be removed, and bony surfaces should be sealed by bone wax to prevent recurrence. In the authors' experience, there are some ankles that continuously produce a significant amount of diffuse ectopic bone around the TAA as if they want to end up in an ankle fusion at any price. In

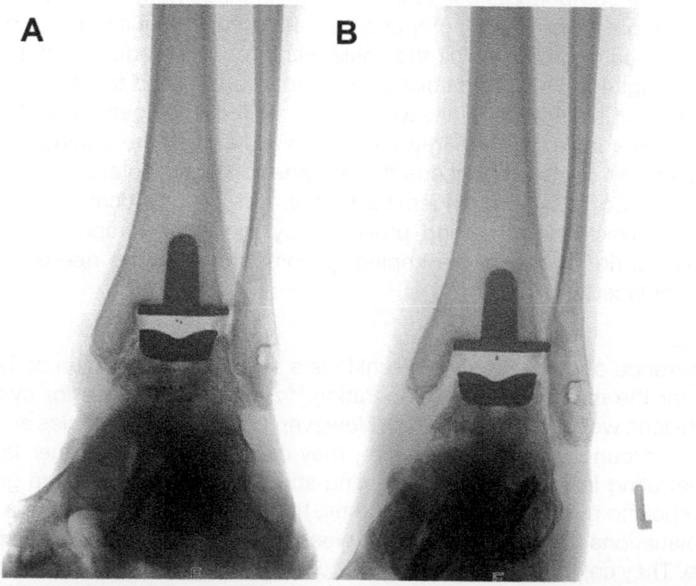

Fig. 2. (*A*) Painful medial malleolar gutter arthrosis 1 year after TAA in a 62-year-old female patient. (*B*) After wide debridement of the medial malleolar gutter, symptoms completely resolved after 6 weeks.

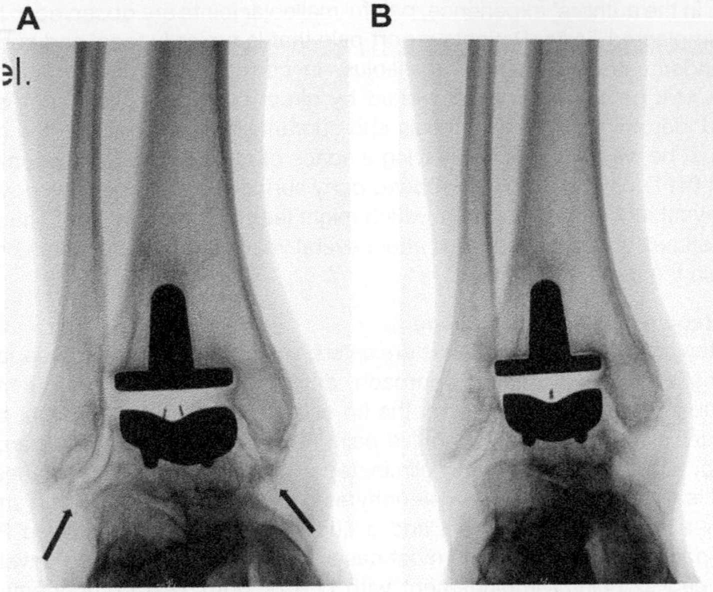

Fig. 3. (*A*) Typical painful osteophytes at the tip of both malleoli (*black arrows*) in a 52-year-old female patient. (*B*) After removal of the osteophytes, symptoms completely resolved.

such cases, removal of ectopic bone is not indicated and take down to fusion is the best option.

Impingement caused by oversized/incorrectly implanted components

Talar and tibial components can lead to painful impingement if they are oversized or incorrectly implanted.[21] Talar components usually impinge with one or both malleoli and lead to localized pain inside the ankle, either on the medial or lateral side or on both sides (**Fig. 4**A). Oversized tibial components usually lead to painful impingement with the fibula. Treatment is always surgical. If the impingement is limited, bone resection at the impingement area can be considered. If the impingement is more pronounced, the component needs to be repositioned or replaced by a smaller one (see **Fig. 4**B). Soft tissue impingement is rare. It is usually located posteromedially (tibial nerve, flexor tendons) and provoked by the tibial component. Soft tissues cannot be debrided; hence, the impinging component always needs to be repositioned or replaced.

Bone cysts

The occurrence of cysts around the ankle is a specific complication of TAA and can account for the main reason of reoperation.[22] The classic cause for cyst formation is polyethylene wear (**Fig. 5**A, **Fig. 6**A). However, polyethylene particles are not always found in or around the cysts; therefore, they can be caused by other factors. Joint fluid penetrating into the bone, preexisting subchondral cysts that are growing, and disease-specific cysts (rheumatoid arthritis, hemochromatosis) are some of the possible explanations for cysts that are not wear induced. Cysts are usually progressing over time. They can remain asymptomatic for a very long period and produce pain only when they have collapsed. Such a collapse can lead to subsidence of the TAA. Once a certain size has been achieved, some cysts become symptomatic without any evidence of collapse, which may be because of pressure changes within the cyst itself

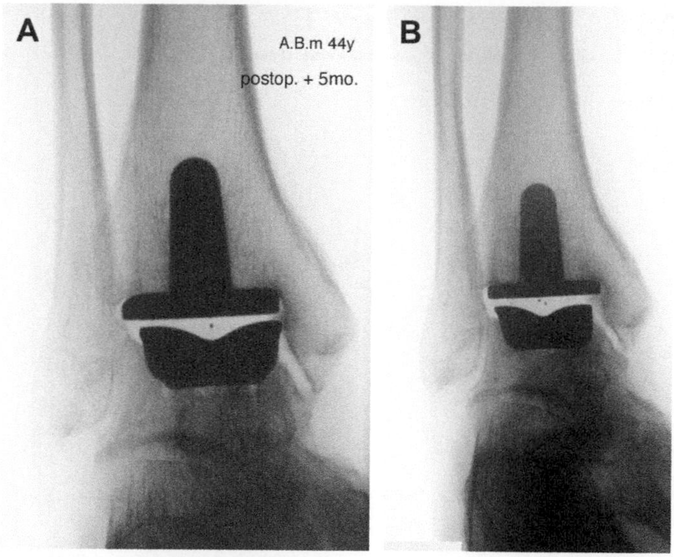

Fig. 4. (*A*) Oversized talar component with painful medial impingement in a 44-year-old male patient 5 months after TAA. (*B*) The talar component has been downsized and the symptoms completely resolved.

(joint fluid). Smaller asymptomatic cysts usually do not require treatment; however, regular radiographic follow-up (twice during the first year of occurrence and then yearly) is recommended. CT scans might be useful to determine the exact size and location. If cysts achieve a critical size that could lead to TAA subsidence, fracture of bone, or induce pain, then surgical revision is indicated. Cysts are curetted and filled with autologous cancellous bone. The polyethylene inlay should also be exchanged. If any reason for early polyethylene abrasion has been identified (eg, tibial or talar malalignment leading to edge loading), then this underlying problem must be addressed at the same time (see **Fig. 5**A–C). If multiple cysts around a TAA occur, treatment is

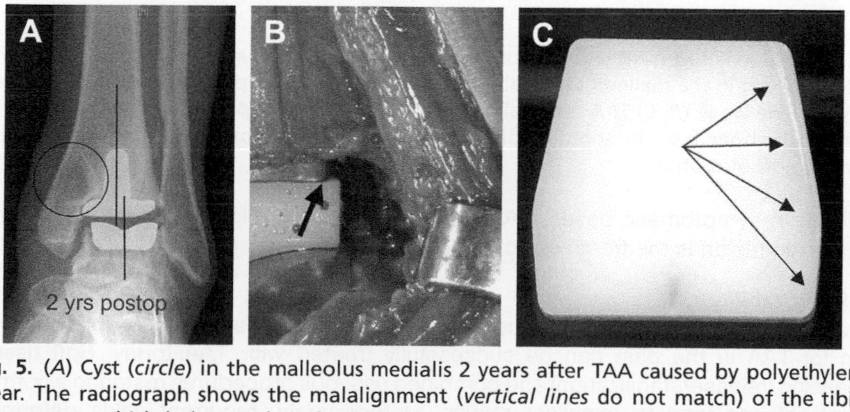

Fig. 5. (*A*) Cyst (*circle*) in the malleolus medialis 2 years after TAA caused by polyethylene wear. The radiograph shows the malalignment (*vertical lines* do not match) of the tibial component, which led to early polyethylene wear (*edge loading*). (*B*) Intraoperative view indicating polyethylene edge loading (*black arrow*) caused by malalignment of the tibial component. (*C*) Polyethylene with very early macroscopic wear (step, *black arrows*) on the medial side related to edge loading.

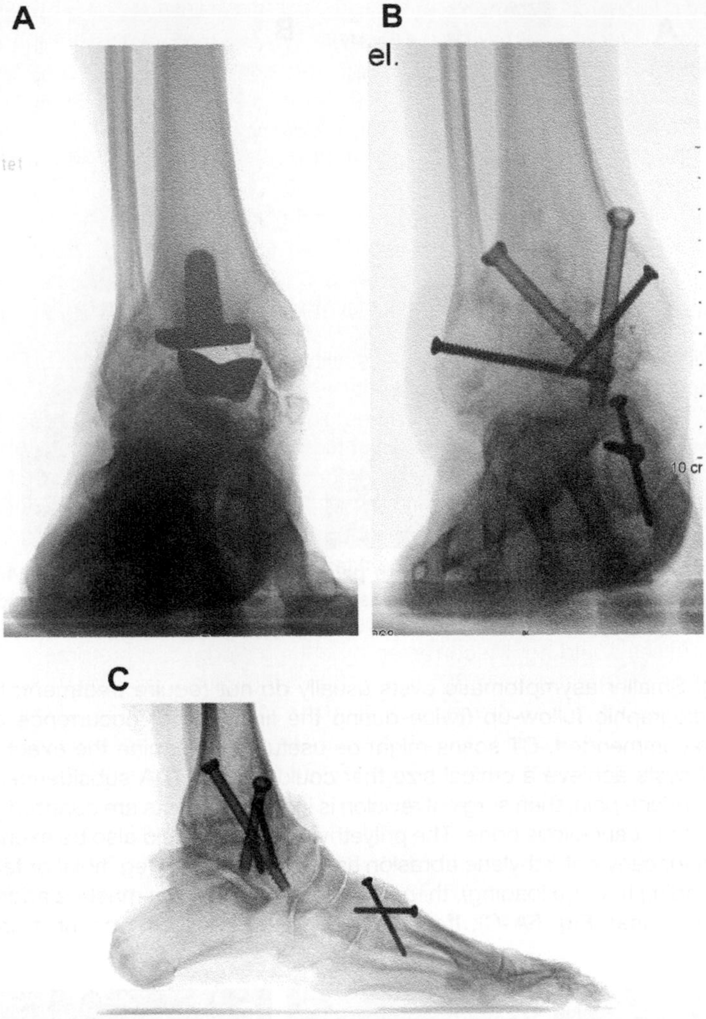

Fig. 6. (*A*) Slowly recurrent varus deformity 3 years after TAA in a 57-year-old male patient. Notice the cyst in the malleolus medialis, which obviously developed because of accelerated polyethylene wear. (*B*, *C*) TAA removal and ankle fusion 2 years postoperatively. Because of limited talar bone loss, the subtalar joint could be preserved, providing important compensatory hindfoot motion.

difficult. In symptomatic cases, TAA-preserving surgery might not be possible and then ankle fusion is the treatment of choice.

Ankle instability

Severe ankle varus/valgus deformities that have been considered to be a contraindication for TAA in the past can be successfully treated with TAA today. Soft tissue balancing (release/stabilization) and combined osseous procedures restoring a normal alignment can lead to excellent results. Unfortunately, recurrent ankle deformity remains a potential risk, especially for valgus deformities.[1,20] Recurrent ankle deformities can be treated by different means (change of one or both components, soft tissue procedures for stabilization, realignment of the foot); but in the authors' experience, a successful outcome is less predictable. One should, therefore, have good reasons to decide to revise an unstable TAA instead of performing an ankle fusion (see **Fig. 6**A–C). Patients with rheumatoid arthritis represent a special entity regarding ankle deformities.[23] Valgus and varus deformities are more frequently observed in this group of patients. The poor quality of the soft tissues is probably the reason for the higher incidence of recurrence after TAA implantation. In the authors' series of 233 consecutively implanted TAAs (Mobility TAR System, DePuy, Leeds, England), they observed 8 recurrent deformities and a new deformity developing in another case.[1] Out of these 9 patients, 8 had rheumatoid arthritis. These recurrent deformities were mostly asymptomatic (mean Visual Analogue Scale [VAS] 0.8, range 0–2.5), and only 1 patient complained about significant pain (VAS 7).[1]

Component loosening

Component loosening is a classic complication after any type of joint replacement and also after TAA. Loosening is either aseptic (wear, mechanical reasons) or caused by low-grade infection and accounts for a considerable number of TAA revisions.[24,25] The diagnosis of TAA loosening can be difficult. Radiolucencies at the bone-component interface are frequently observed in patients with asymptomatic TAA and can, therefore, not be used as a reliable criterion to determine if a component is definitely loose or not.[1,26–28] Bone scintigraphy frequently remains positive for a longer period of time in well-integrated TAAs and is, therefore, also not a reliable criterion. Single-photon emission CT might give additional diagnostic information (ie, to distinguish a component loosening from arthrosis in the malleolar joints or from a component impingement). Biologic markers can probably support the hypothesis of a loosening caused by low-grade infection, but the sensitivity and specificity of these diagnostic tools are still rather low. The diagnosis of symptomatic component loosening is, therefore, essentially based on the history of the patient reporting about diffuse pain deep inside the ankle, provoked on weight bearing and motion, and after the exclusion of other factors as a source of pain. Because of the lack of reliable criteria for confirming the suspicion of a TAA loosening, the decision to revise the TAA can be difficult to make. Loose components can be successfully exchanged. If a low-grade infection is suspected, the diagnosis can only be definitively confirmed postoperatively, after microbiologic culture of tissue samples. TAA revision can be performed either in one operation or in a staged procedure.

Acute infection

Acute infection occurring during the first 6 weeks postoperatively is associated with *Staphylococcus aureus* in most cases. Acutely infected TAAs should be rapidly addressed by open revision, extensive debridement, irrigation, and polyethylene exchange. Repeated arthroscopic irrigation might be an alternative. The authors successfully treated 4 cases with acute infection by early arthroscopic irrigation without polyethylene exchange. Antibiotic therapy has to be immediately started and adapted as soon as the responsible germ has been identified. The authors recommend intravenous antibiotic administration for 3 weeks followed by a period of 4 to 6 months of oral therapy. If acutely infected TAAs are rapidly and adequately treated, component removal is not imperatively necessary and the incidence of infection recurrence is very low. None of the acutely infected TAAs treated in the authors' department required component removal.

Component subsidence/migration

Component subsidence can occur early or late. Early subsidence is usually related to osteoporotic bone that does not provide sufficient support for the implanted components, which is the talar component in most cases.[24,25] Late subsidence is caused by cyst formation underneath the components or to progressive avascular bone necrosis. Depending on the degree of subsidence, observation and regular radiographic follow-ups or surgical revision can be considered. If surgical revision is indicated, it depends on the remaining bone stock if salvage will consist of TAA exchange or ankle fusion. Cases with poor bone stock are better treated by fusion, often requiring bone grafts. The bone graft of choice is the iliac crest, which allows tricortical specimens to be obtained. Homolog bone grafts, such as femoral heads or condyles, are bigger and more convenient to use; but osseous integration is less reliable and requires more time and they also include the risk of partial resorption. The authors do not recommend reconstructing defects exceeding 2 cm in height. For larger defects, shortening of the ankle seems to be a more reliable method to assure fusion. In case of ankle fusion, the subtalar joint should always be preserved if possible, providing important compensatory hindfoot motion. Ankle fusion should be performed using screws (see **Fig. 6**B, C), and additional plates might be required. If the subtalar joint cannot be preserved, ankle fusion can be alternatively performed using an intramedullary nail.

SUMMARY

TAA is a complex procedure that can be associated with different types and severity of complications, which are largely influenced by the skills and the experience of the treating surgeon. Ankle fusion should always be considered as a reasonable option for the salvage of any symptomatic TAA. Depending on the severity of the complication, TAA will be preserved/exchanged or removed for ankle fusion. The decision of revising a symptomatic TAA should be made carefully and only if the reason for the complication is well understood and revision surgery has a reasonable chance of success in relation to its surgical extent. TAAs with poor motion might be better treated by ankle fusion. A further refinement of TAA designs and surgical techniques as well as increasing numbers of implanted TAAs will lead to an improved understanding of this type of surgery and, hence, result in a continuously decreasing incidence of its complications.

REFERENCES

1. Rippstein PF, Huber M, Coetzee JC, et al. Total ankle replacement with use of a new three-component implant. J Bone Joint Surg Am 2011;93:1426–35.
2. Lee KB, Cho SG, Hur CI, et al. Perioperative complications of HINTEGRA total ankle replacement: our initial 50 cases. Foot Ankle Int 2008;29:978–84.
3. Lee KT, Lee YK, Young KW, et al. Perioperative complications of the MOBILITY total ankle system: comparison with the HINTEGRA total ankle system. J Orthop Sci 2010;15:317–22.
4. Schuberth JM, Patel S, Zarutsky E. Perioperative complications of the agility total ankle replacement in 50 initial, consecutive cases. J Foot Ankle Surg 2006;45:139–46.
5. Haddad SL, Coetzee JC, Estok R, et al. Intermediate and long-term outcomes of total ankle arthroplasty and ankle arthrodesis. A systematic review of the literature. J Bone Joint Surg Am 2007;89:1899–905.
6. Bolton-Maggs BG, Sudlow RA, Freeman MA. Total ankle arthroplasty. A long-term review of the London Hospital experience. J Bone Joint Surg Br 1985;67:785–90.
7. Buechel FF Sr, Buechel FF Jr, Pappas MJ. Ten-year evaluation of cementless Buechel-Pappas meniscal bearing total ankle replacement. Foot Ankle Int 2003;24:462–72.

8. Buechel FF Sr, Buechel FF Jr, Pappas MJ. Twenty-year evaluation of cementless mobile-bearing total ankle replacements. Clin Orthop Relat Res 2004;424:19–26.
9. Helm R, Stevens J. Long-term results of total ankle replacement. J Arthroplasty 1986;1:271–7.
10. Kitaoka HB, Patzer GL. Clinical results of the Mayo total ankle arthroplasty. J Bone Joint Surg Am 1996;78:1658–64.
11. Kofoed H. Scandinavian Total Ankle Replacement (STAR). Clin Orthop Relat Res 2004;424:73–9.
12. Naal FD, Impellizzeri FM, Loibl M, et al. Habitual physical activity and sports participation after total ankle arthroplasty. Am J Sports Med 2009;37:95–102.
13. Newton SE 3rd. Total ankle arthroplasty. Clinical study of fifty cases. J Bone Joint Surg Am 1982;64:104–11.
14. Rippstein PF. Clinical experiences with three different designs of ankle prostheses. Foot Ankle Clin 2002;7:817–31.
15. Labek G, Thaler M, Janda W, et al. Revision rates after total joint replacement: cumulative results from worldwide joint register datasets. J Bone Joint Surg Br 2011;93:293–7.
16. Goldberg AJ, Sharp RJ, Cooke P. Ankle replacement: current practice of foot & ankle surgeons in the United Kingdom. Foot Ankle Int 2009;30:950–4.
17. Labek G, Klaus H, Schlichtherle R, et al. Revision rates after total ankle arthroplasty in sample-based clinical studies and national registries. Foot Ankle Int 2011;32:740–5.
18. Myerson MS, Mroczek K. Perioperative complications of total ankle arthroplasty. Foot Ankle Int 2003;24:17–21.
19. San Giovanni TP, Keblish DJ, Thomas WH, et al. Eight-year results of a minimally constrained total ankle arthroplasty. Foot Ankle Int 2006;27:418–26.
20. Spirt AA, Assal M, Hansen ST Jr. Complications and failure after total ankle arthroplasty. J Bone Joint Surg Am 2004;86:1172–8.
21. Kurup HV, Taylor GR. Medial impingement after ankle replacement. Int Orthop 2008;32:243–6.
22. Bonnin M, Gaudot F, Laurent JR, et al. The Salto total ankle arthroplasty: survivorship and analysis of failures at 7 to 11 years. Clin Orthop Relat Res 2011;469:225–36.
23. Rippstein PF, Naal FD. Total ankle replacement in rheumatoid arthritis. Orthopade 2011;40:984–6.
24. Hintermann B, Valderrabano V, Dereymaeker G, et al. The HINTEGRA ankle: rationale and short-term results of 122 consecutive ankles. Clin Orthop Relat Res 2004;424:57–68.
25. Hintermann B, Valderrabano V, Knupp M, et al. The HINTEGRA ankle: short- and mid-term results. Orthopade 2006;35:533–45.
26. Doets HC, Brand R, Nelissen RG. Total ankle arthroplasty in inflammatory joint disease with use of two mobile-bearing designs. J Bone Joint Surg Am 2006;88:1272–84.
27. Ali MS, Higgins GA, Mohamed M. Intermediate results of Buechel Pappas unconstrained uncemented total ankle replacement for osteoarthritis. J Foot Ankle Surg 2007;46:16–20.
28. Knecht SI, Estin M, Callaghan JJ, et al. The agility total ankle arthroplasty. Seven to sixteen-year follow-up. J Bone Joint Surg Am 2004;86:1161–71.

The New Zealand Joint Registry

Report of 11-Year Data for Ankle Arthroplasty

Matthew Tomlinson, MBChB, FRACS*, Matthew Harrison, MD

KEYWORDS

- Ankle arthroplasty • New Zealand Joint Registry • Patient-based questionnaires
- Surgery results

KEY POINTS

- The New Zealand Joint Registry catalogs patient-based questionnaire data in addition to joint specific data.
- Over an 11-year period, 728 primary and 50 revision ankle arthroplasties were performed.
- Unfavorable outcome scores 6 months after the index procedure correlate well with risk of failure.

INTRODUCTION

Large-scale collection and analysis of arthroplasty data are crucial for monitoring, developing, and improving outcomes of joint replacement surgery.[1] Joint registries have collected prosthetic component data as well as patient-related data, with revision as the primary outcome. Over time, they have evolved to a more multidimensional position that includes traditional clinical outcome parameters as well as patient-reported outcome measures.[2] Registries have provided the opportunity for studying large numbers of patients, procedures, and prostheses. They are invaluable for guiding orthopedic surgeons to improve patient care and outcomes of total joint arthroplasty.[3,4]

Implementation of the New Zealand Joint Registry began in 1997. It became fully operational in April of 1999. Initially, only primary and revision hip and knee data were collected. In January of 2000, the database was expanded to include total hip replacements for femoral neck fractures, unicompartmental replacements for knees, total and hemiarthroplasty for shoulders, and total joint replacement for elbows and ankles. Participation in the registry is mandatory for all orthopedic surgeons undertaking arthroplasty surgery, and it is a requirement for recertification. The validated

Middlemore Hospital, Department of Orthopaedics, Otahuhu Manukau 1640, Auckland, New Zealand
* Corresponding author.
E-mail address: matthew.tomlinson@middlemore.co.nz

Foot Ankle Clin N Am 17 (2012) 719–723
http://dx.doi.org/10.1016/j.fcl.2012.08.011 foot.theclinics.com

Oxford 12 questionnaire was available for the shoulder and was adapted but not validated at the time for the elbow and ankle joints. Recently, a Swedish study was presented at the annual meeting of the American Academy of Orthopaedic Surgeons,[5] which tested the construct validity of the New Zealand version of the Oxford 12 questionnaire for the ankle and compared it with Foot and Ankle Outcome Score (FAOS), 36-Item Short Form Health Survey (SF-36), and Euroqol Score (EQ-5D) questionnaires. This group's findings would appear to validate the New Zealand version of the Oxford 12 questionnaire for ankles. The report is currently in press.[5] All ankle arthroplasty patients are sent questionnaires 6 months after surgery and at 5 yearly intervals. Reply rates have been between 70% and 75%.

Analysis of the 6-year data has been previously reported.[4] For this period, the overall failure rate was 7%. An unfavorable Oxford score at 6 months was a good predictor of subsequent failure. Each 1-point increase in the patient score (ie, a poorer outcome) corresponded to a 5% relative increase in the risk of failure. Analysis of results for the different types of arthroplasty implanted in New Zealand during this time period was also performed.

The 11-year data for ankle arthroplasty are presented here. This information is also available online through the Web site of the New Zealand Joint Registry.[6]

ANKLE ARTHROPLASTY REGISTRY DATA

Primary Arthroplasty

The 11-year report includes data for the period from January 2000 to December 2010. Over this time, 728 primary ankle arthroplasties were performed. The number of procedures has steadily increased from 17 in the year 2000 to 125 in 2010. The average age for an ankle replacement was 65.2 years (range 32.3–88.4 years). Most of the patients were men (60.85%). Osteoarthritis was the main indication for surgery (n = 528). One hundred thirty eight patients were diagnosed with post-traumatic arthritis. Other diagnoses included rheumatoid arthritis, other inflammatory arthropathies, and avascular necrosis.

The American Society of Anesthesiologists (ASA) class was collected for each patient beginning in 2005. This system classifies patients on levels of systemic disease. A healthy patient is class 1, and a patient with incapacitating disease is class 4. One hundred four patients were ASA class 1; 314 patients were class 2. Seventy-seven patients were class 3, and 2 patients were class 4. Body mass index (BMI) for patients in 2010 was available for 34 primary ankle replacements. The average BMI was 27.58 kg/m^2 (range 17–37, standard deviation [SD] 4.66).

Logistical data have been collected for each operation. Ninety-six percent of patients received at least 1 systemic antibiotic. Three hundred ninety cases were performed in a conventional operating theater. Three hundred thirty-two cases used laminar flow. One hundred twenty-five cases were done with surgeons using arthroplasty hoods, or space suits. The average operating time was 124 minutes (range 30–290 minutes, SD 36 minutes).

Table 1
All primary ankle arthroplasties and revision statistics

Total Operations	Observed Component Years	Number Revised	Rate/100 Component Years	95% Confidence Interval
728	2497	34	1.36	0.94–1.9

Table 2
Revision statistics for prosthesis type

Prosthesis	Total Operations	Observed Component Years	Number Revised	Rate/100 Component Years	95% Confidence Interval
Agility Tibial Shell	119	820	13	1.58	0.84–2.71
Box	2	3	0	0	0–131.07
Mobility	350	846	11	1.3	0.65–2.33
Ramses	11	61	2	3.3	0.4–11.91
Salto	199	464	1	0.22	0.01–1.20
STAR	47	302	7	2.31	0.93–4.77

Prosthesis type has been collected since 2006. Over the years, the Mobility (Mobility TAR System; DePuy, Leeds, England) and Salto (Tornier SAS, Montbonnot Saint Martin, France) have been the dominant prostheses. In 2010, 76 prostheses were mobility, and 49 were Salto. The Agility (DePuy Orthopaedics, Inc. Warsaw, IN, USA), STAR (Small Bone Innovations, Inc., Morrisville, PA, USA), Ramses (Laboratoire Fournitures Hospitalieres, Heimsbrunn, France), and Box (MatOrtho, Leatherhead, Surrey, UK) prostheses have not been implanted over the last 3 years.

Revision Arthroplasty

Revision arthroplasty is defined by the registry as a new operation in a previously replaced ankle joint during which 1 or more of the components are exchanged, removed, manipulated, or added. It includes arthrodesis or amputation but not soft tissue procedures. Between January 2000 and December 2010, there were 50 registered revision ankle procedures. The average patient age was 65.29 years (range 42.13–83.06 years). Seventy percent of patients were men.

The mean time to revision over the 11-year period was 1196 days (range 21–3325 days, SD 786 days). Pain and loosening of the talar component were the most common reasons for revision (34% each). There were 7 revisions for loosening of the tibial component and 3 revisions for deep infection. Six revisions were done for reasons not otherwise specified. Although revision rates were somewhat higher for male patients, the difference was not statistically significant.

Tables 1 and **2** present revision arthroplasty data with statistical terms that may seem unfamiliar. The observed component years are the number of registered primary procedures multiplied by the number of years each component has been in place. The rate per 100 component years is equivalent to the yearly revision rate, expressed as a percent, and the rate is derived by dividing the number of prostheses revised by the observed component years multiplied by 100. It allows for the number of years of postoperative follow-up in calculating the revision rate. These rates are usually

Table 3
Oxford questionnaire scores

Oxford Score	Number of Patients
>41	137
34–41	183
27–33	112
<27	142

Table 4
Percentage of responses indicating 0 or 1 for each question

Question	% Scoring 0 or 1
Moderate or severe pain from the operated ankle	22
Only able to walk around the house or unable to walk before the pain becomes severe	6
Extreme difficulty or impossible to walk on uneven ground	15
Most of the time or always have to use an orthotic	23
Pain greatly or totally interferes with work	16
Limping most days or every day	34
Extreme difficulty of impossible to climb a flight of stairs	6
Pain from the ankle in bed most or every night	7
Pain from the ankle greatly or totally interferes with usual recreational activities	23
Have swelling of the foot most or all of the time	31
Very painful or unbearable to stand up from a chair after a meal	6
Sudden severe pain from the ankle most or every day	6

very low; hence it is expressed per 100 component years rather than per component year. Statisticians consider that this is a more accurate way of deriving a revision rate for comparison when analyzing data with widely varying follow-up times. It is also important to note the confidence intervals. The closer they are to the estimated revision rate per 100 component years, the more precise the estimate is.

Patient-Reported Outcome Measures

Patients are sent a questionnaire 6 months and 5 years after surgery. It is modeled on the Oxford 12 questionnaire.[7] The new scoring system has been adopted as recommended by the authors of the Oxford paper, and a validation study has recently been presented.[5] Each question is scored from 0 to 4 points, with total scores ranging from 0 to 48. Forty-eight is the best score, indicating normal function. A score of 0 is the worst, indicating the most severe disability. The questionnaire responses were grouped according to the grading system published by Kalairajah.[8] In this system, scores above 41 are considered excellent; scores between 34 and 41 are good. Scores between 27 and 33 are fair, and scores less than 27 are poor.

For the 11-year period, there were 574 primary ankle questionnaire responses at 6 months after surgery. The mean primary ankle score was 33.38 (range 2–48, SD 9.67). Fifty-six percent of patients had a score of good or excellent. **Table 3** shows the numbers for each scoring category. All patients who had a 6-month questionnaire and who had not had a revision were sent a questionnaire at 5 years after surgery. Of the 83 respondents, 64% achieved a good or excellent score. **Table 4** lists each of the questions and the percentage of patients scoring 0 or 1.

There were 26 revision ankle responses, with 46% achieving an excellent or good score. This group includes all revision ankle responses. The mean revision ankle score was 31.04 (range 8–48, SD 11.5).

SUMMARY

This represents the results of the first 11 years of ankle arthroplasty data for the New Zealand Joint Registry. The main purpose is to collect accurate outcome information regarding these procedures and to guide orthopedic surgeons in the care of their patients. Trends can often be identified early, and implants with higher revision rates can be identified. In addition, individual surgeons can be given data that compare their performance with the collective data, providing invaluable feedback. As can be seen, the patient-based questionnaires are highly important for gauging the results of surgery. Patient response rates have been less than optimal, particularly after revision surgery. In the future, it is hoped that the overall quality of the joint registry can be improved by increasing patient involvement. As time goes by, cumulative information and analysis should provide clinicians with further information to optimize the practice of total ankle arthroplasty, both in New Zealand and around the world.

REFERENCES

1. Sedrakyan A, Paxton E, Phillips C, et al. The International Consortium of Orthopaedic Registries: overview and summary. J Bone Joint Surg Am 2011;93(Suppl 3E): 1–12.
2. Rolfson O, Rothwell A, Sedrakyan A, et al. Use of patient-reported outcomes in the context of different levels of data. J Bone Joint Surg Am 2011;93(Suppl 3E):66–71.
3. Macpherson G, Brenkel I, Smith R, et al. Outlier analysis in orthopaedics: use of CUSUM. J Bone Joint Surg Am 2011;93(Suppl 3E):81–8.
4. Hosman A, Mason R, Hobbs T, et al. A New Zealand National Joint Registry Review of 202 total ankle replacements followed for up to 6 years. Acta Orthop 2007;78(5): 584–91.
5. Coster M, Karlsson M, Carlsson A. Validity, reliability, and responsiveness of the Self-reported Foot and Ankle Score (SEFAS). Presented at the annual meeting of the American Academy of Orthopaedic Surgeons. San Francisco, California, February 2012.
6. New Zealand National Joint Registry. Available at: http://www.cdhb.govt.nz/njr/. Accessed February 27, 2004.
7. Dawson J, Fitzpatrick R, Murray D, et al. Questionnaire on the perceptions of patients about total knee replacement. J Bone Joint Surg Br 1998;80:63–9.
8. Kalairajah Y, Azurza K, Hulme C, et al. Health outcome measures in the evaluation of total hip arthroplasties: a comparison between the Harris hip score and the oxford hip score. J Arthroplasty 2005;20(8):1037–41.

Index

Note: Page numbers of article titles are in **boldface** type.

Foot Ankle Clin N Am 17 (2012) 725–749
http://dx.doi.org/10.1016/S1083-7515(12)00103-9

C

D

G

H

I

K

L

M

S

United States Postal Service

Statement of Ownership, Management, and Circulation
(All Periodicals Publications Except Requestor Publications)

1. Publication Title: Foot and Ankle Clinics
2. Publication Number: 0 1 6 - 3 6 8
3. Filing Date: 9/14/12
4. Issue Frequency: Mar, Jun, Sep, Dec
5. Number of Issues Published Annually: 4
6. Annual Subscription Price: $295.00
7. Complete Mailing Address of Known Office of Publication (*Not printer*) (*Street, city, county, state, and ZIP+4®*)
   Elsevier Inc.
   360 Park Avenue South
   New York, NY 10010-1710
   Contact Person: Stephen R. Bushing
   Telephone (Include area code): 215-239-3688
8. Complete Mailing Address of Headquarters or General Business Office of Publisher (*Not printer*)
   Elsevier Inc., 360 Park Avenue South, New York, NY 10010-1710
9. Full Names and Complete Mailing Addresses of Publisher, Editor, and Managing Editor (*Do not leave blank*)
   Publisher (*Name and complete mailing address*)
   Kim Murphy, Elsevier, Inc., 1600 John F. Kennedy Blvd. Suite 1800, Philadelphia, PA 19103-2899
   Editor (*Name and complete mailing address*)
   David Parsons, Elsevier, Inc., 1600 John F. Kennedy Blvd. Suite 1800, Philadelphia, PA 19103-2899
   Managing Editor (*Name and complete mailing address*)
   Barbara Cohen-Kligerman, Elsevier, Inc., 1600 John F. Kennedy Blvd. Suite 1800, Philadelphia, PA 19103-2899
10. Owner (*Do not leave blank. If the publication is owned by a corporation, give the name and address of the corporation immediately followed by the names and addresses of all stockholders owning or holding 1 percent or more of the total amount of stock. If not owned by a corporation, give the names and addresses of the individual owners. If owned by a partnership or other unincorporated firm, give its name and address as well as those of each individual owner. If the publication is published by a nonprofit organization, give its name and address.*)

Full Name	Complete Mailing Address
Wholly owned subsidiary of	1600 John F. Kennedy Blvd., Ste. 1800
Reed/Elsevier, US holdings	Philadelphia, PA 19103-2899

11. Known Bondholders, Mortgagees, and Other Security Holders Owning or Holding 1 Percent or More of Total Amount of Bonds, Mortgages, or Other Securities. If none, check box → None

Full Name	Complete Mailing Address
N/A	

12. Tax Status (*For completion by nonprofit organizations authorized to mail at nonprofit rates*) (*Check one*)
    The purpose, function, and nonprofit status of this organization and the exempt status for federal income tax purposes:
    Has Not Changed During Preceding 12 Months
    Has Changed During Preceding 12 Months (*Publisher must submit explanation of change with this statement*)

PS Form 3526, September 2007 (Page 1 of 3 (Instructions Page 3)) PSN 7530-01-000-9931 **PRIVACY NOTICE**: See our Privacy policy in www.usps.com

13. Publication Title: Foot and Ankle Clinics
14. Issue Date for Circulation Data Below: September 2012

15. Extent and Nature of Circulation			Average No. Copies Each Issue During Preceding 12 Months	No. Copies of Single Issue Published Nearest to Filing Date
a. Total Number of Copies (*Net press run*)			925	871
b. Paid Circulation (By Mail and Outside the Mail)	(1)	Mailed Outside-County Paid Subscriptions Stated on PS Form 3541. (*Include paid distribution above nominal rate, advertiser's proof copies, and exchange copies*)	579	547
	(2)	Mailed In-County Paid Subscriptions Stated on PS Form 3541 (*Include paid distribution above nominal rate, advertiser's proof copies, and exchange copies*)		
	(3)	Paid Distribution Outside the Mails Including Sales Through Dealers and Carriers, Street Vendors, Counter Sales, and Other Paid Distribution Outside USPS®	112	132
	(4)	Paid Distribution by Other Classes Mailed Through the USPS (e.g. First-Class Mail®)		
c. Total Paid Distribution (*Sum of 15b (1), (2), (3), and (4)*) ►			691	679
d. Free or Nominal Rate Distribution (By Mail and Outside the Mail)	(1)	Free or Nominal Rate Outside-County Copies Included on PS Form 3541	69	56
	(2)	Free or Nominal Rate In-County Copies Included on PS Form 3541		
	(3)	Free or Nominal Rate Copies Mailed at Other Classes Through the USPS (e.g. First-Class Mail)		
	(4)	Free or Nominal Rate Distribution Outside the Mail (Carriers or other means)		
e. Total Free or Nominal Rate Distribution (Sum of 15d (1), (2), (3) and (4))			69	56
f. Total Distribution (Sum of 15c and 15e) ►			760	735
g. Copies not Distributed (See instructions to publishers #4 (page #3)) ►			165	136
h. Total (Sum of 15f and g)			925	871
i. Percent Paid (15c divided by 15f times 100) ►			90.92%	92.38%

16. Publication of Statement of Ownership
    If the publication is a general publication, publication of this statement is required. Will be printed in the **December 2012** issue of this publication. Publication not required

17. Signature and Title of Editor, Publisher, Business Manager, or Owner
    Stephen R. Bushing –Inventory Distribution Coordinator
    Date: September 14, 2012

I certify that all information furnished on this form is true and complete. I understand that anyone who furnishes false or misleading information on this form or who omits material or information requested on the form may be subject to criminal sanctions (including fines and imprisonment) and/or civil sanctions (including civil penalties).

PS Form 3526, September 2007 (Page 2 of 3)

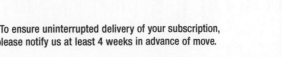

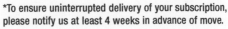

Printed and bound by CPI Group (UK) Ltd, Croydon, CR0 4YY
03/10/2024
01040442-0006